Cancer Therapy

New Trends

Edited by Peter Bannasch

With 76 Figures

Springer-Verlag Berlin Heidelberg New York
London Paris Tokyo Hong Kong

Prof. Dr. PETER BANNASCH
Institut für Experimentelle Pathologie
Deutsches Krebsforschungszentrum
Im Neuenheimer Feld 280
D-6900 Heidelberg

The publication of this book was supported by the Arbeitsgemeinschaft für Grossforschungseinrichtungen (AGF).

Institutions participating in the AGF-Koordinierungsausschuß Krebsforschung

DKFZ Deutsches Krebsforschungszentrum Heidelberg
GBF Gesellschaft für Biotechnologische Forschung Braunschweig
GSF Gesellschaft für Strahlen- und Umweltforschung Neuherberg
KFA Kernforschungsanlage Jülich
KfK Kernforschungszentrum Karlsruhe

ISBN-13: 978-3-540-51034-5 e-ISBN-13: 978-3-642-74683-3
DOI: 10.1007/978-3-642-74683-3

Library of Congress Cataloging-in-Publication Data. Cancer therapy. "Proceedings of a conference held in July 1988 in Heidelberg, Germany; organized by the Committee Coordinating Cancer Research in the Grossforschungseinrichtungen in the Federal Republic of Germany. Includes bibliographies and index. 1. Cancer – Treatment – Congresses. I. Bannasch, Peter. II. AGF-Koordinierungsausschuss Krebsforschung. [DNLM: 1. Neoplasms – therapy – congresses. QZ 266 C2184 1988]
RC270.8.C374 1989 616.99'406 89-11292
ISBN-13: 978-3-540-51034-5

2121/3130-543210 – Printed on acid-free paper

Preface

Cancer is not a uniform disease. A large variety of histological tumor types may be distinguished, and there is considerable cellular heterogeneity in each. The diversity in the pathobiology of tumors is reflected by a multitude of clinical courses and requires a broad spectrum of therapeutic approaches, most of which are addressed in this book.

Although remarkable progress has been made in some areas of tumor therapy, there is still an urgent need to improve cancer treatment, which in the majority of cases is insufficient. To this end all promising new trends in basic and clinical research should be checked carefully and introduced into clinical oncology as rapidly as possible.

It was this aim which prompted the committee coordinating cancer research in the *Großforschungseinrichtungen* in the Federal Republic of Germany to organize a conference on new trends in cancer therapy. The conference was duly held in Heidelberg in July 1988, and this book contains the contributions presented by more than 20 highly competent international speakers. Recent advances in the major fields of clinical oncology are reviewed and critically discussed against the background of established treatment modalities. In eight sections special emphasis is placed on surgical oncology, including photodynamic laser therapy and radiosurgery, new approaches in radiation oncology, hyperthermia, new antineoplastic agents, enzyme-pattern-targeted chemotherapy, drug resistance, biological response modifiers, bone marrow transplantation, antibody-guided therapy, induction of cell differentiation in transformed cells, and the individualization of tumor therapy. The stimulating discussion on each topic is summarized at the end of the respective sections.

I am grateful to all my colleagues, particularly to the members of the Scientific Committee, who provided valuable assistance in drawing up the program of the conference: U. Hagen (Munich, Neuherberg), P. Herrlich (Karlsruhe), M. Matzku (Heidelberg), G. Nagel (Göttingen), D. Schmähl (Heidelberg), K.-H. von Wangenheim (Düsseldorf/Jülich), M. Wannenmacher (Heidelberg), W. Wilmanns (Munich/Neuherberg), and H. zur Hausen (Heidelberg). I am obliged to Drs. T. M. Fliedner, W. Hunstein, F. W. Schildberg, C. G. Schmidt, K. H. von Wangenheim, and M. Wannenmacher for serving as chairmen of the sessions. I am also grateful to the administration of the German Cancer Research Center and to my coworkers, who ensured the smooth running of the meeting. My special thanks go to the speakers, the moderators, and the rapporteurs of the discussions and to all the participants who contributed to the success of the conference. They provided the basis for this book, which should be of interest both to clinicians involved in the treatment of cancer patients and to researchers taking up the challenge to improve cancer therapy. Finally, I am indebted to Heide Zerban for careful editorial help, and to Ute Heilmann and Doris Keidel-Müller of Springer-Verlag for excellent cooperation and much support in achieving rapid publication of the proceedings.

Heidelberg PETER BANNASCH

Contents

List of Contributors

AMMON, A., Abtl. Hämatologie/Onkologie, Medizinische Klinik und Poliklinik, Universität Göttingen, Robert-Koch-Str. 40, D-3400 Göttingen, FRG

BALDWIN, R.W., Cancer Research Campaign Laboratories, University of Nottingham, Nottingham, UK

BARTRAM, C.R., Sektion Molekularbiologie, Universitätskinderklinik, Universität Ulm, Prittwitzstr. 43, D-7900 Ulm, FRG

BARTSCH, H.H., Abtl. Hämatologie/Onkologie, Medizinische Klinik und Poliklinik, Universität Göttingen, Robert-Koch-Str. 40, D-3400 Göttingen, FRG

BERGER, M.R., Institut für Toxikologie und Chemotherapie, Deutsches Krebsforschungszentrum, Im Neuenheimer Feld 280, D-6900 Heidelberg, FRG

BERTINO, J.R., Memorial Sloan-Kettering Cancer Center, 1275 York Avenue, New York, NY 10021, USA

BIHL, H., Zentrum für Radiologie, Universität Heidelberg, Im Neuenheimer Feld 400, D-6900 Heidelberg, FRG

BYERS, V. S., XOMA Corporation, Berkeley, CA 94710, USA

CLEMM, C., Medizinische Klinik III, Klinikum Großhadern, Universität München, Marchioninistr. 45, D-8000 München 70, FRG

DÖRKEN, B., Medizinische Universitäts-Poliklinik, Universität Heidelberg, Hospitalstr. 3, D-6900 Heidelberg, FRG

DRINGS, P., Abtl. Innere Medizin-Onkologie der Thoraxklinik HD-Rohrbach, Amalienstr. 5, D-6900 Heidelberg, FRG

EPENETOS, A.A., ICRF Oncology Group, Royal Postgraduate Medical School, Hammersmith Hospital, Du Cane Road, London W12 0NN, UK

FIEBIG, H., Medizinische Universitätsklinik, Universität Freiburg, Hugstetter Str. 55, D-7800 Freiburg, FRG

FLIEDNER, T.M., Abteilung für Klinische Physiologie, Universität Ulm, Oberer Eselsberg, D-7900 Ulm, FRG

FUJIMORI, K., Theoretical Immunology Section, Laboratory of Mathematical Biology, National Cancer Institute, Bldg. 10, Rm. 4B–56, Bethesda, MD 20892, USA

GERHARTZ, H., Medizinische Klinik III, Klinikum Großhadern, Universität München, Marchioninistr. 15, D-8000 München 70 FRG

GRUNICKE, H., Institut für Medizinische Chemie und Biochemie, Universität Innsbruck, Fritz-Pregl-Str. 3, A-6020 Innsbruck, Austria

HAHN, E.W., Institut für Radiologic und Pathophysiologie, Deutsches Krebsforschungszentrum, Im Neuenheimer Feld 280, D-6900 Heidelberg, FRG

HARTMANN, G., Institut für Radiologie und Pathophysiologie, Deutsches Krebsforschungszentrum, Im Neuenheimer Feld 280, D-6900 Heidelberg, FRG

HELLIGER, W., Institut für Medizinische Chemie und Biochemie, Universität Innsbruck, Fritz-Pregl-Str. 3, A-6020 Innsbruck, Austria

HERFARTH, CH., Chirurgische Universitätsklinik, Universität Heidelberg, Im Neuenheimer Feld 110, D-6900 Heidelberg, FRG

HERRMANN, F., Medizinische Klinik und Poliklinik, Universität Mainz, Langenbeckstr. 1, D-6500 Mainz, FRG

HOFMANN, J., Institut für Medizinische Chemie und Biochemie, Universität Innsbruck, Fritz-Pregl-Str. 3, A-6020 Innsbruck, Austria

HUNSTEIN, W., Medizinische Universitäts-Poliklinik, Universität Heidelberg, Hospitalstr. 3, D-6900 Heidelberg, FRG

ISSELS, R.D., Medizinische Klinik III, Klinikum Großhadern, Universität München und Institut für Klinische Hämatologie, Gesellschaft für Strahlenforschung, Hämatologikum Großhadern, Marchioninistr., D-8000 München 70, FRG

KAICK, G. VAN, Institut für Radiologie und Pathophysiologie, Deutsches Krebsforschungszentrum, Im Neuenheimer Feld 280, D-6900 Heidelberg, FRG

KALOFONOS, H.P., ICRF Oncology Group, Royal Postgraduate Medical School, Hammersmith Hospital, Du Cane Road, London W12 0NN, UK

KEPPLER, B.K., Institut für Anorganische Chemie, Universität Heidelberg, Im Neuenheimer Feld 270, D-6900 Heidelberg, FRG

KIMMIG, B., Zentrum für Radiologie, Universität Heidelberg, Im Neuenheimer Feld 400, D-6900 Heidelberg, FRG

Klenner, T., Institut für Toxikologie und Chemotherapie, Deutsches Krebsforschungszentrum, Im Neuenheimer Feld 280, D-6900 Heidelberg, FRG

Kolb, H.-J., Medizinische Klinik III, Klinikum Großhadern, Marchioninistr. 15, D-8000 München 70, FRG

Körbling, M., Medizinische Universitäts-Poliklinik, Universität Heidelberg, Hospitalstr. 3, D-6900 Heidelberg, FRG

Krieger, K., Institut für Anästhesiologie, Klinikum Großhadern, Universität München, Marchioninistr. 15, D-8000 München 70, FRG

Krönke, K., Klinische Arbeitsgruppe der Max-Planck-Gesellschaft, c/o Abtl. Hämatologie/Onkologie, Medizinische Universitätsklinik, Robert-Koch-Str. 40, D-3400 Göttingen, FRG

Lindemann, A., Medizinische Klinik und Poliklinik, Universität Mainz, Langenbeckstr. 1, D-6500 Mainz, FRG

Lorenz, W. J., Institut für Radiologie und Pathophysiologie, Deutsches Krebsforschungszentrum, Im Neuenheimer Feld 280, D-6900 Heidelberg, FRG

Maly, K., Institut für Medizinische Chemie und Biochemie, Universität Innsbruck, Fritz-Pregl-Str. 3, A-6020 Innsbruck, Austria

Marks, P. A., Memorial Sloan-Kettering Cancer Center, 1275 York Avenue, New York, NY 10021, USA

Matsuda, T., Department of Radiation Therapy, Tokyo Metropolitan Kamagone Hospital, Honkomagome 3-18-22, Bunkyo, Tokyo, 113 Japan

Matsutani, M., Department of Neurosurgery, Metropolitan Komagone Hospital, Honkomagome 3-18-22, Bunkyo, Tokyo, 113 Japan

Matzku, S., Institut für Radiologie und Pathophysiologie, Deutsches Krebsforschungszentrum, Im Neuenheimer Feld 280, D-6900 Heidelberg, FRG

Mertelsmann, R., Medizinische Klinik und Poliklinik, Universität Mainz, Langenbeckstr. 1, D-6500 Mainz, FRG

Möller, P., Zentrum für Pathologie, Universität Heidelberg, D-6900 Heidelberg, FRG

Moldenhauer, G., Institut für Immunologie und Genetik, Deutsches Krebsforschungszentrum, Im Neuenheimer Feld 280, D-6900 Heidelberg, FRG

Nagashima, T., Department of Neurosurgergy, Tokyo Metropolitan Komagome Hospital, Honkomagome 3-18-22, Bunkyo, Tokyo, 113 Japan

Nagel, G. A., Abtl. Hämatologie/Onkologie, Medizinische Klinik und Poliklinik der Universität, Robert-Koch-Str. 40, D-3400 Göttingen, FRG

NAKAMURA, O., Department of Neurosurgery, Tokyo Metropolitan Komagome Hospital, Honkomagome 3-18-22, Bunkyo, Tokyo, 113 Japan

NATSUMEDA, Y., Laboratory for Experimental Oncology, Indiana University School of Medicine, Indianapolis, IN 46223, USA

NIEDERLE, N., Innere Klinik und Poliklinik (Tumorforschung), Universitätsklinikum Essen, Hufelandstr. 55, D-4300 Essen, FRG

O'BRIEN, J. P., Memorial Sloan-Kettering Cancer Center, 1275 York Avenue, New York, NY 10021, USA

OLSSON, I. L., University of Lund, University Hospital, Research Department 2, E-Blocket, S-22185 Lund, Sweden

OSTER, W., Medizinische Klinik und Poliklinik, Universität Mainz, Langenbeckstr. 1, D-6500 Mainz, FRG

OVERGAARD, J., Danish Cancer Society, Department of Experimental Clinical Oncology, Radiumstationen, Noerrebrogade 44, DK-8000 Aarhus C, Denmark

PASTYR, O., Institut für Radiologie und Pathophysiologie, Deutsches Krebsforschungszentrum, Im Neuenheimer Feld 280, D-6900 Heidelberg, FRG

PFIZENMAIER, K., Klinische Arbeitsgruppe der Max-Planck-Gesellschaft, c/o Abtl. Hämatologie/Onkologie, Medizinische Universitätsklinik, Robert-Koch-Str. 40, D-3400 Göttingen, FRG

POSCH, L., Institut für Medizinische Chemie und Biochemie, Universität Innsbruck, Fritz-Pregl-Str. 3, A-6020 Innsbruck, Austria

POSSINGER, K., Medizinische Klinik III, Klinikum Großhadern, Universität München, Marchioninistr. 15, D-8000 München 70, FRG

PUSCHENDORF, B., Institut für Medizinische Chemie und Biochemie, Universität Innsbruck, Fritz-Pregl-Str. 3, A-6020 Innsbruck, Austria

RICHARD, F., Université Catholique de Louvain, Cliniques Universitaires St.-Luc, Avenue Hippocrate, B-1200 Bruxelles, Belgium

RIFKIND, R. A., Memorial Sloan-Kettering Cancer Center, 1275 York Avenue, New York, NY 10021, USA

ROMANINI, A., Memorial Sloan-Kettering Cancer Center, 1275 York Avenue, New York, NY 10021, USA

ROTHER, K., Institut für Immunologie und Serologie, Universität Heidelberg, Im Neuenheimer Feld, D-6900 Heidelberg, FRG

SANTOS, G. W., The Johns Hopkins Oncology Center, 600 N. Wolfe Street, Baltimore, MD 21205, USA

SAUER, H., Medizinische Klinik III, Klinikum Großhadern, Universität München, Marchioninistr. 15, D-8000 München 70, FRG

Schabbert, S., Institut für Radiologie und Pathophysiologie, Deutsches Krebsforschungszentrum, Im Neuenheimer Feld 280, D-6900 Heidelberg, FRG

Schlag, P., Chirurgische Universitätsklinik, Sektion Chirurgische Onkologie, Universität Heidelberg, Im Neuenheimer Feld 110, D-6900 Heidelberg, FRG

Schlegel, W., Institut für Radiologie und Pathophysiologie, Deutsches Krebsforschungszentrum, Im Neuenheimer Feld 280, D-6900 Heidelberg, FRG

Schletterer, C., Institut für Medizinische Chemie und Biochemie, Universität Innsbruck, Fritz-Pregl-Str. 3, A-6020 Innsbruck, Austria

Schmähl, D., Institut für Toxikologie und Chemotherapie, Deutsches Krebsforschungszentrum, Im Neuenheimer Feld 280, D-6900 Heidelberg, FRG

Sivolapenko, G. B., Department of Immunology, Royal Postgraduate Medical School, Hammersmith Hospital, Du Cane Road, London W12 0NN, UK

Streffer, C., Institut für Medizinische Strahlenbiologie, Universitätsklinikum Essen, Hufelandstr. 55, D-4300 Essen, FRG

Sturm, V., Abteilung Neurochirurgie/Stereotaxie, Universität zu Köln, Josef-Stelzmann-Str. 9, D-5000 Köln 41, FRG

Talasz, H., Institut für Medizinische Chemie und Biochemie, Universität Innsbruck, Fritz-Pregl-Str. 3, A-6020 Innsbruck, Austria

Tanaka, Y., Department of Radiation Therapy, Tokyo Metropolitan Komagone Hospital, Honkomagome 3-18-22, Bunkyo, Toyko, 113 Japan

Trott, K.-R., Department of Radiation Biology, Medical College of Bartholomew's Hospital, Charterhouse Square, London EC1M 6BQ, UK

Überall, F., Institut für Medizinische Chemie und Biochemie, Universität Innsbruck, Fritz-Pregl-Str. 3, A-6020 Innsbruck, Austria

Unger, C., Abtl. Hämatologie/Onkologie, Medizinische Klinik und Poliklinik der Universität, Robert-Koch-Str. 40, D-3400 Göttingen, FRG

Unsöld, E., Zentrales Laserlaboratorium, Gesellschaft für Strahlen- und Umweltforschung, D-8042 Neuherberg

Wambersie, A., Université Catholique de Louvain, Cliniques Universitaires St.-Luc, Avenue Hippocrate, B-1200 Bruxelles, Belgium

Wannenmacher, M., Zentrum für Radiologie, Universität Heidelberg, Im Neuenheimer Feld 400, D-6900 Heidelberg, FRG

Weber, G., Laboratory for Experimental Oncology, Indiana University School of Medicine, Riley Cancer Wing, Barnhill Drive, Indianapolis, IN 46223, USA

Weinstein, J. N., Theoretical Immunology Section, Laboratory of Mathematical Biology, National Cancer Institute, Bldg. 10, Rm. 4B–56, Bethesda, MD 20892, USA

Weiss, G., Institut für Medizinische Chemie und Biochemie, Universität Innsbruck, Fritz-Pregl-Str. 3, A-6020 Innsbruck, Austria

Wieser, M., Medizinische Klinik und Poliklinik, Universität Mainz, Langenbeckstr. 1, D-6500 Mainz, FRG

Wilmanns, W., Medizinische Klinik III, Klinikum Großhadern, Universität München und Institut für Klinische Hämatologie, Gesellschaft für Strahlen- und Umweltforschung, Marchioninistr. 15, D-8000 München 70, FRG

Wowra, B., Neurochirurgische Universitätsklinik, Universität Heidelberg, Im Neuenheimer Feld 400, D-6900 Heidelberg, FRG

Yamada, Y., Laboratory for Experimental Oncology, Indiana University School of Medicine, Riley Cancer Wing, Barn Hill Drive, Indianapolis, IN 46223, USA

SESSION 1

Surgery

Chairman: F. W. Schildberg

Advances in Surgical Oncology

CH. HERFARTH and P. SCHLAG

Important advances in surgical oncology have been of various kinds. The principle of radicality in the surgical treatment of carcinoma is still valid for a great number of tumors. A truly radical operation is the decisive factor in the attainment of cure for gastrointestinal carcinoma more than for any other type, as is documented by analyses of follow-up data collected in patients treated for gastric carcinoma and colorectal tumors (Jeekel 1987; Maruyama et al. 1987).

Not everyone interprets the concept of radical surgery in the same way, even now. The term refers to the tumor, to the organ bearing the tumor, and also to the lymph drainage area affected, with the lymph nodes of the first three orders. Restrictions on the degree of radicality of surgery can be imposed by the organ itself, for example the breast (Fisher et al. 1985) or the stomach (Herfarth and Schlag 1979), or by the lymph nodes involved, as in the case of rectal carcinoma (Heberer et al. 1987). The data recorded in Japanese patient populations (Maruyama et al. 1987) and from our department (Schlag et al. 1982) suggest, for example, that in the case of gastric carcinoma, dissection of lymph node groups 1 and 2 is of decisive importance for successful outcome. Our own results show that after radical surgery of gastric cancer the 5-year survival rates are nearly double those in centers not using the typical radical lymph node surgery (Herfarth et al. 1981). In the case of carcinoma of the breast, it seems possible to restrict the extent of surgery performed on the breast itself, but the loss of radicality then needs to be compensate for by substituting radiotherapy (Fisher et al. 1985; Veronesi 1987).

The inference that radical surgery is the logical treatment for carcinoma has not gone uncontested, however. The classic example is carcinoma of the breast. Local surgery, or operations that are less radical in extent, have also increased in significance for carcinoma of the rectum, but strict determination of and adherence to the indications are essential. In rectal carcinoma, preoperative endosonography helps to define the extent of the tumor invasion and to plan local treatment (Feifel et al. 1985).

The combination of operation with perioperative adjuvant measures is an attractive approach to improving the results of curative surgery and preventing local relapse. There are three kinds of adjuvant therapy for carcinoma that can be helpful in this regard: preoperative, intraoperative and postoperative. Preoperative adjuvant therapy has been tried mainly in esophageal carcinoma (Kelsen 1984; Kelsen et al. 1986) and in carcinoma of the anus and rectum (Papillon et al. 1983; Papillon 1988). The use of radiotherapy and chemotherapy preoperatively in the treatment of anal cancer may make surgery unnecessary or enable it to be limited to local excision of the lesion in a situation where the only alternative would be extirpation of the rectum and definitive colostomy (Nigro 1987).

Further, combined modality treatment means higher resection rate for some tumors which are not always suitable for surgery without such an approach. Preoperative chemo-radiotherapy increases resectability, for instance, in esophageal cancer. Radical or ultraradical surgery alone, however, significantly influences the survival of patients with this cancer (Schlag et al. 1988).

In carcinoma of the rectum, preoperative radiotherapy has an effect on the frequency of recurrence, but no significant influence on survival has been documented (Gerard et al. 1988).

Oncologists' assessment of intraoperative adjuvant therapy is positive. The modalities being tested are intraportal chemotherapy in colorectal carcinoma and radiotherapy in carcinoma of the stomach and of the pancreas. Really convincing results are, however, not yet available. At this time, intraoperative chemotherapy and radiotherapy are only justified within the context of clinical trials. Isolated chemotherapeutic perfusion of an extremity can be performed to reduce the radicality of surgery. Using this method in the treatment of soft-tissue sarcomas and of malignant melanoma and its in-transit metastases, amputations can be avoided in a great number of patients without compromising survival (Schraffordt Koops et al. 1981; Schraffordt Koops et al. 1987).

The concept of postoperative adjuvant chemotherapy also seems logical from the oncological viewpoint; however, final clinical results that might document the benefit of this therapy are still lacking in most cases. Only in breast cancer are positive results to be gleaned from the literature, mainly by compiling statistics. One of the main fields of interest is complementary stimulation of the immune system. This has led to the coining of new terms, for examples "immunochemosurgery" (Kim 1987). The studies published must be assessed carefully and critically.

In view of the altogether unsatisfactory sensitivity of gastrointestinal tumors to cytostatic drugs and the inherent problems, it was turned to specific active immunotherapy. This approach seems to be promising, because it was shown that modified autologous tumor cells induce a specific immunological response at the cellular and humoral levels in patients. The concept of specific active immunization will therefore be investigated in a randomized prospective study comprising patients subjected to curative operation for advanced or metastatic colorectal carcinoma (Lehner et al. 1989).

Surgical treatment of locoregional recurrences following resection of tumors in the gastrointestinal tract continues to yield results that are not particularly encouraging (Herfarth et al. 1987). It is of benefit in the resection of liver metastases if they are localized to the area of the liver and can be totally resected by surgical means. This is assumed if such metastases do not exceed four in number.

Resection of solitary or singular liver metastases in patients suffering from colorectal cancer can increase survival time so that one third of all patients live for 5 years. Recently this has become evident from the reduced complication rate for surgical interventions in the liver, to which improved operative techniques such as intraoperative sonography and resection of liver segments using an ultrasound knife also contribute. It is important to stress that in treatment of metastases the resection of liver segments yields survival similar to that after hemihepatectomy, if sufficient safety margins are observed. Further discriminating factors for prognosis have been elaborated for patients with liver metastases from colorectal cancer. Especially important seem to be the tumor stage at the time of the first operation and the number of metastases in the liver. In the case of endocrine tumors, however, resection even of multiple metastases is feasible; not only symptoms but also total survival time can be influenced positively, and even cures can be achieved (Hohenberger et al. 1988).

Surgical treatment is even indicated for lung metastases of some tumor types. A recommended approach is median sternotomy. The pleural cavity and the lungs can be exposed from all sides, and any hitherto unsuspected metastases can be resected as well. The results of operative treatment of lung metastases are favorable in the case of soft-tissue sarcomas and hypernephromas (Merkle and Vogt-Moykopf 1989).

Multiple metastatic spread into one organ imposes natural limits on resectability. Local chemotherapy has increasingly been promoted for multiple metastases of the liver in colorectal carcinoma. Its principal advantages are high local concentration of the cytotoxic drugs, direct attack on the tumor and almost complete avoidance of systemic toxicity. Modern advances in catheters, ports, pumps and injection methods have increased the interest in these therapeutic methods (Herfarth and Hohenberger 1987). However, a large number of problems are still unsolved and can hardly be investigated in patients. We therefore developed an animal model to find solutions to the open questions. Of particular interest was identification of the most adequate route of administration – intra-arterial or intraportal, bolus or continuous infusion. In the model intra-arterial infusion proved the most effective route of administration. Continuous intra-arterial infusion achieved the greatest inhibition of tumor growth.

The results obtained in animal experiments have meanwhile been confirmed in part in humans, as detected by NMR spectroscopy. It was demonstrated that intra-arterial long-term infusion was more effective than bolus administration and intravenous administration of 5-FU with reference to formation of metabolites.

The clinical therapeutic situation is additionally complicated by the differing sensitivity of individual tumors to cytostatic drugs. Attempts to predict the sensitivity for cytostatics in the colony-forming assay have failed. More successful seem to be trials in which the absorption and metabolism of radioactively labeled 5-FU are investigated in humans by means of spectroscopy. This method not only permits distinction between chemoresistant and chemosensitive tumors but at the same time allows one to determine whether the cytostatic effect can be changed or enhanced chemically. The combination of folenic acid as pretreatment and subsequent 5-FU chemotherapy seems interesting. Despite these possibilities, the clinical benefits of regional chemotherapy are still marginal, and the results available thus far do not justify recommendation of this technique for routine use. Substantial increases in survival have not yet been recorded, so that the use of regional chemotherapy will have to be restricted to clinical studies for some time to come.

The chances for early diagnosis of recurrences and metastases have become better with the increasing improvements in imaging methods and the regular use of endoscopy in tumor follow-up. Here the so-called tumor markers are of particular relevance, because they might give early evidence of recurrent tumors. It is not impossible for the recurrence to manifest itself by increased tumor marker levels in serum, even if the tumormarkers were negative before the primary operation. Of particular importance in the diagnosis of recurrent colorectal carcinoma is carcinoembryonal antigen (CEA); however, CEA does not permit localization of the recurrence. Hopes have been aroused by immunoscintigraphy with radioactively labeled monoclonal antibodies to the tumor-associated antigens used at the target for diagnostic localization. Despite a few positive reports, however, the own results with this diagnostic technique have been disappointing. Both sensitivity and specificity of immunoscintigraphy with Fab fragments of anti-CA 19-9 were poor in detecting local recurrences and no better than conventional diagnostic methods in detecting organ metastases. In contrast, positron emission tomography proved to be effective in differentiating tumor tissue in the case of suspicion of tumor on computer tomography in the presacral region after anterior resection or abdominoperineal extirpation. This method permits one to carry out metabolic investigations in vivo using radioactively labeled substrates. Tumor tissue has distinctly higher metabolic activity than scar tissue. The alterations could be differentiated with high sensitivity and specificity. This was not possible by immunoscintigraphic methods (Schlag et al. 1987).

The advances in diagnosis have not solved the problem of definitely excluding or proving recurrent diseases when the level of serum tumor markers is elevated. The situation calls for a second-look operation. This procedure has proved its worth, evidence of recurrent disease being found in more than 90% of cases. It is important that the rate of resectability was decisively increased compared to recurrences detected by other diagnostic methods. In a prospective study on colorectal carcinoma we came to the interesting conclusion that strict CEA-supported follow-up, including second-look operation, resulted in significant prognostic benefit for the patient. Patients subjected to second-look operation survive significantly longer than patients in whom the recurrence is diagnosed by other methods or symptomatically. This finding refers to colorectal carcinomas only and cannot be applied to other tumors (Quentmeier et al. 1986).

Surgical oncology provides a number of interesting sidelights on therapy with regard to radicality of surgery, perioperative adjuvant treatment, and operative treatment of locoregional recurrences and metastases. Locoregional chemotherapy may complement this strategy.

Surgical oncology embraces a great many potentially therapeutic activities, whose ultimate value has not yet been adequately demonstrated by objective scientific means. Thus, surgical oncology, with its many fields, is still a strictly academic discipline encompassing a multitude of scientific tasks. Only some of the procedures supplementing surgery can already be said to be part of the standard therapeutic regimen. Nonetheless, a multidisciplinary clinical and experimental approach to oncological problems in surgery is necessary. This approach distinguishes the surgical oncologist from the cancer surgeon.

References

Abe M, Shibamoto Y, Takahashi M, Manabe T, Tobe T, Inamoto T (1987) Intraoperative radiotherapy in carcinoma of the stomach and pancreas. World J Surg 11:459

Douglass HO Jr (1987) Adjuvant treatment in colorectal cancer: an update. World J Surg 11:478

Feifel G, Hildebrandt U, Dhom G (1985) Die endorectale Sonographie beim Rectumcarcinom. Chirurg 56:398

Fisher B, Bauer M, Margolese R, et al (1985) Five-year results of a randomized clinical trial comparing total mastectomy and segmented mastectomy with or without radiation in the treatment of breast cancer. N Engl J Med 312:665

Gerard A, Berrod JL, Pene F, Loygue J, Laugier A, Bruckner R, Camelot G, Arnaud JP, Metzger U, Buyse M, Dalesio O, Duez N (1988) Preoperative radiotherapy and radical surgery as combined treatment in rectal cancer. Recent Results Cancer Res 110:130
Heberer G, Denecke H, Demmel N, Wirsching R (1987) Local procedures in the management of rectal cancer. World J Surg 11:499
Herfarth C, Hohenberger P (1987) Catheters, ports and pumps in surgery. Lecture, Société Internationale de Chirurgie, Sydney
Herfarth C, Schlag P (1979) Gastric cancer. Springer, Berlin Heidelberg New York
Herfarth C, Merkle P, Schlag P (1981) Das Magencarcinom. Chirurg 52:193
Herfarth C, Schlag P, Hohenberger P (1987) Surgical strategies in locoregional recurrences of gastrointestinal carcinoma. World J Surg 11:504
Hohenberger P, Schlag P, Schwarz V, Herfarth Ch (1988) Leberresektion bei Patienten mit Metastasen colorectaler Carcinome. Ergebnisse und prognostische Faktoren. Chirurg 59:410
Jeekel J (1987) Can radical surgery improve survival in colorectal cancer? World J Surg 11:412
Kelsen DP (1984) Chemotherapy of esophageal cancer. Semin Oncol 9:159
Kelsen DP, Fein R, Coonley C, Heelan R, Bains M (1986) Cisplatin, vindesine, and methyl-glyoxal bis (guanylhydrazone) chemotherapy of esophageal cancer. Cancer Treat Rep 70:155
Kelsen DP (1987) Preoperative chemotherapy in esophageal carcinoma. World J Surg 11:433
Kim JP (1987) The concept of immunochemosurgery in gastric cancer. World J Surg 11:465
Lehner B, Liebrich W, Schlag P, Herfarth Ch, Mechtersheimer G, Schirrmacher V (1989) Charakterisierung und erste Ergebnisse einer aktiven spezifischen Immuntherapie bei Patienten mit colorectalem Carcinom. Chirurgisches Forum. Springer, Berlin Heidelberg New York London Paris Tokyo (in press)
Maruyama K, Okabayashi K, Kinoshita T (1987) Progress in gastric cancer surgery in Japan and its limits of radicality. World J Surg 11:418
Merkle NM, Vogt-Moykopf I (1989) Chirurgische Therapie von Lungenmetastasen. In: Rothmund M (ed) Metastasenchirurgie. Thieme, Stuttgart (in press)
Metzger U (1988) Adjuvant portal infusion chemotherapy in colorectal cancer. Recent Results Cancer Res 110:95
Nigro ND (1987) Multidisciplinary management of cancer of the anus. World J Surg 11:446
Papillon J (1988) Current therapeutic concepts in management of carcinoma of the anal canal. Recent Results Cancer Res 110:146
Papillon J (1988) The true role of external-beam in the initial treatment of cancer of the rectum. Recent Results Cancer Res 110:114
Papillon J, Mayer M, Montbaron J, Gerard J, Chassard J, Bailly C (1983) A new approach to the management of epidermoid carcinoma of the anal canal. Cancer 51:1830
Quentmeier A, Schlag P, Herfarth Ch (1986) Schlüsselrolle des CEA-Testes für die Diagnostik und chirurgische Therapie des rezidivierten colorectalen Carcinoms. Chirurg 57:83
Schlag P, Schreml W, Gaus W, Herfarth C, Linder MM, Queisser W, Trede M (1982) Adjuvant 5-fluorouracil and BCNU chemotherapy in gastric cancer: 3 years' results. Recent Results Cancer Res 80:277
Schlag P, Hölting Th, Steinbächer M, Kretzschmar U, Georgi P (1987) Zur derzeitigen Rolle der Immunszintigraphie für die operative Rezidivtherapie colorectaler Carcinome. Chirurg 58:594
Schlag P, Herrmann R, Raeth U, Lehner B, Schwarz V, Herfarth C (1988) Preoperative (neoadjuvant) chemotherapy in squamous cell cancer of the esophagus. Recent Results Cancer Res 110:14
Schraffordt Koops H, Beekhuis H, Oldhoff J, Oosterhuis JW, van der Ploeg E, Vermey A (1981) Local recurrence and survival in patients with (Clark's level IV/V and over 1.5 mm thickness) stage I malignant melanoma of the extremities after regional perfusion. Cancer 48:1952
Schraffordt Koops H, Oldhoff J, Oosterhuis JW, Beekhuis H (1987) Isolated regional perfusion in malignant melanoma of the extremities. World J Surg 11:527
Veronesi U (1987) Rationale and indications for limited surgery in breast cancer: current data. World J Surg 11:493

Photodynamic Laser Therapy of Photosensitized Tumors

E. Unsöld

Introduction

Lasers have proved their feasibility as a valuable instrument in many fields of invasive and operative medicine. Surgical techniques using the laser for coagulation, denaturation, ablation, or cutting of tissue can generally be summarized from a physical viewpoint as thermal methods. The application is guided by the physical properties of the laser radiation (wavelength, power, and energy density) and of the tissue (absorbance, scattering, and *thermal* conductivity). In contrast the therapeutic methods to be described here are based on primarily *nonthermal* phenomena of light-induced biochemical reactions of photosensitizing drugs (Unsöld and Jocham 1987, 1988).

Photosensitization

The photosensitizing drug most commonly used today is a hematoporphyrin derivative (HpD), which to a large extent consists of ether- and/or ester-linked hematoporphyrin molecules (DHE) (Fig. 1) (Kessel et al. 1985; Truscott 1985). Due to their imperfect synthesis, up to about 25 further porphyrins can be detected in commercially available HpD fractions. Synergism of these many components cannot be excluded. Several other sensitizers, e.g., of the group of phthalocyanines (van Lier et al. 1984; Biolo et al. 1987; Milanesi et al. 1987), purpurines (Garbo et al. 1987), or antibody- (Wat et al. 1984) and liposome-bound dyes (Reddi et al. 1985) are under investigation. All substances commercially available today are not admitted for general clinical use but only for experimental application.

The photosensitizing drug is administered systemically, is selectively stored in tumorous tissue, and provides a transient marking of malignant tissue. Ratios of concentration of sensitizer in tumorous versus normal tissue of between 2 and 30 have been determined, depending on the individual organ (Eckhauser et al. 1987; Tralau et al. 1987a, b). Those involved in metabolizing the sensitizer, e.g., liver and kidney, do not show a significant contrast. Inflamed or highly proliferating tissues, however, seem to have a remarkable affinity for porphyrin-based marker (Moan et al. 1984). Visual controls, biopsies, and subsequent histopathological investigations must be performed to substantiate the discrimination of photosensitized normal and tumorous tissue.

The fluoroscopic diagnosis of sensitizer-marked tumors is of high clinical relevance, but has to be omitted in this review (Baumgartner et al. 1986, 1987; Baumgartner and Unsöld 1987; Unsöld et al. 1987; Unsöld 1988).

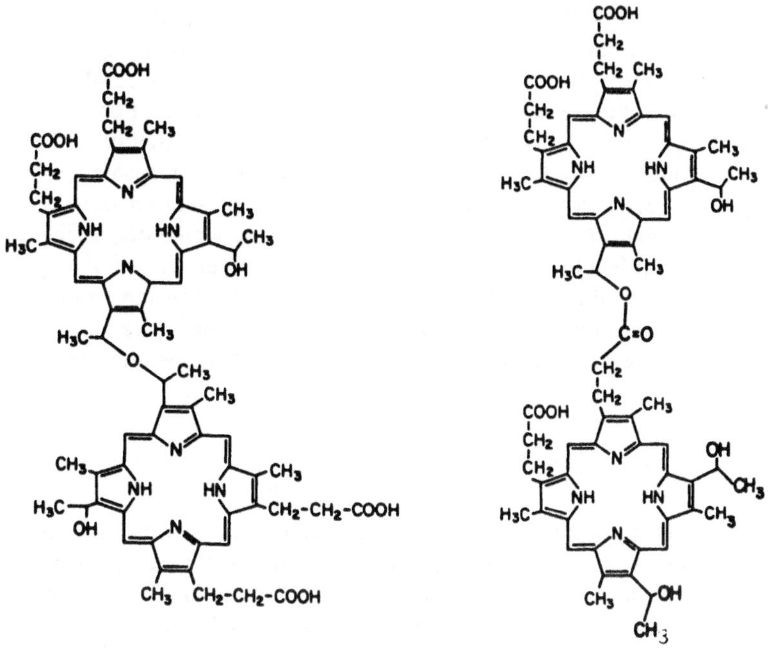

Fig. 1. Structural formulae of dihematoporphyrin ether *(left)* and ester *(right)* (after Kessel et al. 1985), but three or more hematoporphyrin molecules may also be combined (Truscott 1985)

The physiological and chemical mechanisms involved in selectively marking tumors with HpD are not unambiguously known. The reduced lymphatic drainage of tumors, the increased permeability of their blood vessels, and the increased phagocytosis of HpD in malignant tissue are assumed mainly to induce the selective storage of HpD in tumors.

A preferred storage of HpD only in tumorous cells in vitro (Ambesi-Impiombato et al. 1984) could not reproducibly be affirmed (Berns et al. 1983; Weinsheimer 1985). Normal and malignant cells show about the same rates in their HpD uptake, but the rate of release of the drug seems to be reduced for tumorous cells as compared with normal cells (Unsöld 1988).

A selective but photodynamic destruction of malignant tumors of the skin, eye, ENT/head and neck, lung gastrointestinal tract, cervix uteri, and urinary bladder has been proved in a total of over 5000 patients worldwide.

Photodynamic Therapy

Photoactivation of singlet oxygen is claimed as the basic mechanism underlying photodynamic therapy (PDT) of tumors. This effect can only be induced by light sufficiently absorbed by the photosensitizer but little screened by the overlaying tissue in order to obtain a remarkable effect in depth.

Hemoglobin (oxygenated and deoxygenated) is the main optical absorbent in tissue. According to Fig. 2 (Welch et al. 1977), a wavelength of 630 nm has been chosen as the best compromise for DHE excitation. Argon ion laser-pumped dye laser are well introduced as a light source and allow for irradiation of hollow organs also endoscopically (Fig. 3). Also gold vapor laser, flashlamp-, excimer laser-, and copper vapor laser-pumped dye laser are used experimentally. Even incoherent light sources seem to be applicable under certain circumstances for photodynamic therapy (PDT). At present, fully developed irradiation systems with satisfactory and safe performance do not exist. Especially the light applicators existing at present ensure a complete and sufficient irradiation of a tumor-bearing area or the whole organ only in few fields of application (Unsöld and Jocham 1987). For example, the use of a light-scattering medium and special twin-balloon catheters for introduction and fixation of the laser light fiber seems to be a good approach for homogeneously irradiating the whole inner surface of the urinary bladder (Jocham et al. 1986; so-called integral PDT).

Dosimetry

The light dose absorbed by the sensitizer and consequently the quantity of photo-oxidants produced seems to be essential for success or failure of PTD. Depending on the organ to be treated, the tumor size and distribution, and the HpD dose applied (usually i.v. injection of 2–5 mg/kg body weight), irradiances of 20–600 mW/cm^2 and radiant exposures of 15–360 J/cm^2 are required at the site of treatment (Wilson and Jeeves 1987).

Several factors, especially of the irradiation system, have to be taken into account to ensure a reliable dosimetry. Control of the output power of the laser, i.e., "light mode control" or monitoring of the light power transmitted to the area to be irradiated do not guarantee sufficient treatment. Small isotropic detectors, coupled to

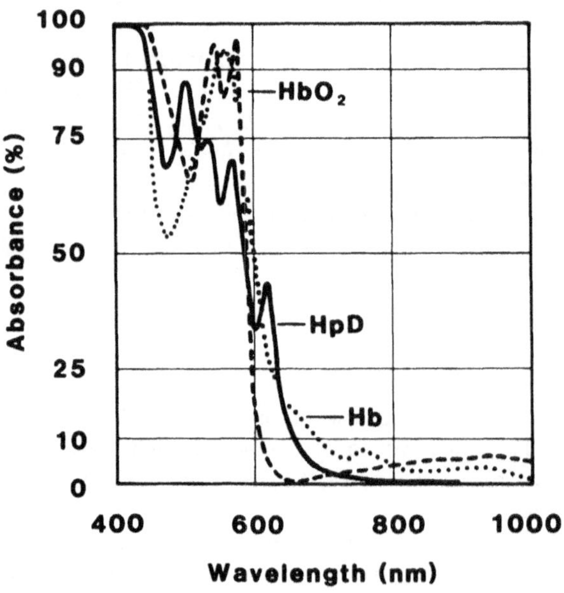

Fig. 2. Absorbance of oxygenated and deoxygenated hemoglobin solution (150 mg/ml, optical path length, 0.1 mm) and HpD in NaCl/FCS (1:1, 1.25 mg/ml, optical path length, 1 mm)

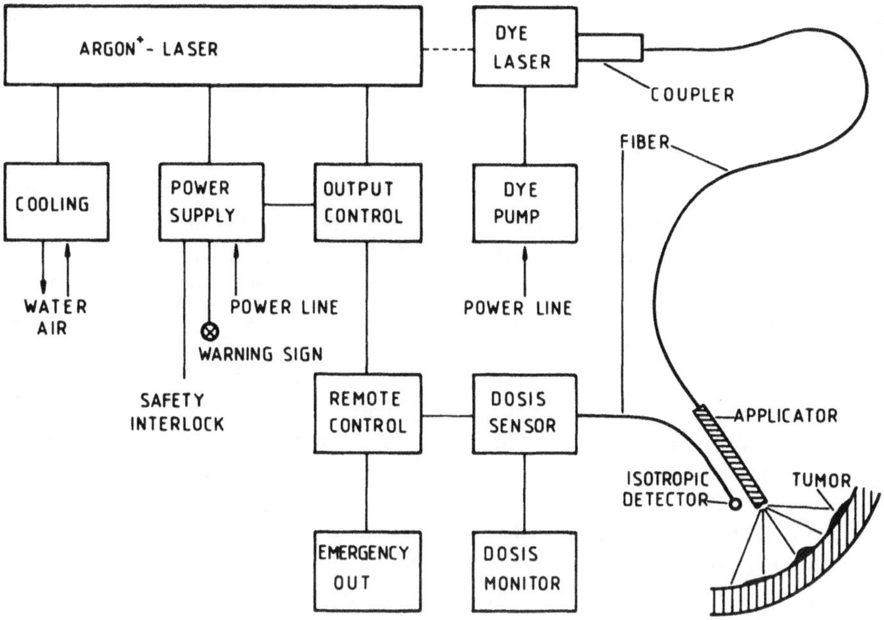

Fig. 3. Schematic diagram of a PDT laser system with integrated isotropic detector

separate sensor fibers and placed at different sites of the area to be treated with PDT (Fig. 3), may serve to reliably control the light dose applied (van Gemert et al. 1987; Marijnissen and Star 1987; Star and Marijnissen 1988). These detectors should, of course, be integrated in the light applicators and devices for irradiation wherever possible to provide a compact system for safe and easy handling.

Side Effects

General photosensitization especially of the skin and the retina is the most striking side effect after administration of HpD. One has to bear in mind that 12–15 min of sun irradiation provides about the same dose of light as a therapeutic irradiation to understand the importance of light protection for patients treated with HpD (Unsöld and Jocham 1988). The sensitivity of skin remains up to 3 months after treatment and hinders the use of HpD for routine administration in tumor diagnosis. Other sensitizers, e.g., aluminum-sulfonated phthalocyanine (A1SPc), seem to overcome the problem of skin photosensitization and add support to their future use in PDT (Tralau et al. 1987b).

Final Remark

The problems briefly outlined above must be satisfactorily solved before photodynamic treatment will be applicable in daily clinical work. But PDT with its "reversible" and repetitively applicable capabilities promises to supplement classical "final" surgical treatment of tumors.

Summary

Several drugs are known to be stored in malignant tissue as compared with normal tissue for a prolonged time after systemic administration. Today this transient marking of tumorous tissue is usually performed with hematoporphyrin derivatives (HpD), enabling photosensitization of malignant tissue and, thus, photodynamic therapy to be carried out. Photoinduced production of singlet oxygen is assumed to be the initial cytotoxic process.

Argon ion laser-pumped dye lasers, or more recently gold vapor lasers, coupled to optic fibers seem to be the most suitable light sources and open up the possibility of endoscopic applications. The light delivery system and dosimetry, however, has to be adapted individually to the different sites of irradiation.

The sensitization method used for therapy can be adapted for use in diagnosis, that is for detection of fluorescing photosensitized tumors.

So far over 5000 patients have been treated worldwide, but further efforts are necessary to improve the sensitizers and the modalities of light application.

Acknowledgments. The work was supported in part by the Bundesministerium für Forschung und Technologie, Bonn, the Wilhelm-Sander-Stiftung, Neustadt, and the Deutsche Krebshilfe, Mildred-Scheel-Stiftung, Bonn.

References

Ambesi-Impiombato FS, Andreoni A, Cubeddu R, Esposito M, Mastrocinque M, Tramontano D (1984) Effects of HpD and laser on transformed and corresponding normal cultured cells: differential cytotoxicity as an in vitro model for tumor photochemotherapy. In: Andreoni A, Cubeddu R (eds) Porphyrins in tumor phototherpay. Plenum Press, New York London, pp 143–155

Baumgartner R, Unsöld E (1987) High contrast fluorescence imaging using two-wavelength laser excitation and image processing. J Photochem Photobiol B: Biol 1:130–132

Baumgartner R, Feyh J, Götz A, Jocham D, Schneckenburger H, Stepp H, Unsöld E (1986) Experimental study on laser-induced fluorescence of hematoporphyrin derivative (HpD) in tumor cells and animal tissue. Laser 2:4–9

Baumgartner R, Fisslinger H, Jocham D, Lenz H, Ruprecht L, Stepp H, Unsöld E (1987) A fluorescence imaging device for endoscopic detection of early stage cancer – instrumental and experimental studies. Photochem Photobiol 46:759–763

Berns MW, Wile AG, Dahlmann A, Johnson F, Burns R, Sperling D, Guiltinan M, Siemens A, Walter R, Hammer-Wilson M (1983) Cellular uptake, excretion, and localization of hematoporphyrin derivative (HpD) In: Kessel D, Dougherty TJ (eds) Porphyrin photosensitization. Plenum Press, New York London, pp 139–151

Biolo R, Spada A, Reddi E, Milanesi C, Jori G (1987) TPPS and Zn-phthalocyanine as photodynamic agents in vivo: pharmacokinetic and toxicological studies. In: 2nd Congr Europ Soc Photobiol, Sept 6–10, 1987, Padova, Italy, Abstracts. Elsevier Sequoia, Lausanne, C 163, p 148 and in: Douglas RH et al (eds) Light in biology and medicine. Plenum Press, New York London, vol 1 (in preparation)

Eckhauser ML, Persky J, Bonaminio A, Crespin J, Imbembo AL, Holt S (1987) Biodistribution of the photosensitizer dihaematoporphyrin ether. Lasers Med Sci 2:101–105

Garbo GM, Keck RW, Selman H, Morgan AR (1987) Comparison of two delivery systems for a hydrophobic photosensitizer in photodynamic therapy of rat bladder tumors. In: 2nd Congr

Europ Soc Photobiol, Sept 6–10, 1987, Padova, Italy, Abstracts. Elsevier Sequoia, Lausanne, C 124, p 126 and in: Douglas RH et al (eds) Light in biology and medicine. Plenum Press, New York London, vol 1 (in preparation)

Gemert MJC van, Cheong WF, Welch AJ, Star WM (1987) Light delivery for whole-bladder photodynamic therapy. Lasers Med Sci 2:273–284

Jocham D, Schmiedt E, Baumgartner R, Unsöld E (1986) Integral laser photodynamic treatment of multifocal bladder carcinoma photosensitized by hematoporphyrin derivative. Eur Urol [Suppl 1] 12:43–46

Kessel D, Chang CK, Musselman B (1985) Chemical, biologic, and biophysical studies on hematoporphyrin derivative. In: Kessel D (ed) Methods in porphyrin photosensitization. Plenum, New York, pp 213–227

Lier JE van, Ali H, Rousseau J (1984) Phthalocyanines labeled with gamma-emitting radionucleides as possible tumor scanning agents. In: Doiron DR, Gomer CJ (eds) Porphyrin localization and treatment of tumors. Liss, New York, pp 315–319

Marijnissen JPA, Star WM (1987) Quantitative light dosimetry in vitro and in vivo. Lasers Med Sci 2:235–241

Milanesi C, Cavallini L, Reddi E, Biolo R, Jori G (1987) TPPS and Zn-phthalocyanine as photodynamic agents in vivo: studies on the mechanism of photoinduced tumor necrosis. In: 2nd Congr Europ Soc Photobiol, Sept 6–10, 1987, Padova, Italy, Abstracts. Elsevier Sequoia, Lausanne, C 164, p 148 and in: Douglas RH et al (eds) Light in biology and medicine. Plenum Press, New York London, vol 1 (in preparation)

Moan J, Christensen T, Jacobsen PB (1984) Porphyrin-sensitized photoinactivation of cells in vitro. In: Doiron DR, Gomer CJ (eds) Porphyrin localization and treatment of tumors. Liss, New York, pp 419–442

Reddi E, Valduga G, Jori G (1985) Photosensitizing properties of liposome-bound hematoporphyrin. In: Jori G, Perria C (eds) Photodynamic therapy of tumors and other diseases. Libreria Progetto, Padova, pp 67–69

Star WM, Marijnissen JPA (1988) Quantitative light dosimetry in vitro and in vivo. In: Siomos K (ed) Lasers in medicine. Pelekanakis, Chania, pp 74–87

Tralau CJ, Baar H, Sandemann DR, Barton T, Lewin MR, Bown SG (1987a) Aluminum sulfonated phthalocyanine distribution in rodent tumors of the colon, brain and pancreas. Photochem Photobiol 46:777–781

Tralau CJ, Young AR, Wacker NPJ, Brown SB, Brown SG (1987b) A comparison of the skin photosensitizing potentials of dihematoporphyrin ether (DHE) and aluminum sulphonated phthalocyanine (AlSPc) in mice. In: 2nd Congr Europ Soc Photobiol, Sept 6–10, 1987, Padova, Italy, Abstracts. Elsevier Sequoia, Lausanne C 129, p 129 and in: Douglas RH et al (eds) Light in biology and medicine. Plenum Press, New York London, vol 1 (in preparation)

Truscott TG (1985) Photochemistry of porphyrins and bile pigments in homogeneous solution. In: Bensasson RV et al (eds) Primary photo-processes in biology and medicine. NATO-ASI Series A: Life sciences, vol 85. Plenum, New York, pp 309–320

Unsöld E (1988) Lasergestützte Diagnose selektiv markierter und photosensibilisierter Tumoren. Fortschr Med 106:48/520

Unsöld E, Jocham D (1987) Therapie photosensibilisierter Tumoren. In: Meyer HJ et al (eds) Der Laser in der operativen Medizin. VCH-Verlagsgesellschaft, Weinheim, p 11

Unsöld E, Jocham J (1988) Grundlagen photodynamischer Laser-Therapieverfahren. Chirurg 59: 76–80

Unsöld E, Baumgartner R, Jocham D, Stepp H (1987) Application of photosensitizers in diagnosis and therapy. Laser 3:210–214

Wat CK, Mew D, Levy JG, Towers GHN (1984) Photosensitizer-protein conjugates: potential use as photoimmunotherapeutic agents. In: Doiron DR, Gomer CJ (eds) Porphyrin localization and treatment of tumors. Liss, New York, pp 351–359

Weinsheimer W (1985) Experimente zur Diagnostik und Therapie photosensibilisierter Harnblasentumoren. Thesis, University of Munich

Welch H, Birngruber R, Boergen K-P, Gabel VP, Hillenkamp F (1977) The influence of scattering on the wavelength-dependent light absorption in blood. GSF-Bericht BPT 5, GSF Neuherberg-München, p 14/1–8

Wilson BC, Jeeves WP (1987) Photodynamic therapy of cancer. In: Ben-Hur E, Rosenthal I (eds) Photomedicine, vol 2. CRS Publisher, Boca Raton, pp 127–177

Radiosurgery with a Linear Accelerator: Method, Indications and Preliminary Results

V. Sturm, W. Schlegel, B. Kimmig, B. Wowra, S. Schabbert, G. Hartmann, O. Pastyr, and W. J. Lorenz

Introduction

The term "radiosurgery" has been introduced by Leksell in the early fifties (Leksell 1951) for stereotactically guided percutaneous single dose irradiations of small intracranial lesions. For this purpose, Leksell has developed a Cobalt-60 irradiation unit and a cross fire-technique, yielding extremely steep dose gradients. Drawbacks of this very precise system are the limitation of its use to small irradiation fields with maximal diameters of 2–2.5 cm as well as its high costs.

Along with different other groups (Betti and Derechinski 1983; Colombo et al. 1985) we have developed a radiosurgical method for stereotactically guided convergent beam irradiation with photons form conventional linear accelerators (Hartmann et al. 1985).

Material and Method

A 15 MeV linear accelerator (Mevatron 77, Siemens AG) has been mechanically adjusted and the isocenter stabilised with respect to the rotation of both gantry (vertical plane) and the patient's couch (horizontal plane), the possible deviations being less than 0.5 mm. The isocenter corresponds exactly to the crossing-point of localisation-laser beams in the lateral and frontal plane.

The target-point, i.e. the center of the treatment-volume, is determined using stereotactic CT-information and special computer programs, developed by our group (Sturm et al. 1983, Schlegel et al. 1981) and adjusted to the isocenter.

Extreme beam-convergence is achieved by rotation of the linear accelerator's gantry in a vertical plane, while the patient is rotated horizontally around the isocenter.

Using tungsten-collimators with burr holes of various widths spherical volumes of 6–54 mm in diameter can be irradiated with highest precision, the overall-accuracy being ± 0.5 mm. The beam convergence provides steep dose gradients of 10–15%/mm distance from the surface of the target volume and allows the application of high irradiation doses (in our practice 10–50 Gy) in a single session with optimal sparing of the surrounding tissue.

Localisation and Treatment Planning

After fixation of the patient's head in a modified Riecher-Mundinger stereotaxic frame (Fischer Co., Freiburg), a stereotactic angiography or computerized tomography is

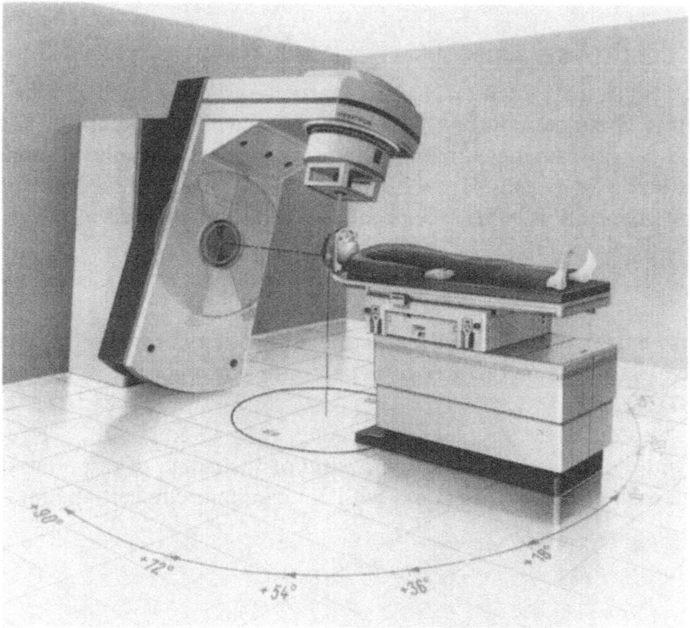

Fig. 1. Linear accelerator for stereotactic convergent beam-irradiation. The gantry is rotated in a vertical plane, the patient horizontally. The target point is adjusted to the isocenter

performed with a special localisation phantom, which provides landmarks for the establishment of a stereotactic coordinate-system with the base ring of the stereotaxic frame as reference-level.

The landmarks, detectable in each transversal CT-slice, are the basis for computerized 3-dimensional treatment planning (Schlegel et al. 1981).

After outlining the borders of the target area in each transversal CT-slice and indication of the desired irradiation dose at the tumour-surface, the target point, the width of the opening of the collimator and the depth dose distribution are calculated with special computer programs. The dose distribution is visualised 3-dimensionally in the form of isodose-surfaces together with the tumour and the surrounding brain. Using a special localisation-device, the couch of the linear accelerator is moved until the target point exactly fits the isocenter. Thereafter, the irradiation is performed.

Indications and Treatment Parameters

Linac-radiosurgery is indicated in inoperable or only partially resectable arteriovenous malformations, small inoperable benign tumours such as solid cranipharyngiomas, pituitary adenomas and basal meningiomas. In addition to these well established indications we have used this method for treatment of not resectable brain metastases with low radiosensitivity. The diameter of the treated lesions ranged between 8 and 54 mm, single doses of 8–35 Gy have been given.

Results

Since 1983, 41 arterio-venous malformations have been treated. 17 cases had a follow-up of at least 18 months. These patients have been controlled with angiography after this interval, which is considered the minimal time span between irradiation and obliteration of the pathological vessels. Total obliteration has been achieved in 6 of the 17 patients, partial obliteration in 5/17. No changes could be observed in the remaining 6 patients.

In 20% of the whole collective (41 patients) transient vasogenic edema has been observed.

Excellent results have been obtained in the treatment of solitary brain metastases with low radiosensitivity, such as metastases of hypernephromas, adenocarcinomas etc. (Sturm et al. 1987).

From 36 patients, treated so far with single doses between 10 and 35 Gy, 28 responded favourably with definitive stop of growth, and/or shrinkage of the tumour as well as a rapid decrease of the brain edema with concomitant clinical amelioration.

Discussion

The linear accelerator-system for radiosurgery with photons, developed by our group, as well as the treatment planning and the stereotactic localisation-system, briefly described above, are precise and reliable. Possible errors in the 3d-localisation of the precalculated isodose-surfaces in the intracranial space are less than 1 mm. The dose gradients are extremely steep and for equal field diameters comparable to the gradients achieved with the Stockholm "Gamma-Unit" or the Proton-unit of Harvard Medical School in Boston.

Compared with Leksell's Gamma-Unit our system has the disadvantage of a more difficult use, which makes the collaboration with a medical physicist indispensible. On the other hand, the system is extremely flexible, allowing the treatment of volumes between 6 and 54 mm in diameter. Our methods of treatment planning have proved safe and precise. Another advantage is the possibility to use any conventional linear accelerator in time-sharing with radiotherapy-units with relatively low additional costs for the necessary modifications.

The reliability of this system has been demonstrated in clinical routine use since 1983.

In our angioma series, the number of patients as well as our observation periods are much smaller than in the series of Steiner (1986) and Kjellberg et al. (1983). Thus, direct comparison of our results with these series is not possible.

The fact, that in about ⅓ of our patients complete and in ⅓ partial obliterations of the treated arterio-venous malformations could be achieved, whereas the rest of the patients did not respond, demonstrates, that the method can be highly effective, if proper treatment parameters have been chosen. The better results of Steiner (1986) may be due to the smaller size of the angiomas treated by him and correspondingly to the fact, that higher irradiation doses have been given than in most of our cases.

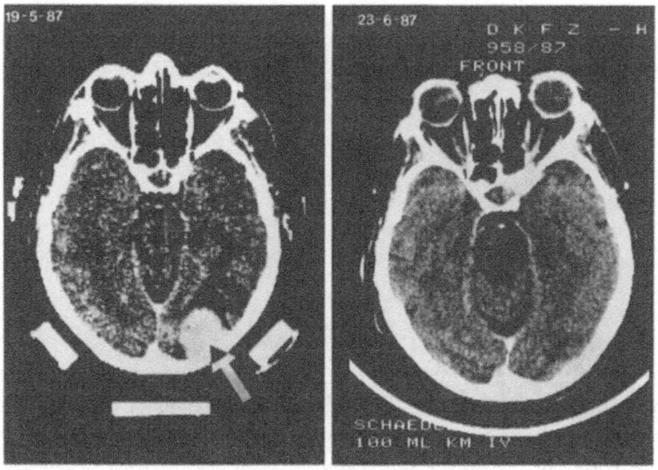

Fig. 2. Brain metastasis (primary cancer: adenocarcinoma of the lung), indicated by arrow, before *(left pannel)* and 5 weeks after stereotactic singe dose irradition with 20 Gy *(right pannel)*. Complete tumour regression has been achieved

The results, achieved in inoperable brain metastases with low radiosensitivity, are very favourable (Fig. 2). The short hospitalisation-time (2–3 days) and the good tolerance of this procedure are of special importance with regard to the limited life expectation of patients with metastatic disease.

References

Betti O, Derechinski V (1983) Irradiation stéréotaxique multifasceoux. Neurochirurgie 29:295–298

Colombo F, Benedetti A, Pozza F, Avanzo RC, Marchetti C, Chierego G, and Zanardo A (1985) External stereotactic irradiation by linear accelerator. Neurosurgery 16(2):154–160

Hartmann GH, Schlegel W, Sturm V, Kober B, Pastyr O, Lorenz WJ (1985) Cerebral radiation surgery using moving field irradiation at a linear accelerator facility. Int J Radiation Oncology Biol Phys 11:1185–1192

Leksell L (1951) The stereotaxic method and radiosurgery of the brain. Acta Chir Scand 102:316–319

Kjellberg RN, Hanamura T, Kenneth RD, Lyons SL, and Adams RD (1983) Bragg-peak proton-beam therapy for arteriovenous malformations of the brain. New Engl J Med 309(5):269–274

Schlegel W, Scharfenberg H, Sturm V, Penzholz H, and Lorenz WJ (1981) Direct visualization of intercranial tumours in stereotactic and angiographic films by computer calculation of longitudinal CT-sections: a new method for stereotactic localization of tumour outlines. Acta Neurochirurgica 58:27–35

Steiner L (1986) Radiosurgery in arteriovenous malformations of the brain. In: Fein J, Flamm E (eds) Textbook of cerebro-vascular surgery, vol IV. Springer-Verlag, New York

Sturm V, Pastyr O, Schlegel W, Scharfenberg H, Zabel HJ, Netzeband G, Schabbert S, Berberich W (1983) Stereotactic computer tomography with a modified Riechert-Mundinger device as the basis of integrated stereotactic neuroradiological investigations. Acta Neurochir 68:11–17

Sturm V, Kober B, Höver KH, Schlegel W, Boesecke R, Pastyr O, Hartmann GH, Schabbert S, zum Winkel K, Kunze S, Lorenz WJ (1987) Stereotactic percutaneous single dose irradiation of brain metastases with a linear accelerator. Int J Radiation Oncology Biol Phys 13:279–282

Summary of Discussion: Session 1

P. Schlag

Today, operative therapy is still the only method which offers the possibility of cure in most patients with solid tumors. In past decades the aim of cure was pursued only by radical surgical intervention. However, in recent years new developments have arisen. Using multimodal therapy, attempts were made to decrease morbidity and mortality after surgical procedures and at the same time improve therapeutic prospects in general. Here, operative tumor therapy has acquired new significance as part of a complete concept of cancer therapy. This development has came about particularly as a result of progress in diagnostic and therapeutic techniques. For example, it is possible that at the time of operation one can better assess tumor stage with the aid of endoscopic and intraoperative sonography or immunodetection, and the extent of surgical intervention can thus be individually adjusted.

Technical developments such as those in endoscopic microsurgery or in tissue transsection (CUSA: Cavitron Utrasonic Surgical Aspirator) have been the chief contributors to this progress. Special interest is being shown in the field of photodynamic therapy. By means of light-irritable substances, e.g., hematoporphyrins or phthalocyanines, which selectively accumulate in tumor tissues, it may be possible to destroy a tumor by laser therapy. The light conductor can be introduced by endoscopy or applied directly during surgery. Most experience has been gained in bladder tumors, but it appears that there is big future potential for the treatment of tumors of many different types and statuses – not only those for which good methods of operative treatment already exist today, but also those in which operations using conventional methods can be undertaken only with difficulty or at high risk. A similar development has been introduced in interstitial radiotherapy for brain tumors. These tumors, which previously could not be treated by conventional operative methods, can now be treated with high precision. The methods of the new field of radiosurgery include additionally very sharply focused single-dose radiation, which depends on highly precise planning of radiotherapy. This kind of treatment strategy has mainly been used in the treatment of brain tumors; in future, it will also be applied in the therapy of other solid tumors which have been difficult to treat.

One addition already made to operative tumor therapy is intraoperative radiotherapy. Radiation therapy is gaining importance especially in case of tumor remnants left after surgery or tumor recurrence. With this, operative measures and operative techniques will be increasingly used in the treatment of tumor recurrence or metastasis. At least for some tumors, it is already apparent in roughly what cases operative treatment as a local therapeutic measure is superior to radiation or chemotherapy only, both in regard to morbidity and prognosis. Cytostatic treatments too will make increased use of regional treatment possibilities such as operative catheter implantation or isolated organ perfusion. These forms of treatment do in part reduce operative measures, which improves preservation of organ function. At the same time, more operative techniques have been developed in recent years which provide adequate organ substitutes, e.g., in stomach or colon operations. This techniques thus have a positive influence on patients' quality of life.

SESSION 2

Radiation

Chairman: M. Wannenmacher

New Trends in Radiation Therapy: Fast Neutrons and New Particles

A. Wambersie and F. Richard

Introduction

The efficiency of radiation therapy can be improved first by increasing the physical selectivity of the irradiation, i.e., the absorbed dose to the target volume relative to the absorbed dose to the normal tissues. In that respect, introduction of new types of radiation, such as protons or helium ions, is probably the most promising approach. However, this trend cannot be separated from continuous efforts for improving dosimetry, treatment planning, patient-beam positioning, or more accurate identification of the target volume by computed tomography (CT) or nuclear magnetic resonance (NMR).

The efficiency of radiation therapy can also be improved by enhancing the biological differential effect, i.e., at a given dose level, increasing the effect on the tumors and/or reducing the effects on normal tissues. As a matter of fact, even with the best available physical selectivity, irradiation of the normal tissues cannot be totally avoided. The first method for enhancing the differential effect was fractionation, and its benefit was universally recognized since the beginning of radiation therapy.

More recently, other approaches have been tried such as: hyperbaric oxygen, radiosensitizers (or protectors), hyperthermia, and high-LET radiation. Of these, this paper will concentrate only on the present place and prospects of high-LET radiation in cancer therapy; it is still a subject of much controversy.

Low-LET Radiation and Improvement in Physical Selectivity

One has to keep in mind that the major improvement of the efficiency of radiation therapy in the 1950s and 1960s was the progressive replacement of 200-kV X-rays by high-energy photons (and electrons). The gain in physical selectivity resulted in a clinical benefit which was rapidly evident for all (or most of) the patients. This point is now universally recognized.

We are coming close to taking a further step: the introduction of proton beams (or helium-ion beams). Proton beams are superior to photon beams from the point of view of physical selectivity. No difference in the biological effect is to be expected: for the energy used in proton beam therapy (or in helium ion beam therapy), we stay in the field of low-LET radiation. Proton beams were initially applied for tumor types or sites for which physical selectivity is essential; a clinical benefit has indeed been demonstrated. The best example is the uveal melanoma, and more than 3000 patients have so far been treated at the Harvard cyclotron (Austin-Seymour et al.

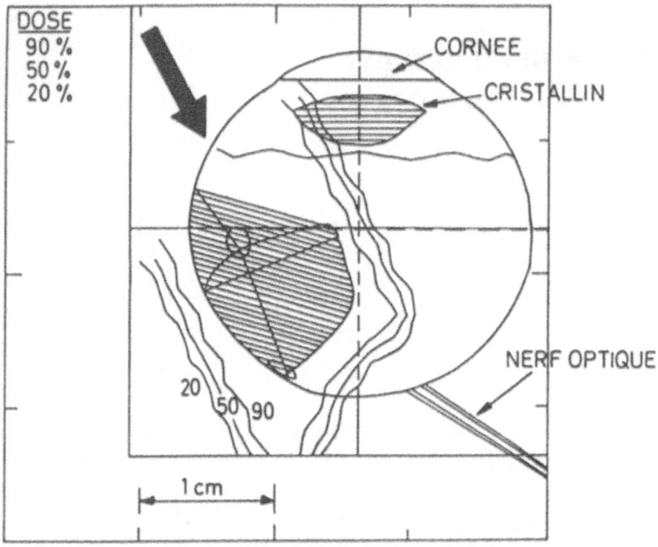

Fig. 1. Proton therapy of uveal melanoma. Dose distribution for 60-MeV proton beam; the Bragg peak has been spread out by modulating the energy from 0 to 46 MeV. The tumor *(hatched area)* as well as some normal structures (cornea, lens, optic nerve) are indicated. The *thick arrow* corresponds to the beam axis and the 90%, 50%, and 20% isodoses are drawn. Proton beams enable a homogeneous irradiation or the target volume with a maximum sparing of the normal tissues to be achieved. However, accurate patient positioning is required. (Courtesy of Ch. Perret, PSI-Villigen, p. 239 in Tubiana et al. 1986)

1989). An active program (Ophthalmology Proton Therapy Instruction Systems) is also being carried out at the Paul-Scheerer-Institut Villigen in Switzerland (Fig. 1) and two proton therapy programs for uveal melanoma are in preparation in Europe using neutron therapy machines, i.e., at Clatterbridge (United Kingdom), and Louvain-la-Neuve (Belgium) (Vynckier et al. 1984). The high degree of physical selectivity of the proton beams has also been exploited for other localizations such as paraspinal tumors, chordomas, or chondrosarcomas of the base of the skull (Austin-Seymour et al. 1989).

Furthermore, there is an increasing number of new projects which aim at treating with protons many other tumor types, and large numbers of patients (Table 1). As a matter of fact, since an improved physical selectivity is in itself always a benefit, all photon patients are, in principle, potential candidates for proton treatment.

The most impressive project is the Loma Linda project at Los Angeles, where a variable-energy synchrotron (70–250 MeV) and three treatment rooms with an isocentric rotating gantry will be the "core" of a large oncology department. An additional horizontal fixed beam will be reserved for eye and brain irradiation. The facility is scheduled for completion by the end of 1989; once all the treatment rooms are fully operational the center is expected to have a capacity of 1000 new proton beam patients/year (Slater and Miller 1987). This kind of project really aims at systematically substituting proton to photon beams. However, it raises a least three types of problem:

Table 1. Proton therapy programs

Location	Type of machine	Energy to be used clinically (MeV)
Harvard (USA)	Cyclotron	160
Loma-Linda (USA)	Synchroton	70–250
Tsukuba (Japan)	Synchroton	250
PSI-Villigen (Switzerland)	Synchroton OPTIS	250 60
Orsay (France)	Synchrocyclotron	200
Uppsala (Sweden)	Synchrocyclotron	187
Dubna (USSR)	Synchrocyclotron	90–200
Moscow (USSR)	Synchrocyclotron	70–200
Gatchina-Leningrad (USSR)	Synchrocyclotron	–
Clatterbridge (UK)	Cyclotron	65
Louvain-la-Neuve (Belgium)	Cyclotron	90

1. To what extent will the clinical benefit justify the increased cost and efforts involved?
2. Such programs imply, in the more or less near future, a redefinition of the radiotherapy network, and a progressive replacement of several small photon therapy units (or departments) by huge proton therapy facilities.
3. Finally, the full advantage of the high physical selectivity of the proton beams will be obtained only to the extent that the proton beam generators are as reliable as the modern electron linear accelerators, and that patient-beam positioning and dosimetry reach the same level of accuracy as for photons.

It is the task of the teams who have access today to high-energy proton machines to provide, as quickly as possible, a clear answer to the problem. It would be indeed a significant improvement if one could, for example, deliver with protons high-doses (60–70 Gy) to bronchial or esophageal tumors, or treat a Hodgkin's patient, with a minimum dose to the spinal cord.

High-LET Radiation and the Differential Effect

Of the types of high-LET radiation, fast neutrons were and are the most widely used. More than 15000 patients have been treated so far, at least partly, with fast neutrons, throughout the world at more than 20 facilities.

Radiobiological Considerations

The rationale for introducing fast neutrons was the existence of hypoxic cancer cells and a reduction in oxygen enhancement ratio with increasing LET. However, high-LET radiation exhibits other differences in its biological properties when compared with low-LET radiation (Tubiana et al. 1986; Wambersie et al. 1986).

- A reduction in the differences between intrinsic cell radiosensitivities, or even an inversion of the relative intrinsic radiosensitivities (Fertil et al. 1982).
- A reduction in the differences in radiosensitivity related to the position of the cells in the mitotic cycle.
- Less repair phenomena, thus a reduced importance of fractionation (consequently limited possibility of enhancing the differential effect by selecting the optimum fraction sizes).

As a result, all cell populations, in all conditions, tend to respond in a more similar way when exposed to neutrons compared with photons.

A reduction in OER is always an advantage, since the normal tissues are in general well oxygenated. By contrast, a reduction in the differences between intrinsic radiosensitivities, or radiosensitivities related to cell position in the mitotic cycle, or a reduction in the repair phenomena could bring an advantage or a disadvantage depending on the characteristics of the tumor cell population and of the normal tissue(s) at risk for a given clinical situation. In clinical situations where the cancer cell population is more resistant than the normal population to X irradiation, a reduction in the difference in radiosensitivity brings a therapeutic gain.

Two practical consequences can be derived:

1. The importance of patient selection. An absence of (or a wrong) selection of the patients for neutron therapy could lead to erroneous conclusions about the value of fast neutrons. This maybe explains at least some of the discrepancies between the reported clinical results. Selection between low- and high-LET radiation according to the individual characteristics of the tumor appears to be a promising approach. Several predictive tests have been proposed: micronuclei (Streffer), chromosome aberrations (Barendsen), and cell cultures (Brock) (Mitchell 1988).

2. The need for a high physical selectivity with high-LET radiation. When large differences in radiosensitivity are observed between the cancer and normal cell populations, a poor physical selectivity is of limited consequence. In typical cases, such as seminomas or lymphomas, where the dose prescribed to the target volume lies below the tolerance dose, irradiation of a few additional cubic centimeters of normal tissue is of little clinical importance (in chemotherapy, there is obviously no physical selectivity at all, and the therapeutic gain depends only on biological selectivity). By contrast, when the differences in radiosensitivity are reduced, as observed with high-LET radiation, the therapeutic efficiency rests mainly on a high level of physical selectivity; sparing a few cubic centimeters of normal tissues then becomes of real importance.

Clinical Data

As far as the clinical data are concerned, the superiority of fast neutrons compared with photons is recognized for well-selected types of tumors. This was first recognized for locally extended salivary gland tumors, and Table 2 summarizes the results reported worldwide (Griffin et al. 1988). In the series presented in Table 2, patients treated de novo and for gross disease after a postsurgical recurrence are included, but not patients who were treated postoperatively for microscopic residual disease. The overall local control rate is 68%; it is superior to the overall local control rate of 28% currently observed with conventional photon (electron, interstitial) therapy techniques.

The benefit of applying fast neutrons was also demonstrated for locally extended prostatic adenocarcinoma (Fig. 2). A randomized trial carried out by the RTOG (Russell et al. 1987) confirmed the results of several pilot studies (e.g. Richard et al. 1986).

There is also evidence that neutrons are superior to photons for well-differentiated soft tissue sarcomas (G1) (Table 3), osteosarcomas and chondrosarcomas. For

Table 2. Summary of local control rates for malignant salivary gland tumors treated with neutron radiotherapy (Griffin et al. 1988)

	No. of patients	Local control
Saroja et al.	113	71 (63%)
Catterall and Errington	65	50 (77%)
Duncan et al.	22	12 (55%)
Ornitz et al.	8	3 (38%)
Batterman and Mijnheer	32	21 (66%)
Maor et al.	9	6 (67%)
Eichhorn	5	3 (60%)
Skolyszewski	3	2 (67%)
University of Washington	32	26 (81%)
Overall	267	182 (68%)[a]

[a] Overall local control rate after photon (or electron) irradiation was 52/188, i.e., 28%

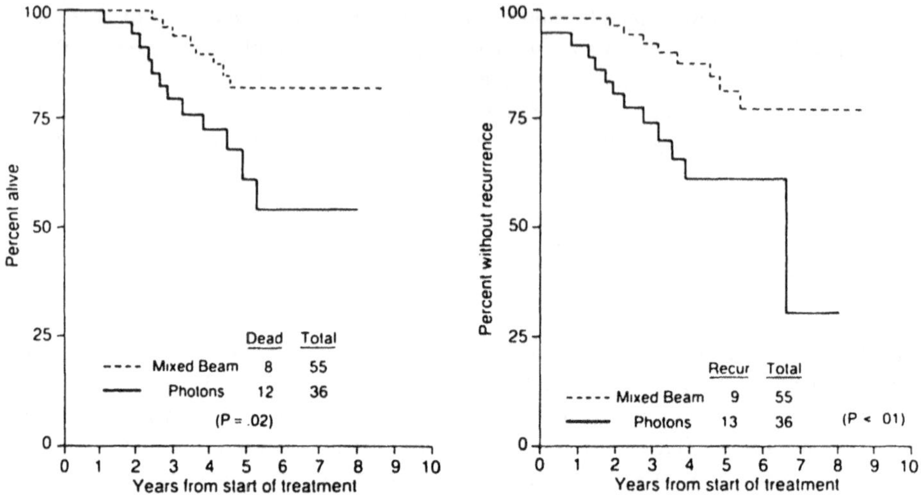

Fig. 2. Radiation therapy oncology group randomized trial comparing a combination of fast neutrons and photons ("mixed-beam") and conventional photon irradiation alone. *On the left-hand side,* the actuarial survivals at 8 years are indicated, adjusted by exclusion of intercurrent noncancer death ("determinental" survival rates). *On the right-hand side,* the local control rates are indicated. Clinical and biopsy criteria are combined. (Russell et al. 1987)

soft tissue sarcomas, Laramore et al. (Laramore et al. in press), combining the different neutron series reported worldwide, obtained an average local control rate of 53%, which is superior to the average local control rate of 38% achieved with conventional photon/electron techniques. However, as discussed elsewhere, the differences in the reported local control rates mainly reflect differences in patient recruitment, which makes any comparison very difficult (Richard et al. 1989). In general, well-differentiated slowly growing tumors are good indications for fast neutrons.

Table 4 summarizes the tumor types for which clinical experience has shown the superiority of fast neutrons. It is, of course, difficult today to evaluate the exact proportion of patients suitable for high-LET therapy; a proportion between 10% and 20% of the radiotherapy patients has been indicated (Wambersie 1988). Assuming the lower value of 10%, it would imply that one neutron generator is needed for every ten linear accelerators or cobalt units. The cost cannot be taken as a major argument against the development of fast neutron therapy. The proportions of patients treated with other special radiotherapy techniques (such as electron beams, intracavitary or interstitial therapy) are not higher, and, nevertheless, these techniques are well-accepted radiotherapy modalities, although they are also expensive.

Heavy Ions: Combination of High-LET and Improved Physical Selectivity

The physical selectivity which can be achieved with heavy ions is similar to that achieved with proton beams. To the extent that some tumors are better treated with

Table 3. Neutron therapy of soft tissue sarcomas (Laramore et al. 1989)

Facility	Local control	Percentage
Hammersmith	26/50	52
NIRS[a]	7/12	58
Fermilaboratory	13/26	50
MANTA[b]	4/10	40
TAMVEC[c]	18/20	62
Edinburgh	5/12	42
Hamburg/Eppendorf	27/45	60
Heidelberg and Essen	31/60	52
Louvain-la-Neuve	4/19	21
Amsterdam	8/13	61
Seattle[d]	15/21	71
Overall[e]	158/297	53

Summary of local control rates for soft-tissue sarcomas treated definitively with fast neutrons. Patients treated de novo or for gross disease after surgery are included but not patients treated postoperatively for microscopic residual disease or for limited macroscopic residual disease

[a] NIRS, National Institut Radiology Science (Qiba)
[b] MANTA, Middle Atlantic Neutron Therapy Association (Washington)
[c] TAMVEC, Texas A + M University Variable Energy Cyclotron (Houston)
[d] Two-year actuarial data
[e] Overall local control rate after photon/electron irradiation was 49/128, i.e., 38%

Table 4. Clinical indications for fast neutron therapy (summary)

1. Salivary gland tumors
   Locally extended
2. Prostatic adenocarcinomas
   Locally extended (C, D)
3. Soft tissue sarcomas
   Especially slowly growing well-differentiated G1 (G2)
4. Paranasal sinuses
5. Some tumors of the head and neck area
   Locally extended, metastatic adenopathies
6. Melanomas
   Inoperable/recurrent (palliative treatment)

high-LET radiation, and that the physical selectivity required with high-LET radiation is at least as high as that required with low-LET radiation, there is a place for heavy-ion beams in radiation therapy (Castro et al. 1987; Wambersie 1989).

There are at present two heavy-ion therapy projects in Europe: the GSI-Darmstadt project in the Federal Republic of Germany, and the EULIMA project (European Light Ion Medical Accelerator). For any program of that size, the investment in money and effort is so high that rigorous planning and collaboration at an international level is essential. Recruitment of a sufficient number of patients, who could fully benefit from heavy ions, also requires international collaboration.

Summary

Of the new trends in radiation therapy, the introduction of new types of ionizing radiation is one of the most promising. Low-lineal energy transfer (LET) particle beams, such as protons, aim at improving the physical selectivity of the irradiation. The clinical benefit has been demonstrated for selected tumor types or sites (e.g., uveal melanoma). High-LET radiation (e.g., fast neutrons or heavy ions) exhibits different radiobiological properties compared with low-LET radiation. Historically, the rationale for introducing high-LET radiation was a reduction in oxygen enhancement ratio. However, radiobiological evidence indicates that all cell populations, in all conditions, tend to respond in a more similar way when exposed to high-LET compared with low-LET radiation. A reduction in the differences in radiosensitivity can be an advantage or disadvantage depending on the tumor characteristics and on the normal tissues at risk. This raises the important problem of patient selection. Fast neutrons are the most widely used type of high-LET radiation. They were proven to be superior to photons for the treatment of some well-defined tumor types such as locally extended salivary gland tumors, and prostatic adenocarcinoma, or some types of sarcoma. Slowly growing well-differentiated tumors are, in general, an indication for fast neutrons (or high-LET radiation). Development of heavy-ion therapy programs is justified for some types of tumor requiring a combination of high-LET radiation and a high degree of physical selectivity.

References

Austin-Seymour M, Urie M, Muzenrider J, Willett C, Goitein M, Verhey L, Gentry R, McNulty P, Koehler A, Suit H (1988) Considerations in fractionated proton radiation therapy: clinical potential and results. Radiother Oncol (in press)

Castro JR, Gademann G, Collier JM, Linstad D, Pitluck S, Woodruff K, Gauger G, Chard D, Gutin Ph, Phillips ThL, Chu W, Henderson Sh (1987) Strahlentherapie mit schweren Teilchen am Lawrence Berkeley Laboratory der Universität von Kalifornien. Strahlenther Onkol 163:9–16

Fertil B, Deschavanne JP, Gueulette J, Possoz A, Wambersie A, Malaise EP (1982) In vitro radiosensitivity of six human cell lines. II. Relation to the RBE of 50-MeV neutrons. Radiat Res 90: 526–537

Griffin BR, Laramore GE, Russell KJ, Griffin TW, Eenmaa J (1988) Fast neutron radiotherapy for advanced malignant salivary gland tumors. Radiother Oncol 12:105–111

Laramore GE, Griffeth JT, Boespflug M, Pelton JG, Griffin TW, Griffin BR, Russell KJ, Koh W (in press) Fast neutron radiotherapy for sarcomas of soft tissue, bone, and cartilage

Mitchell JB (1988) Potential applicability of non clonogenic measurements to clinical oncology. Radiat Res 114:401–414
Richard F, Renard L, Wambersie A (1986) Current results of neutron therapy at the UCL, for soft tissue sarcomas and prostatic adenocarcinomas. Bull Cancer 73:562–568
Richard F, Renard L, Wambersie A (1989) Neutrontherapy of soft tissue sarcoma at Louvain-la-Neuve (Interim results 1987) Strahlentherapie 165:306–308
Russell KJ, Laramore GE, Krall JM, Thomas FJ, Maor MH, Hendrickson FR, Krieger JN, Griffin TW (1987) Eight years experience with neutron radiotherapy in the treatment of stages C and D prostate cancer: updated results of the RTOG 7704 randomized clinical trial. Prostate 11:183–193
Slater JM, Miller DW (1987) Loma Linda University Proton Therapy facility. In: Kraft G, Grundinger U (eds) Third workshop on heavy charged particles in biology and medicine. GSI, Darmstadt, Report 87-11, ISSN 0171-4546, K-2
Tubiana M, Dutreix J, Wambersie A (1986) Radiobiologie. Hermann, Paris
Vynckier S, Meulders JP, Robert P, Wambersie A (1984) The protontherapy program at the cyclotron "Cyclone" of Louvain-la-Neuve (first dosimetric results) Eur J Radiat Oncol 5:245–247
Wambersie A (1989) Is there any future for high-LET radiation? Strahlentherapie 165:348–356
Wambersie A, Bewley DK, Lalanne CM (1986) Prospects for the application of fast neutrons in cancer therapy: radiobiological bases and survey of the clinical data. Bull Cancer 73:546–561

Altered Fractionation in Radiotherapy

K.-R. Trott

Radiotherapy has developed through clinical experience. This means that data regarding numerous different patients were collected, averages estimated, and standardized treatments designed. Standardized field arrangements and dosage schedules are in common use today, and departure from the standardized schedules is only allowed if excessive acute reactions in the patient force the radiotherapist to change his plan.

For the individual patient this standardized treatment means that, at best, he receives the optimal average treatment – optimized, maybe, in randomized clinical trials by averaging responses from a large number of similar but not identical patients. He does not get the treatment which is best for him and his illness, but that which is best for the type of cancer he has been diagnosed as having.

Advances in diagnostic radiology, especially computed axial tomography, led to profound changes in the practice of radiotherapy by individualizing field arrangements and dose distribution in the patient. Standard field arrangements are less frequently used in curative radiotherapy today. Individual planning according to the extension of the malignant growth and the topography of the critical normal tissues adjacent to it is now common clinical practice.

The dosage schedule, however, still follows the old, time-honored way of standardization. Most radiotherapists are not even aware (nor are chemotherapists) how crudely their treatment prescription levels out individual differences in tumor biology which could be exploited to give more efficient treatment by adapting schedules to the particular features of each individual tumour.

Until recently, it was impossible to evaluate the biological data important for optimizing the treatment schedule for the individual patient. But radiobiological research has brought us closer to that aim by elucidating the biological mechanisms which determine success and failure in fractionated, curative radiotherapy. New approaches to measure the intrinsic radiosensitivity of the tumor cells in each patient are being developed (Peters et al. 1988). My paper will concentrate on the dynamic processes which go on in tumors and critical normal tissues during the course of fractionated radiotherapy. These are commonly labelled the four Rs of radiotherapy: redistribution, reoxygenation, repair, and repopulation (Withers 1975; Trott 1982).

Redistribution is associated with the differences in radiosensitivity of cells in the different phases of the cell cycle. Early in the course of radiotherapy, sensitive cells will be killed preferentially, and in a static tumor or in non-proliferating tissue, overall radiosensitivity will decrease as radioresistant cells survive preferentially. However, progression of surviving cells through the cell cycle will lead to redistribution of the cells over the various phases of the cell cycle between dose fractions. Redistribution may be of some importance especially in acute responses of rapidly proliferating tissues to accelerated fractionation treatment. But no solid data exist; redistribution is thus largely a speculative mechanism.

Reoxygenation was assumed 10 years ago to be the most important determining factor in the effectiveness of radiotherapy. This idea has recently given way to a more balanced view. Due to differences in their microenvironment, tumor cells display great differences in radiosensitivity, hypoxic cells being three times more radioresistant than cells exposed to oxygen concentrations above 10 mmHg. In a static tumor model, the proportion of hypoxic cells should increase as radiotherapy progresses, due to selective elimination of radiosensitive oxygenated cells. However, in all but one rodent tumor studied so far, the previous ratio of hypoxic to oxic cells, i.e. *the hypoxic fraction,* is back to the original value within a few hours (Kummermehr et al. 1981). No data in human tumors are available, but the experimental data in rodent tumors consistently show that reoxygenation

- occurs in the majority of tumors,
- is a fast process and complete within one day, and
- is not dependent on regression of the tumor.

Since even the mere existence of hypoxic tumor stem cells in human cancers has been disputed (Trott et al. 1984), and since clinical evidence suggesting that the failure to cure certain cancers by radiotherapy was due to insufficient reoxygenation is far from convincing, reoxygenation, despite its great importance in fractionated radiotherapy of rodent tumors, must be regarded as a speculative mechanism as regards the cure of human tumors. In any case, it does not play any role in the design of new or individualized treatment schedules in radiotherapy today.

Repair is usually associated with the restitution of the shoulder in a cellular survival curve as first described by Elkind and Sutton (1960). Since this can take place after every new dose fraction, cell survival curves after fractionated irradiation with equal doses per fraction are strictly exponential and the relative effect of each dose fraction is identical from the first to the last dose of a multifractionated course of radiotherapy.

This concept is, however, somewhat misleading since repair – even much more repair – occurs in tissues where clonogenic survival of stem cells is not the primary cellular mechanism leading to functional or structural failure of the irradiated organ. Repair can be precisely measured in cells, in tissues, in tumors but we do not know what repair actually is; moreover, it probably reflects very different molecular and cellular mechanisms in different tissues of the body. I just cannot believe that the increased tolerance of the brain to fractionated radiotherapy should be due to the same molecular DNA repair mechanism which allows irradiated bacteria to continue proliferating rapidly.

In tissues, repair is determined by the increase in radiation dose necessary to produce the same effect when radiation is given in multiple fractions as when it is given in a single dose (Reisner 1933). The increase in skin tolerance with increased fractionation can be explained as being due to the fact that part of the dose effect is repaired and that only the unrepaired dose effect accumulates.

More recent models assume that part of the radiation effect is altogether nonrepairable and this effect accumulates in proportion to the accumulation of the radiation dose. Another part of the radiation effect develops by interaction of repairable lesions. This is the basis for the linear-quadratic model, which is essentially just another way of looking at fractionation data in radiobiology and radiotherapy without necessarily implying any underlying molecular or cellular mechanism.

Each dose of the same size say, 2 Gy, has exactly the same effect; these effects are additive, i.e. 10 fractions of 2 Gy have exactly 10 times the effect of a single fraction of 2 Gy. This is very different from what happens in chemotherapy. The effect of each of the 2 Gy fractions is a composite of two effects, one contributing in proportion to the dose (α-effect) and another one contributing with the square of the dose (β-effect). The relative contributions of the linear and of the quadratic dose effects at different fraction sizes determine the relative sensitivity of a given tissue to changes in dose fractionation. Usually this fractionation sensitivity is described by the ratio of the exponents α/β. The greater α/β, the less sensitive the tissue to small changes in fraction size; the lower the α/β the more the tissue is spared as the dose per fraction is decreased (for a thorough discussion see Thames and Hendry 1987). Since tumors in general have a higher α/β value than most critical late-reacting normal tissues, significant improvements in therapeutic ratio can be expected by decreasing fractional doses even below the standard 2 Gy (Thames et al. 1983). In any case, there is no justification, no excuse, for giving dose fractions higher than about 2 Gy in curative radiotherapy.

Data on α/β values for various responses of normal tissues and tumors in experimental animals have been published frequently during the last few years, but there is still a great lack of data on α/β values in human tumors, especially of radioresistant human tumors. Overgaard (1986) has suggested that the relative radioresistance of malignant melanomas may be associated with their surprisingly low α/β value, but his conclusions have not been generally accepted. Xenografts of human tumors are an attractive experimental model for the study of this question (Lindenberger et al. 1986). Of special interest would be more data on malignant melanoma, glioblastoma, osteosarcoma, etc.; even more interesting would be data on the variability of the fractionation sensitivity (i.e., α/β values) between different tumors of the same histopathological type, so that this information could be taken into consideration when decisions about the treatment schedule are made for the individual patient. The greatest source of uncertainty with regard to apparent α/β values and fractionation sensitivity of tumors and normal tissues is the virtual absence of systematic investigations about the influence of chemotherapy on the fractionation response or repair in tumors and critical normal tissues.

Although we do not understand the molecular mechanisms of repair in tissues, we can measure its kinetics with good precision in normal tissues and in tumors of experimental animals. It is usually expressed as the exponential decrease of repairable dose with time, the repairable dose being a function of the dose per fraction and the α/β value. Repair half-times have been measured in different tissues to range from about 20 to about 200 min. Thus, repair kinetics become critical and the limiting factor in the design of accelerated treatment schedules, because a minimum of three half-times has to be allowed to elapse before the next dose of radiation is inflicted, so as to avoid the risk of accumulating unrepaired repairable damage which easily may convert the gain from the application of reduced fraction sizes into loss due to incomplete repair between insufficiently spaced fractions.

Although data on repair kinetics are rapidly accumulating now, we do not yet have enough information to decide whether there are systematic differences in repair half-times between tumors, acutely responding normal tissues, and late responding normal tissues. Moreover, it has been suggested that the repair half-time may depend on the dose per fraction, which would be of considerable practical interest. What is even more important, no data exist about the influence of chemotherapy on the kinetics of repair.

Repopulation describes the increase of the number of surviving tumor stem cells during the course of radiotherapy by cell proliferation. The importance of this factor was overlooked for a long time, since tumor volume doubling times are usually within the range of the duration of a course of radiotherapy. One doubling of tumor cells during treatment would be roughly equivalent to the effect of one additional dose fraction of 2 Gy. However, recent analysis of clinical data (Trott and Kummermehr 1985; Withers et al. 1988) has demonstrated that repopulation in lymphomas and in squamous cell carcinomas may be much faster, with doubling times close to the potential doubling time (a measure of the cell production rate in a tumor). This has lead to the suggestion that the potential doubling time, which can easily be measured within 1 day from human tumor biopsies (Wilson et al. 1985), might be a useful predictor of the repopulation potential of the individual tumor and might be used in the individual design of treatment strategies. This is especially interesting for squamous cell carcinomas, which have a median potential doubling time of about 4 days, ranging from less than 3 days to more than 20 days. This means that, provided repopulation continues throughout radiotherapy at the rate of the potential doubling time, between 2 and 13 doublings may occur, which would increase the curative radiation dose by between 4 and 26 Gy.

There are no data available which demonstrate that repopulation to such a degree does not occur during the long intervals of the chemotherapy cycles. The disappointing results of chemotherapy in squamous cell carcinomas may, at least in part, be due to efficient tumor stem cell repopulation during the bone marrow recovery/repopulation phase.

Nevertheless, so far, repopulation is nothing more than an interesting working hypothesis, and more definitive information will only come from the analysis of the present clinical trials on head and neck cancer treated either with accelerated or conventional fractionation (in which individual determination of the potential doubling time of every single tumor is included in the study protocol). Animal experiments, however, suggest that repopulation is not constant throughout the course of radiotherapy and, especially in squamous cell carcinomas, may be considerably accelerated as the radiation dose accumulates. This is also consistent with experimental data on repopulation in irradiated oral mucosa and skin. The analysis by Withers et al. (1988) of a large body of published clinical data suggests a period of little repopulation in the first 2–3 weeks of radiotherapy followed by a burst of rapid repopulation at a rate of two stem cell doublings per week. The start of stimulated repopulation is different in skin and mucosa and may differ between different tumor types, and, even more importantly, between different patients having the same type of carcinoma.

Acceleration of radiotherapy is the most appropriate method to decrease the negative effect of repopulation on tumor curability. However, accelerated treatment during the period of slow tumor repopulation will not improve results; accelerated irradiation during a period when the mucosa has already started stimulated repopulation but the tumor is still slow (maybe the 2nd and 3rd week of radiotherapy) may make things even worse! Therefore, it is of considerable practical interest to find methods to determine the nature or the time of the stimulus which could be used to start accelerated irradiation only when accelerated tumor cell repopulation begins.

Another attractive possibility to overcome the problems arising from rapid or stimulated repopulation is to develop a combination of radiotherapy and drug treatment, e.g., chemotherapy to block or suppress effective tumor stem cell repopulation. This approach may have less effect on repopulation of normal tissue stem cells than accelerated irradiation.

In any case, the concept of a continuous course of accelerated fractionation for all tumors, or for all tumors of the same type, is as gross an oversimplification and leveling out of individual differences between tumors and patients as the traditional treatment giving 30 fractions in 6 weeks to 60 Gy total dose – *which still has to be regarded as the best average treatment in curative radiotherapy.* Research should concentrate on developing parameters which define the optimal adaptation of treatment scheduling to the dynamic changes occurring in tumors and critical normal tissues. The resulting treatment schedules are unlikely to be the same for every patient with the same tumor type, unlikely to be constant throughout the course of treatment, and unlikely to give all patients treatment-free weekends.

References

Elkind MM, Sutton H (1960) Radiation response of mammalian cells grown in culture. I. Repair of X-ray damage in surviving Chinese hamster cells. Radiat Res 66:401–426

Kummermehr J, Fink R, Preuss-Bayer G, Trott KR (1981) Reoxygenierung in einem transplantablen Fibrosarkom der Maus. Strahlentherapie 157:272–276

Lindenberger J, Hermeking H, Kummermehr J, Denekamp J (1986) Response of human xenografts to fractionated X-irradiation. Radiother Oncol 6:15–27

Overgaard J (1986) The role of radiotherapy in recurrent and metastatic malignant melanoma: a clinical radiobiological study. Int J Radiat Oncol Biol Phys 12:867–872

Peters LJ, Brock WA, Chapman JD, Wilson G, Fowler JF (1988) Response predictors in radiotherapy. Megavoltage radiotherapy 1937–1987. Br J Radiol [Suppl] 22:96–108

Reisner A (1933) Hauterythem und Roentgenstrahlung. Ergeb Med Strahlenforsch 6:1–60

Thames HD, Hendry JH (1987) Fractionation in radiotherapy. Taylor and Francis, London

Thames HD, Peters LJ, Withers HR, Fletcher GH (1983) Accelerated fractionation vs hyperfractionation: rationales for several treatments per day. Int J Radiat Oncol Biol Phys 9:127–138

Trott KR (1982) Experimental results and clinical implications of the four R's in fractionated radiotherapy. Radiat Environ Biophys 20:159–170

Trott KR, Kummermehr J (1985) What is known about tumour proliferation rates to choose between accelerated fractionation and hyperfractionation? Radiother Oncol 3:1–9

Trott KR, Maciejewski B, Preuss-Bayer G, Skolyszewski J (1984) Dose-response curve and split dose recovery in human skin cancer. Radiother Oncol 2:123–130

Wilson GD, McNally NJ, Dunphy E, Karcher H, Pfragner R (1985) The labelling index of human and mouse tumours assessed by bromodeoxyuridine staining in vitro and in vivo and by flow cytometry. Cytometry 6:641–647

Withers HR (1975) The four R's of radiotherapy. In: Lett JT, Adler H (eds) Advances in radiation biology, vol 5. Academic, New York, pp 241–271

Withers HR, Taylor JMG, Maciejewski B (1988) The hazard of accelerated tumor clonogen repopulation during radiotherapy. Acta Oncol 27:131–146

New Trends in Computer-Assisted Radiotherapy with Conventional Radiation

W. Schlegel

Introduction

Radiotherapy as a local treatment modality aims at the treatment of localized tumors. As local or locoregional failure of therapy is the cause of death in about one-third of all tumor patients, the development of methods for improved local tumor control is still expected to dominate research activities in the next 5–10 years (de Vita 1983; Kuttig 1987). The other important aspect of these research and development activities, of course, is to reduce side effects in normal tissue and to improve the quality of life of tumor patients after treatment.

There are different directions within the field of radiotherapy research which can be followed in order to reach these goals. Examples are the combination of radiotherapy with surgery, hyperthermia, or chemotherapy, the alteration of fractionation schemes, or the use of radiolabeled antibodies.

Our working hypothesis is, that there is still *room for improvement of radiotherapy* by the optimization of the *physical dose distribution*.

Two ways are suited to improve the physical dose distribution. Proton beams, pi-mesons, or heavy ions produce dose distributions in tissue which are superior to the conventional treatment modalities with electrons or photons (Castro 1987; Kraft 1987; Munzenrider et al. 1987; Greiner and Blattmann 1987). Unfortunately, these particle beams are very expensive to produce and only available at some large nuclear research centers, so in order to guarantee the broad clinical applicability of the developments, we put the priority of our efforts into the alternative: conventional radiation as photons or electrons. Fortunately, the past decade has been an era of exciting advances not only in particle accelerators, but also in several other technologies which will influence how radiation therapy with conventional beams is practiced within the next years.

Figure 1 gives an overview of the chain of radiotherapy, reaching from localization of target volumes, treatment planning, patient fixation and positioning, to treatment and its verification. On the left hand side are listed some recent technological innovations which are not yet implemented in routine radiotherapy, but probably will have strong impact to radiotherapy within the next decade. For example, composite imaging with CT, MRI, PET, and digital radiography, followed by three-dimensional image correlation, will increase our ability to determine target volumes more accurately than before (Kessler 1987; Schad et al. 1988).

Having three-dimensional anatomical models of the individual patient at hand, methods of three-dimensional graphics (Bauer-Kirpes et al. 1987; McShan and Fraass 1987), accurate mathemathical methods of three-dimensional dose calculation

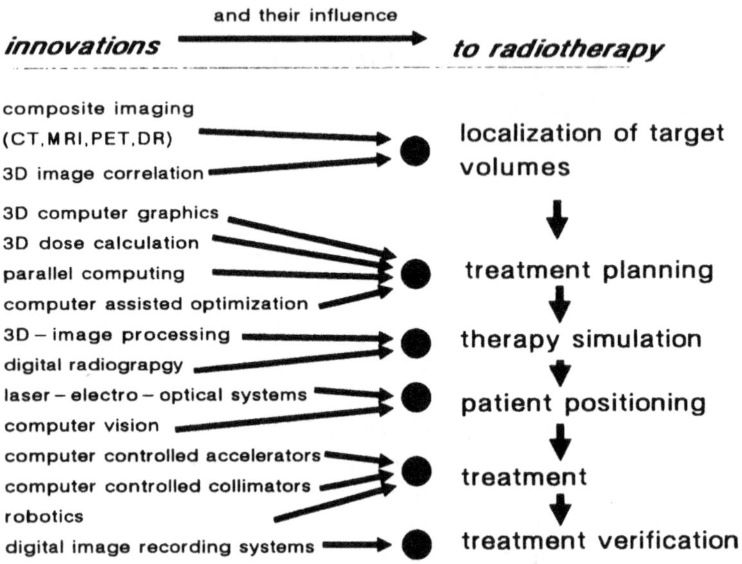

Fig. 1. Possible influence of modern technology on radiotherapy

(Schlegel et al. 1984), parallel computing, and computer-assisted optimization (Werner et al. 1987) treatment planning will be improved.

Image processing and digital radiography (Sherouse et al. 1987; Smith 1987), stereotactic techniques (Sturm et al. 1983), laser electro-optical systems and computer vision could support the radiotherapist during patient fixation and positioning under the treatment unit.

Computer-controlled linear accelerators (Smith 1986; Chin et al. 1983), computer-controlled collimators (Pastyr et al. 1987; Boesecke et al. 1988), and probably also robots (Doll et al. 1987; Kwoh et al. 1987) will enable more complex and more precise treatment modalities with superior physical dose distributions.

Digital verification systems such as multiwire proportional chambers or diode arrays could be used for on line verification and monitoring of individual dose delivery (Morton and Swindell 1987; von Herk and Meertens 1987).

New concepts of quality assurance, e.g., those adapted from flight technology, will have to be implemented in order to assure the security and safety of complex treatments with radiation (Jacky and Kalet 1987).

In this paper, I am not able to go into all details of this list of future possibilities of computer-assisted radiotherapy. In order to present some facets of the application of computers in conventional radiation in oncology, and some examples of progress, I will restrict myself to computer-assisted treatment planning and computer-controlled treatment techniques.

Computer-Assisted Treatment Planning

Besides the definition of the target volume, three steps are involved in computer-assisted treatment planning. First, the treatment technique and the related irradia-

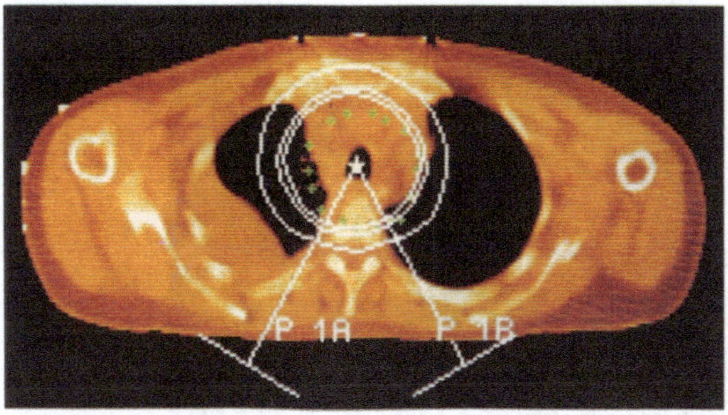

Fig. 2. Two-dimensional treatment plan for a patient with cancer of the esophagus using a moving beam treatment technique: CT image through the central plane of the target volume with 50%, 80% and 90% isodose curves

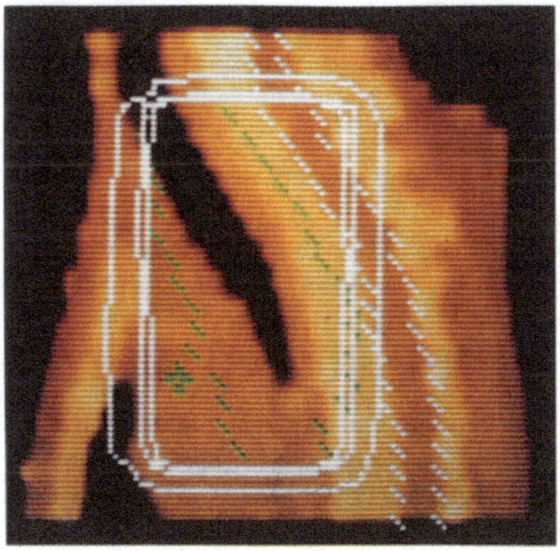

Fig. 3. Multi-planar-reconstruction of a sagittal section through the set of 21 CT images and the three-dimensional dose distribution of the treatment plan in Fig. 2. The target volume *(green dots),* the organ at risk (spinal cord, *white dots*) and the 50%, 80% and 90% isodose curves are shown

tion parameters have to be selected, the dose has to be calculated, and the resulting dose distribution has to be evaluated, either visually or numerically. These steps have to be repeated until an acceptable dose distribution is found.

In clinical routine, the calculation and visualization is performed in two dimensions, i.e. in the midline cross section through the target volume. Figure 2 illustrates this two-dimensional technique of treatment planning. After the definition of the target volume, in this case cancer located in the middle part of the esophagus, a moving beam treatment technique has been selected. It will be seen that the target volume is covered by the therapeutic dose, and that the spinal cord (the organ at risk) is beyond the critical dose.

It is often sufficient to have such a two-dimensional plan and to deliver the dose to the patient as it is planned, in two dimensions. In other cases, however, where the target volume is of irregular shape, or the critical organs (in this example the spinal

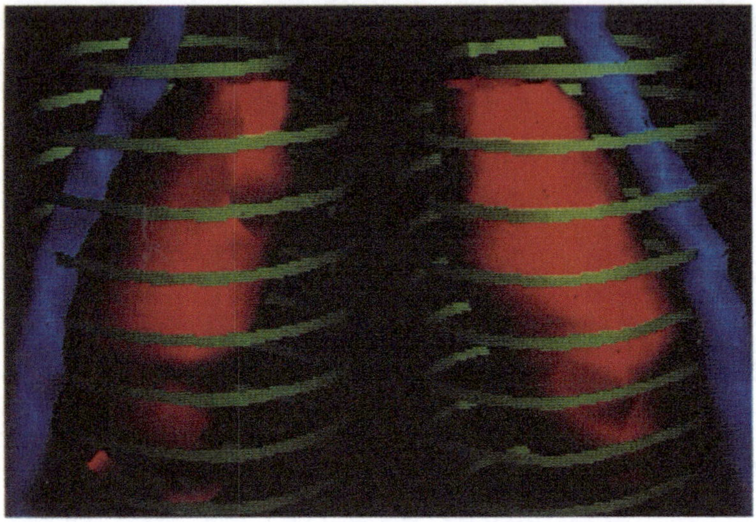

Fig. 4. Three-dimensionally shaded object representation of the target volume *(red)*, spinal cord *(blue)*, and 80% isodose surface *(green ribbons)* of the treatment plan shown in Fig. 2. Right lateral and left lateral views

cord) are very close to the target volume, it is very important to perform the dose calculation in three dimensions.

Figure 3 shows the three-dimensional dose calculation in a reconstructed sagittal plane through the midline of the patient. What could not recognized in the two-dimensional plan is obvious in this reconstructed section: if this treatment plan is implemented, there will be overdosing of the spinal cord in the upper region, possibly causing for side effects.

Figure 4 shows that it is possible to visualize the three-dimensional dose distribution even better with the help of three-dimensional computer graphics. The overdosing of the spinal cord, and in this case also underdosage of a small part of the target volume, can be clearly recognized.

Dynamic Therapy

The question now arises: what techniques might be available in order to improve the radiotherapy for this patient.

One prerequisite for the improvement of the physical dose distribution in such a situation is the combination of tomographic imaging and computer graphics, which today provide us with new methods of geometrical optimization. After outlining the interesting organ structures in a series of CT images, it is possible to match radiation field orientations and field forms from the so-called "beam's eye view" to the contour of the target volume. Thus, having the three-dimensional data of the patients anatomy stored in the computer, prior to dose calculation, a geometrical simulation of the treatment can be performed, equivalent to the conventional radiographic treatment simulation.

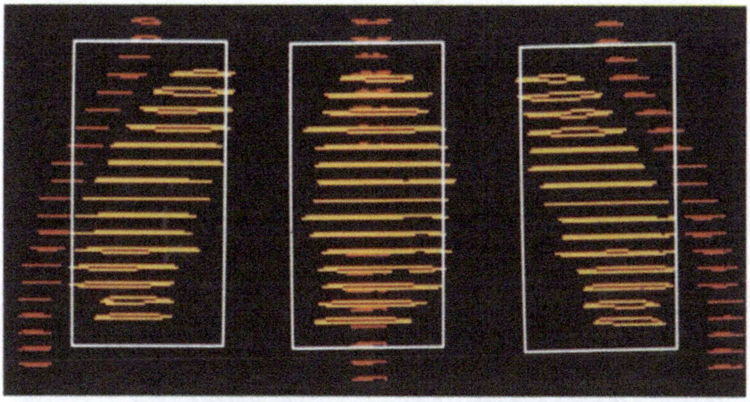

Fig. 5. Beam's eye view projections for three gantry angles (right lateral, anterior and left lateral) for the treatment plan shown in Fig. 2

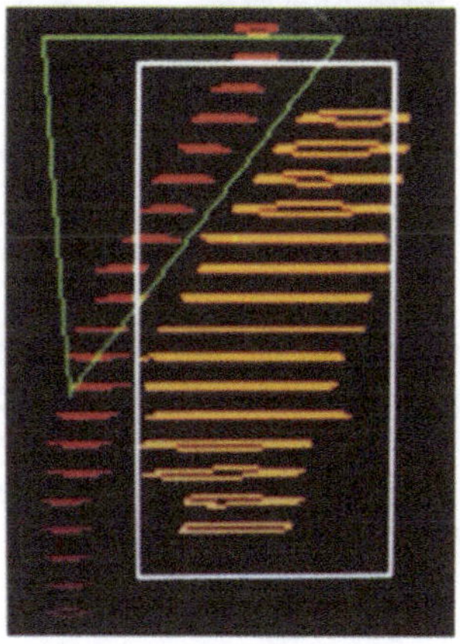

Fig. 6. Graphic design of a lead block for shielding the spinal cord using the beam's eye view technique for the treatment plan shown in Fig. 2. Right lateral view. Target volume *(yellow)*, spinal cord *(red)*, the outlines of the irradiation field *(white rectangle)*, and the outlines of the shielding block *(green)* are shown

Figure 5 shows an example of the beam's eye view projections of the target volume and of the organ at risk for the patient with the esophageal tumour. Without having performed any dose calculation, it is already possible to anticipate the problems that will arise when the moving beam irradiation technique with rectangular fields is applied to this patient: because of the kyphosis in the upper region of the body, parts of the spinal cord are completely covered by the irradiation field. In order to avoid this overdosage, the critical part of the spinal cord has to be shielded with a lead block, indicated by the green outline in this beam's eye view projection in Fig. 6.

Blocking of critical organs raises no problems when a stationary beam treatment technique is intended. However, for a therapy with a moving gantry, it is also necessary to move the shielding block to the appropriate position for each angle of beam incidence. This form of radiation with permanent change of one or several beam parameters is called dynamic therapy. Dynamic therapy can only be carried out with the help of sophisticated mechanics which is under complete computer control.

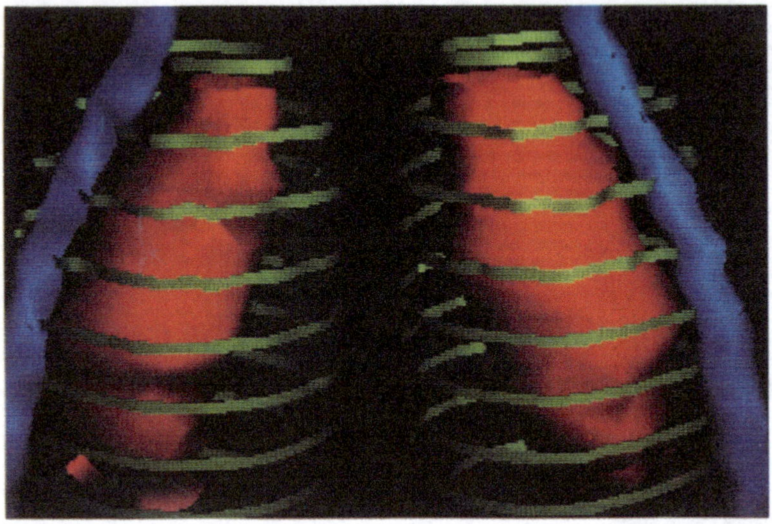

Fig. 7. Three-dimensionally shaded object representation of the target volume *(red)*, spinal cord *(blue)*, and 80%-isodose surface *(green ribbons)* of the treatment plan shown in Fig. 2, using a dynamic shielding technique to protect the spinal cord. Right lateral and left lateral views

The group at the radiation clinics of the University of Freiburg has developed a device for dynamic shielding of the spinal cord (Bruggmoser et al. 1983). When this is introduced into treatment planning and dose calculation, as can be seen from the sagittal section (Fig. 7), the dose distribution is improved as far as the sparing of the spinal cord is concerned. The three-dimensional presentation of the 60% isodose shows that, using the Freiburg method of dynamic therapy, the spinal cord is completely protected from the critical dose.

Conformation Therapy

While the device for dynamic shielding developed at Freiburg is a special system for the treatment of esophageal cancer, several other groups started with a more general approach, the use of multiple leaf collimators. The principle of this old idea (Takahashi 1964) is shown in Fig. 8. The collimator consists of two sets of thin steel or tungsten leaves which can be moved independently and adjusted in such a way that the opening in the collimator matches the outline of the target volume from the beam's eye view. The first multi-leaf collimators had to be adjusted manually, which was a cumbersome task and hampered the practical applicability of these systems. A completely computer-controlled multi-leaf collimator is under development at the mechanical workshop of the German Cancer Research Center (Pastyr et al. 1987), in which the leaves of the collimator will be driven by stepping motors which are under complete computer control and interfaced to the three-dimensional treatment planning system.

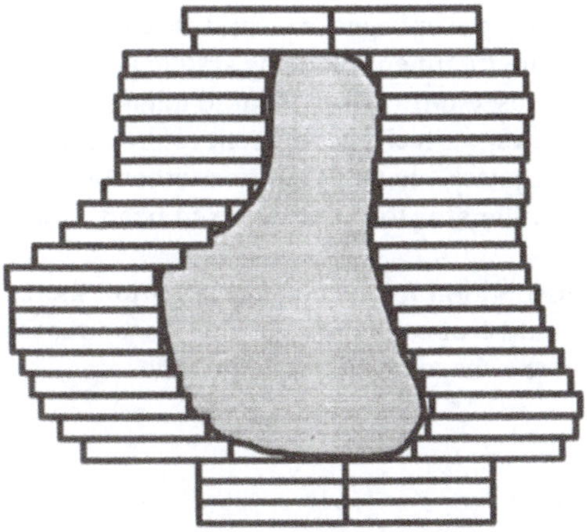

Fig. 8. Principle of the multi-leaf collimator

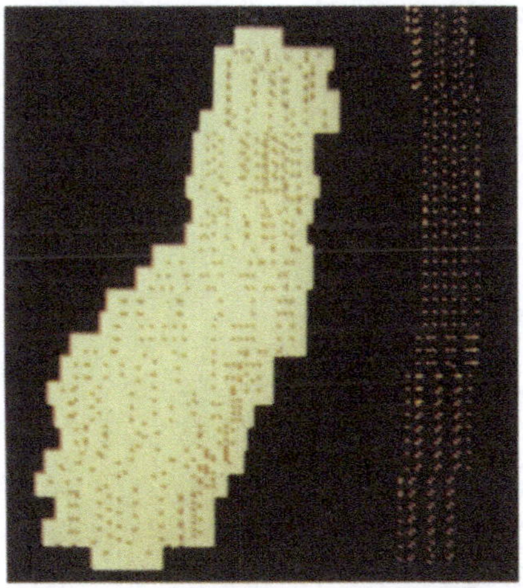

Fig. 9. Beam's eye view projection (left lateral view) of a multi-leaf collimator irradiation field for treatment of a target volume in a patient with esophageal cancer

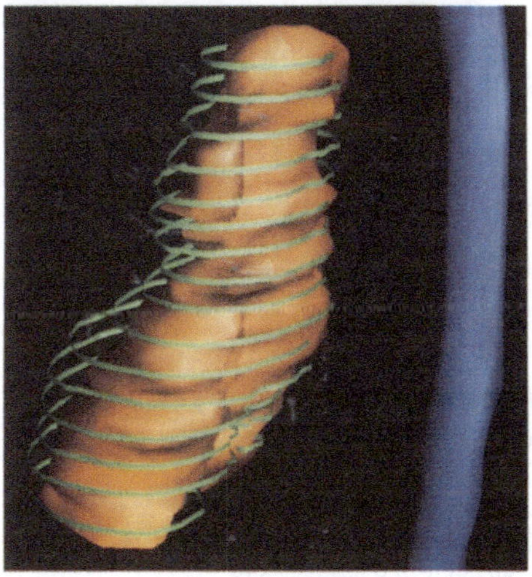

Fig. 10. Three-dimensionally shaded object representation of the target volume *(red)*, the spinal cord *(blue)* and the 80%-isodose surface *(green ribbons)* for a dynamic treatment technique using dynamic field matching with a multi-leaf collimator. Left lateral view

As is shown in Fig. 9 for another example of esophageal cancer, the leaf positions for a given gantry angle are calculated by the treatment planning system and the positions stored in a control file which can be used during treatment to adjust the positions of the leaves in order to form a field shape which is congruent to the outline of the target volume. Switching from one irregularly shaped field to another takes less than 30 seconds, which allows use of the collimator for multiple fixed beam conformation therapy.

Figure 10 shows the resulting dose distribution for such a conformation therapy with the use of the computer-controlled multi-leaf collimator. It can be seen that the dose distribution really can be tailored to the shape of the target volume.

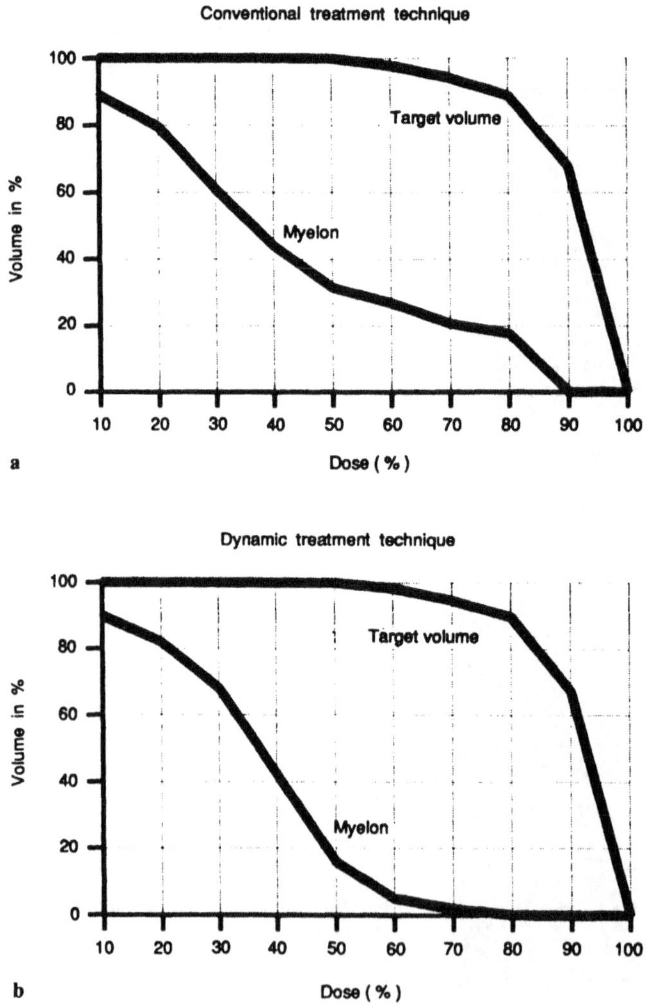

Fig. 11 a, b. Dose-volume histograms of the target volume and the spinal cord for the treatment plan shown in Fig. 2, (**a**) without and (**b**) with dynamic shielding of the spinal cord

Computer-Assisted Methods of Dose Evaluation

While the isodose presentations shown in normal treatment plans (Figs. 2–4, 7, 10) are qualitative means of evaluation of spatial dose distributions, quantitative methods of evaluation of three-dimensional dose distributions are now also becoming important.

For each volume which has been defined, either target volume or organ at risk, it is possible to calculate the percentage of the volume which is covered by a certain dose. A plot of the volume against the relative dose is called a "dose-volume histogram". An example is shown in Fig. 11. Defining a certain critical dose level, in this case 60%, the amount of improvement can be directly extracted from the dose-volume histograms: while in the conventional plan about 40% of the spinal cord receives a dose higher than 60%, the dynamic technique reduces this overdosed volume to about 10%. Our feeling is that the tools of quantitative evaluation of three-dimensional dose distributions will become very important in high precision radiotherapy.

Optimization of Treatment Plans

The straightforward approach of geometrical optimization of the dose distribution works very well as long as the target volumes are convex, but when there are target volumes with concave surfaces, as is the case, for example, in the pelvic or lymphatic region, the geometrical approach fails (Fig. 12). At first glance it seems nearly impossible to solve the dose optimization problem for target volumes of such complex shape with conventional irradiation such as photon or electron beams.

However, in connection with computer-controlled radiation therapy, one approach has recently been published (Brahme 1988) which seems to be a most efficient way to handle even such difficult situations. It is an analytical approach to solving the dose optimization problem for a multiple beam irradiation technique. The

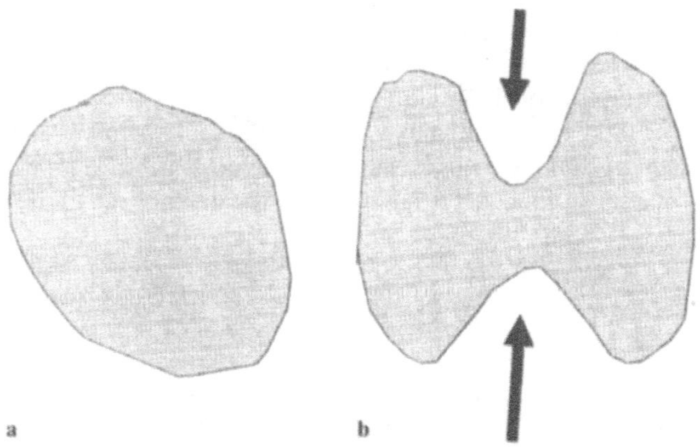

Fig. 12a, b. Shapes of target volumes in radiation therapy. Convex target volumes (**a**) can easily be covered by conformation therapy, but problems arise in the "bays" of target volumes with concave surfaces

first step is to specify the shape of the desired dose distribution; in a second step this desired distribution is deconvolved, the deconvolution function being the dose distribution of a multiple pencil beam irradiation, and then the fluence distribution of the primary beams is calculated.

The analytical method of Brahme is a general solution of the dose optimization problem. Though it is still not applicable, it may in a few years replace the cumbersome trial-and-error method which today exists in treatment planning.

Though this approach is very promising, there remains one severe restriction. If this method is to be carried out with a conventional linear accelerator, there arises the difficulty that beams with nonuniform dose distribution within the radiation field have to be applied. Therefore, this attractive optimization and treatment technique is currently restricted to accelerators with computer-controlled scanning beams. Nevertheless, one could imagine that specially designed collimators could be constructed and used to perform dynamic conformal radiotherapy at every linear accelerator.

Conclusion

While reporting my expectations concerning the development of radiotherapy within the next decade, I am of course aware of the fact that a lot of other more fundamental problems of radiotherapy have still to be solved. Currently, we are faced with the following problems to mention only the most severe ones (Smith 1986):

- In daily clinical routine, the tools with which to plan the results of complex treatments with reasonable accuracy in reasonable times are not yet available.
- It is not possible to detect and correct for motion of the patient during treatment.
- Mechanical and electronic limitations of today's accelerators prevent the introduction of dynamic techniques under normal clinical conditions.

These practical constraints mean that the full potential of external beam radiotherapy cannot yet been reached. On the other hand, there are estimates indicating that a significant fraction of cancer patients would benefit from better dose localization, to the extent that either less complications or better local control, or both, would be seen (Matsuda 1984; Smith 1986; Rosengren 1988).

Our hope is that new technologies will make it possible to implement new dynamic conformal treatment techniques which will make it possible to optimize physical dose distributions of conventional external radiotherapy towards the desired level.

References

Bauer-Kirpes B, Schlegel W, Boesecke R, Lorenz WJ (1987) Display of organs and isodoses as shaded 3D objects for 3D therapy planning. Int J Radiat Oncol Biol Phys 13: 135–140

Boesecke R, Doll J, Schlegel W, Lorenz WJ (1988) A multileaf collimator. Strahlenther Onkol 164: 151–154

Brahme A (1988) Optimization of stationary and moving beam radiation therapy techniques. Radiother Oncol 12: 129–140

Bruggmoser G, Hodapp N, Kuphal K, Nanko N (1983) Apparative Anwendung zur Ausblendung des Rückenmarkkanals bei Rotationsbestrahlung individuell angepaßter Zielvolumina. In: Schütz J (ed) Medizinische Physik 1983. Hüthig, Heidelberg, pp 537–541

Castro JR (1987) Strahlentherapie mit schweren Ionen am Lawrence Berkeley Laboratory. In: zum Winkel K (ed) Wirkungssteigerung der Strahlentherapie maligner Tumoren. Springer, Berlin Heidelberg New York, pp 136–145

Chin LM, Kijewski PK, Sensson GK, Bjarngard BE (1983) Dose optimization with computer controlled gantry rotation, collimator motion and dose rate variation. Int J Radiat Oncol Biol Phys 9:723–729

deVita VT (1983) Progress in cancer management. Keynote address. Cancer 51:24012–24019

Doll J, Schlegel W, Pastyr O, Sturm V, Maier-Borst W (1987) The use of an industrial robot as a stereotactic guidance system. In: Lemke H (ed) Computer assisted radiology 87. Springer, Berlin Heidelberg New York, pp 374–378

Greiner R, Blattmann H (1987) Strahlentherapie mit negativen Pi-Mesonen. In: zum Winkel K (ed) Wirkungssteigerung der Strahlentherapie maligner Tumoren. Springer, Berlin Heidelberg New York, pp 136–145

Jacky J, Kalet I (1987) Assuring the quality of critical software. In: Bruinvis IAD, van der Giessen PH, van Kleffens HJ, Wittkämper FW (eds) The use of computers in radiation therapy. North-Holland, Amsterdam, pp 49–52

Kessler M (1987) Computer techniques for correlating NMR and X-ray CT-imaging for radiotherapy treatment planning. In: Bruinvis IAD, van der Giessen PH, van Kleffens HJ, Wittkämper FW (eds) The use of computers in radiation therapy. North-Holland, Amsterdam, pp 441–444

Kraft G (1987) Biologische Effekte schwerer Ionen. In: zum Winkel K (ed) Wirkungssteigerung der Strahlentherapie maligner Tumoren. Springer, Berlin Heidelberg New York, pp 126–135

Kuttig H (1987) Klinische Aspekte. In: zum Winkel K (ed) Wirkungssteigerung der Strahlentherapie maligner Tumoren. Springer, Berlin Heidelberg New York, pp 17–35

Kwoh YS, Jonckheere E, Hayati S (1987) An improved absolute positioning accuracy robot for stereotactic brain surgery. In: Lemke H (ed) Computer assisted radiology 87. Springer, Berlin Heidelberg New York, pp 899–904

Matsuda T (1984) Clinical significance of computer controlled conformation radiotherapy – from seven years experience. In: Cunningham JR (ed) Proceedings of the 8th international conference on the use of computers in radiation therapy. IEEE Computer society, Silver Spring, pp 474–478

McShan DL, Fraass BA (1987) 3D-Treatment planning: II. Integration of gray scale images and solid surface graphics. In: Bruinvis IAD, van der Giessen PH, van Kleffens HJ, Wittkämper FW (eds) The use of computers in radiation therapy. North-Holland, Amsterdam, pp 41–44

Morton EJ, Swindell W (1987) A digital system for the production of radiotherapy verification images. In: Bruinvis IAD, van der Giessen PH, van Kleffens HJ, Wittkämper FW (eds) The use of computers in radiation therapy. North-Holland, Amsterdam, pp 375–377

Munzenrider JE, Austin-Seymour M, Gragoudas ES, Seddon JM, Verhey L, Goitein M, Suit HD, Koehler AM (1987) Radiotherapie mit Protonen. In: zum Winkel K (ed) Wirkungssteigerung der Strahlentherapie maligner Tumoren. Springer, Berlin Heidelberg New York, pp 58–68

Pastyr O, Schlegel W, Boesecke R, Alandt K, Meenenga D, Maier-Borst W, Lorenz WJ (1987) Ein Lamellen-Kollimater für die Konformations-Strahlentherapie. In: Bergmann H (ed) Medizinische Physik 87. DGMP, Nürnberg, pp 665–669

Rosengren B (1988) Trends in treatment modalities. Computer Assisted Radiation Therapy 10:6–8

Schad L, Boesecke R, Schlegel W, Hartmann GH, Sturm V, Strauss L, Lorenz WJ (1988) 3D-Image correlation of CT, MRT and PET in radiotherapy treatment planning of brain tumors. J Comput Assist Tomogr 11:948–954

Schlegel W, Scharfenberg H, Doll J, Hartmann G, Sturm V, Lorenz WJ (1984) Three-dimensional dose planning using tomographic data. In: Cunningham JR (ed) Proceedings of the 8th international conference on the use of computers in radiation therapy. IEEE Computer society, Silver Spring, pp 191–196

Sherouse GW, Rosenamn J, Harris L, McCurry MS, Pizer SM, Chaney EL (1987) Automatic digital contrast enhancement of radiotherapy films. Int J Radiat Oncol Biol Phys 13:801–806

Smith AR (1986) Radiotherapy in the year 2000: dynamic conformal therapy. In: Proceedings of the 11th Varian users meeting. Varian, Palo Alto, pp 31–35

Smith V (1987) Routines for enhancement of radiation therapy images. In: Bruinvis IAD, van der Giessen PH, van Kleffens HJ, Wittkämper FW (eds) The use of computers in radiation therapy. North-Holland, Amsterdam, pp 37–40

Sturm V, Pastyr O, Schlegel W, Scharfenberg H, Zabel HJ, Netzteband G, Schabbert S, Berberich W (1983) Stereotactic computer tomography with a modified Riechert Mundinger device as the basis for integrated stereotactic neuroradiological investigations. Acta Neurochir 68: 11–17

Takahashi S (1964) Conformation therapy: Rotation techniques as applied to radiography and radiotherapy of cancer. Acta Radiol Supplement, p 242

von Herk M, Meertens H (1987) A digital imaging system for portal verification. In: Bruinvis IAD, van der Giessen PH, van Kleffens HJ, Wittkämper FW (eds) The use of computers in radiation therapy. North-Holland, Amsterdam, pp 371–373

Werner T, Herrmann G, Schlegel W, Lorenz WJ (1987) Parallel processing in radiotherapy treatment planning. In: Bruinvis IAD, van der Giessen PH, van Kleffens HJ, Wittkämper FW (eds) The use of computers in radiation therapy. North-Holland, Amsterdam, pp 21–24

Intraoperative Radiation Therapy for Glioblastoma – Indications and Treatment Results

M. Matsutani, O. Nakamura, T. Nagashima, Y. Tanaka, and T. Matsuda

Introduction

Glioma, a neoplasm of neuroectodermal origin, is oncopathologically defined as carcinoma in the brain. The most poorly differentiated glioma, glioblastoma multiforme, usually grows in the deep white matter of cerebrum and rapid invasion in multiple directions along the white matter has already occurred by the time of diagnosis. Infiltrated tumor cells into the surrounding brain tissue were observed at least 2 cm apart from the margin of the enhanced tumor area on computed tomography (CT) scan (Burger et al. 1983). In advanced stages, the tumor infiltration in the white matter extends into the contralateral hemisphere, and finally to the brain stem or the cerebellum through the cerebral peduncle. On surgery for such an invasive glioblastoma, most cases are beyond the stage for desirable removal of tumors, because of the risk of damage to the normal function of surrounding brain tissue. With surgery alone followed by best conventional care, patients have a uniformly fatal course with a median survival of 17.0 weeks (Walker et al. 1978). The restriction of the surgical treatment has inevitably required postoperative radiation therapy, which has been the most important treatment modality following surgery.

The results of phase III studies for malignant glioma showed that radiation therapy and chemotherapy together were slightly more effective than radiation therapy alone, but that the median survival did not greatly exceed 50 weeks (Edwards et al. 1980; Takakura et al. 1986). Histologic analysis of glioblastoma after radiation therapy revealed that radiation effects depended upon the degree of ischemic necrosis, and that tumor cells around the ischemic necrosis were quite viable in spite of irradiation of 60 Gy, and became the source of recurrent tumors (Burger et al. 1983; Matsutani et al. 1985).

On the other hand, it was strongly suggested by Salazar et al. (1979) and Walker et al. (1979) that survivals extended in proportion to target absorbed doses. In order to sterilize the remaining malignant remnants after surgery and conventional radiation therapy, a localized high-dose irradiation is ideal (Hochberg and Pruitt 1980) and a high-energy electron beam is most suitable for this purpose (Fig. 1). Intraoperative radiation therapy (IORT) with a high-energy election beam has the advantages of precise demarcations of the target volume, minimum damage to surrounding normal tissues, and a high absorbed target dose with 15–25 Gy in 5–10 min, using a Shimadzu 20 MeV betatron with an excellent energy conversion capability ranging from 4–20 MeV (Fig. 2) (Matsutani et al. 1986). By selecting the proper delivering energy, and by choosing either a round or oval-shaped radiation cone as well as its specific size, it becomes possible to limit the area of high-dose radiation to conform to the unique tumor size in each case.

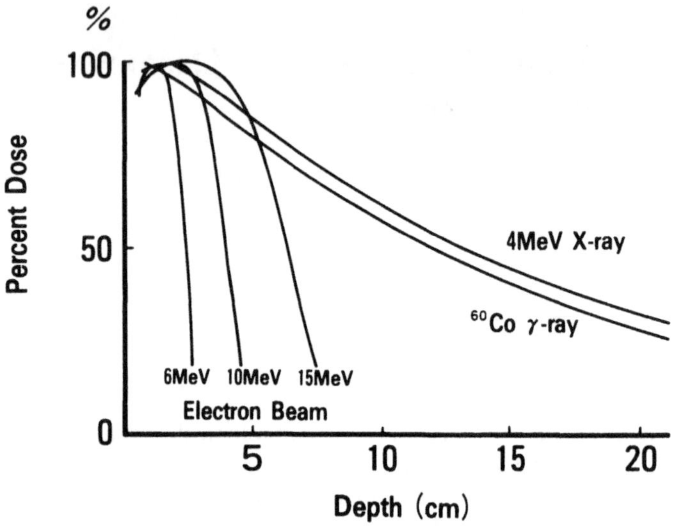

Fig. 1. Percentage dose-depth curves delivered by different accelerators

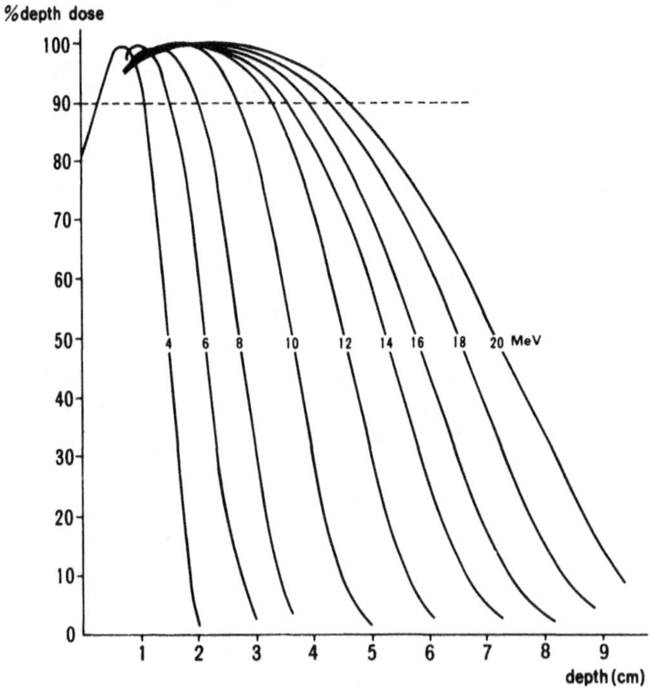

Fig. 2. Isodose curves generated by Shimadzu 20-MeV betatron. An optional target volume can be obtained by selecting a proper energy

Two steps of pilot studies of IORT for malignant gliomas indicated that the dose delivered during operation should be less than 25 Gy, and that IORT should be applied as a boost therapy for minimum residual tumor (Matsutani et al., in press). As a clinical approach to maximizing resectability and intensive irradiation of the tumor area, intraoperative radiation therapy combined with wide re-resection of the remnant tumor after conventional radiation therapy and intensive conformative irradiation controlled by computer has been developed for treatment of glioblastoma (Matsutani et al. 1986).

Patients and Method

Ninety-five adult patients with cerebral glioblastoma were treated according to the treatment course, which was selected from the results of the preceding therapy (Fig. 3). After conservative surgery and conventional external radiation therapy, wide re-resection of the tumor combined with or without IORT was applied to expected resectable cases. Conformation radiation therapy with a total of 60–80 Gy was finally submitted to cases obtaining marked reduction of tumors.

When the tumor is smaller than 3 cm in diameter, cone-shaped resection of tumor with overlying brain tissue is possible, and the tumor tissue and tumor infiltrative area are observed at the bottom of the resected region. In these cases, bleeding from the epidural space or CSF from the brain tissue are drained continuously by using a ventricular drainage tube in order to keep the area dry, because the treatment volume is 1–2 cm below the marginal wall. When the tumor is large, wide resection of overlying tissue is impossible because of the risk of sacrificing the surrounding normal brain. Minimal removal of overlying tissue and intratumoral resection is the usual procedure, and the tumor tissue remains beneath the surgical margin. Saline-

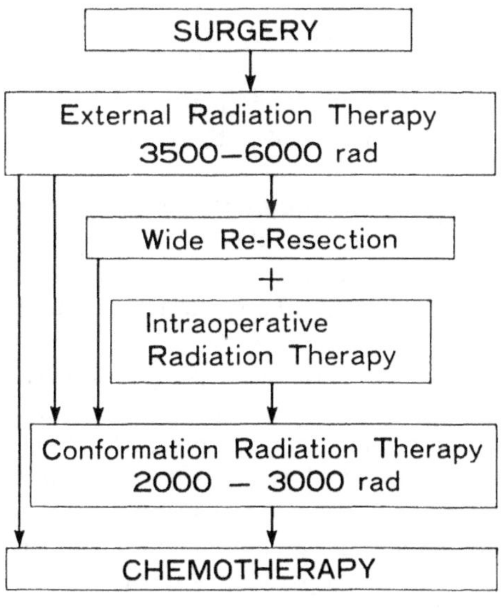

Fig. 3. Treatment course. After the surgery and following external radiation therapy, wide re-resection of the remaining tumor combined with or without intraoperative radiation therapy is performed

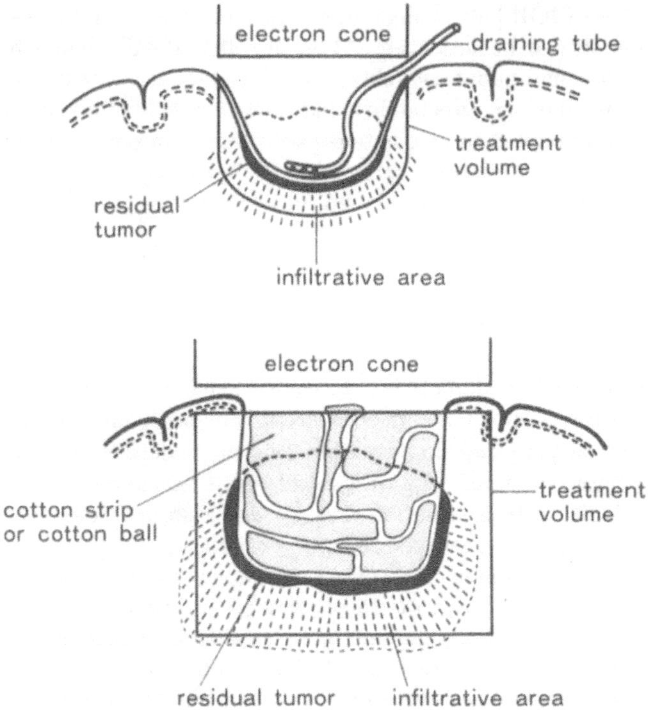

Fig. 4. For a smaller tumor, cone-shaped resection of the tumor with overlying brain tissue is performed, and the treatment volume is designed as 1–2 cm below the marginal wall *(top)*. For a larger tumor, intratumoral resection is the usual procedure and the tumor tissue remains beneath the surgical margin. Saline-saturated cotton strips are inserted into the surgical deficit as tissue-compensating material to maintain dose homogeneity *(bottom)*

saturated cotton strips or cotton balls are inserted into the U-shaped surgical deficit as tissue-compensating material to maintain dose homogeneity (Fig. 4). The cone size was determined to give a 1-cm perimeter of "normal" brain tissue. The electron beam energy was selected so that the 90% isodose line fell at lest 1–2 cm below the deepest aspect of the tumor.

One of the major problems in performing IORT is to transport patients from the operating theater to the radiation therapy department (Matsutani et al., to be published). In the operation room on the first basement, a patient who receives preparatory management there is moved, while still under general anesthesia, to the third basement where the betatron apparatus is.

The patient is laid on the removable operative bed. An anesthesic gas tank with nitrous oxide and oxygen (1 : 1) is attached to the bed for transportation. In the radiation treatment room, electrocardiography, respiration rate, blood pressure, and airway pressure of patients are monitored by closed-circuit television. After irradiation, the patient is returned to the operation room again, for original surgery. In close cooperation with neurosurgeons, anesthesiologists, radiotherapists, and nurses, the average time required is less than 30 min, until the final operation is started.

Results

According to the treatment protocol, 95 patients with nonrecurrent glioblastoma were treated. Twenty-two patients were selected for IORT. The delivered dose of IORT was 10–25 Gy (mean, 11.4 ± 3.8 Gy) with a range from 8 to 20 MeV. All patients received external radiation therapy with a dose of 35–80 Gy (mean, 59.4 ± 12.5 Gy). Fourteen patients have died and eight patients are alive. The median time to tumor progression from the first operation was 60 weeks, and the 1-year and 2-year survival rates were 100% and 61.1%, respectively (Table 1). In 13 patients, the recurrent tumor developed at the primary site, and at the remote site in 3. Seven patients have now been disease free for 26–192 weeks.

Seventeen patients received tumor re-resection after external radiation therapy. IORT, however, was not applied to their deep-seated tumors, because there would be mechanical damage to surrounding tissues by insertion of a radiation cone. The median time to tumor progression was 56 weeks and the 2-year survival rate was 35.9% (Table 1).

External radiation therapy alone was performed in 56 patients with a total of 50–80 Gy (mean, 59.0 + 11.6 Gy). Their tumors were too large for the wide re-resection and IORT. The median time to tumor progression was 26 weeks and the 2-year survival rate was 6.8% (Table 1).

Table 1. Treatment results

	External radiation		Intraoperative radiation therapy
	Partial resection	Wide resection	
No. of patients	56	17	22
Age (mean ± SD)	49.0 ± 17.3	43.9 ± 14.6	46.2 ± 15.3
ERT dose (Gy)	59.0 ± 11.6	62.1 ± 9.2	59.4 ± 12.5
IORT dose (Gy)	–	–	17.4 ± 3.8
Median TTP (weeks)	26.0	56.0	60.0
Median survival (weeks)	40.0	92.0	>104
% Survival (Kaplan-Meier)			
6 months	71.7	100	100
12 months	36.1	81.6	100
18 months	18.1	62.7	94.4
24 months	6.8	35.9	61.1

ERT, external radiation therapy; IORT, intraoperative radiation therapy; TTP, time to tumor progression

Discussion

The biological significance of exposing tumors to large doses of radiation is not fully understood. However, it may be useful to discuss the dose survival curve for rat glioma cells inoculated into the rat brain and to use these data to predict what may occur in a human tumor under similar conditions (Fig. 5). When we assume the residual tumor after surgery is 4 cm in diameter with 1 cm depth, the number of cells would be 1.2×10^{10} cells. The 4 log cell kill effect by one exposure to high-dose irradiation would reduce the number of cells to 1.2×10^{6} cells. This reduction in cell number may allow host defense mechanisms to control the tumor. The dose for 4 log cell kill would be 26 Gy in intracerebral glioma models of rats. This is the theoretical basis for intraoperative radiation therapy.

The results of treatment comparisons in this protocol have demonstrated that the significant difference between a 2-year survival of 35.9% for wide re-resection and that of 6.8% for conventional external irradiation is closely correlated to the extent to which the tumor mass was surgically removed. The difference in survival between IORT of patients with this indication and those with wide re-resection might be related to the intensive dose absorbed in the operation. The results apparently indicate that areas adjacent to the margin of almost complete removal should be irradiated with a sufficient dose to sterilize the remaining malignant remnants. It can be said that IORT is the best treatment modality available at present for glioblastoma.

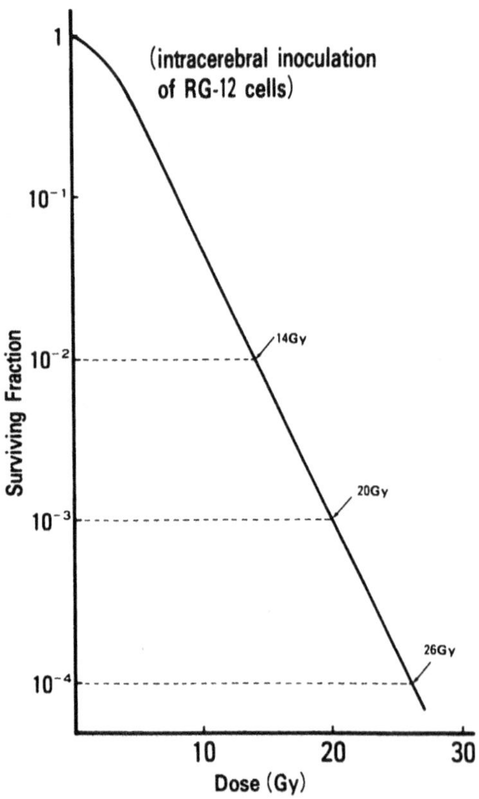

Fig. 5. Survival curves of irradiated rat glioma cells. Four log cell kill is obtained by irradiation of 26 Gy

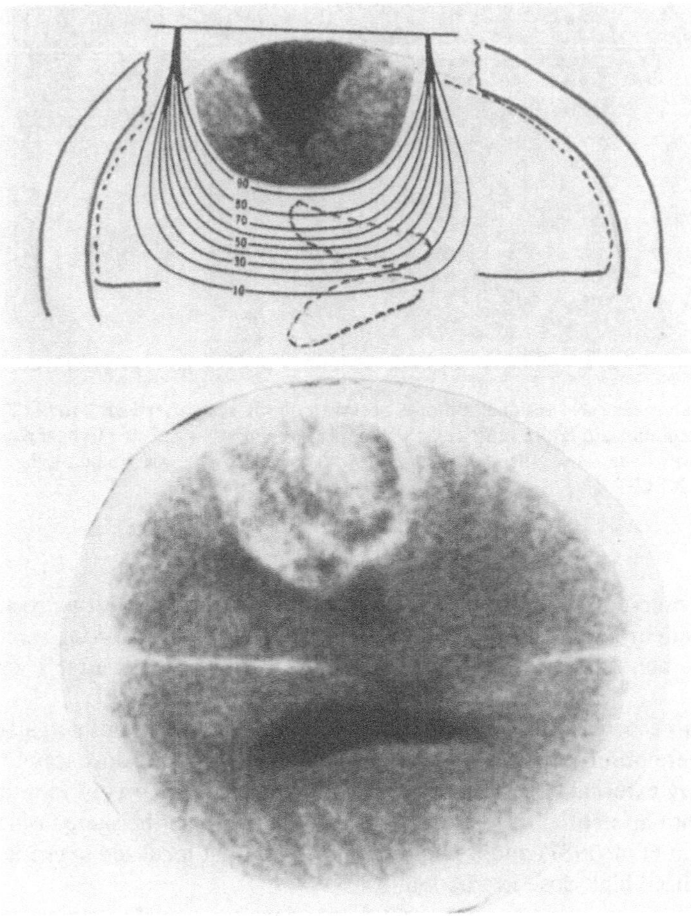

Fig. 6. An illustrative case. The CT scan is presented *at the bottom*. Isodose curves delivered by the 14-MeV betatron (6-cm cone) are superimposed on the schematic drawing of the CT scan *(top)*. The cone size was determined to give a 1-cm perimeter of "normal" brain tissue, and the electron beam energy was selected so that the 90% isodose line fell at least 1–2 cm below the deepest aspect of the tumor

Three important problems developed in performing IORT for malignant gliomas. The first problem was a male patient with posterior temporal glioblastoma who underwent IORT with a dose of 20 Gy against maximally resected tumor margin (Fig. 6). By using a 6-cm radiation cone with 14 MeV electron beam energy, the 90% isodose line fell 2 cm below the tumor margin. The calculated isodose line demonstrates precise demarcation of the target volume and minimum damage to surrounding normal tissue. But the patient deteriorated 45 weeks after the first operation and underwent a second operation for suspected local recurrence. The histology showed wide-spread coagulation necrosis with scattered heavily damaged tumor cells, giving a diagnosis of no viable recurrent tumor. In another male patient, an enhanced high-

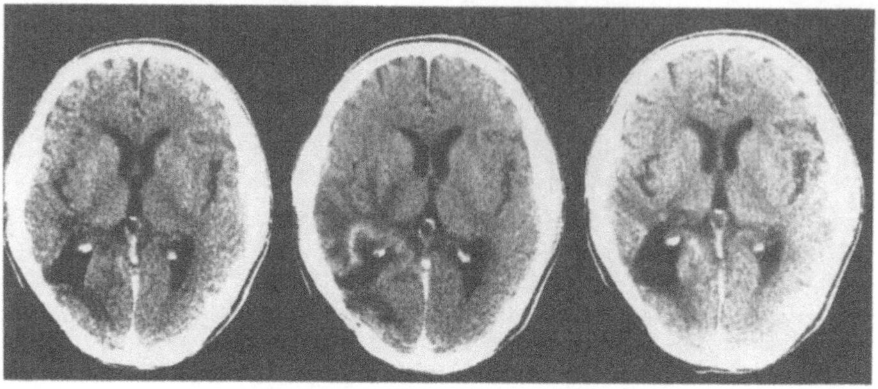

Fig. 7. Another illustrative case. No residual tumor is observed on CT scan after IORT *(left)*. Two years later, an enhanced mass along the ventricular wall appeared and was suspected to be a recurrent tumor *(center)*. But, 1 year later, the abnormal shadow disappeared and was thought to be the tumor necrosis due to IORT *(right)*

density area was observed along the surgical defect 2 years later, suggesting recurrent tumor. The patient had headache, which was not complained of during remission. However, the abnormal shadow remained stable and diminished after 1 year (Fig. 7).

These localized necroses with contrast enhancement on CT scan and surgically verified necrosis were observed in six patients. The median delivered dose was 17.5 Gy IORT and 70 Gy external dose. The median period after IORT was 14 months. In the treatment with interstitial irradiation, a localized necrosis in the same fashion was reported (Gutin et al. 1987) and it might be inevitable that localized necrosis is introduced by localized high-dose irradiation.

The second problem was that the recurrent tumor developed at the primary site in most patients. In intraoperative irradiation, the size of the radiation cone was determined to give a 1-cm perimeter of normal brain tissue, and the treatment volume was designed as 1–2 cm below the surgical margin. Since glioblastoma cells generally infiltrate into areas at least 2 cm apart from the margin of tumor bulk (Burger et al. 1983), this treatment volume might be inadequate. The pathological examination of autopsy cases revealed the localized necrosis in the area included in a 90% isodose line of the treatment volume, and suggested the possible severe damage to the normal brain by enlarging the treatment volume of IORT. From the analysis of autopsy cases and suspected necrosis on CT scan, the treatment volume should be limited to the area immediate to the margin of the tumor area.

The third problem is that the number of patients suitable for IORT is restricted, only 22 out of 95 patients (23%) in our study.

Generally, IORT has been applied in cases of inoperable cancer, such as advanced pancreatic cancer. The IORT used in glioblastoma is in response to this category. The goal of IORT in such invasive cancer is the prolongation of survival of patients, and treatment results of IORT for glioblastoma are most remarkable among cancers where this therapy is indicated.

Summary

Intraoperative radiation therapy (IORT) with a high-energy election beam has the advantages of precise demarcation of the target volume, minimum damage to surrounding normal tissues, and a high absorbed target dose with 15–25 Gy in 5 min. It has been developed in order to sterilize the remaining malignant remnants after surgery and radiation therapy.

In the treatment of glioblastoma, wide re-resection of the tumor combined with IORT was applied to expected resectable cases after radiation therapy. The delivered dose was between 10 and 25 Gy with a range form 8–20 MeV. Twenty-two patients were selected to receive IORT, and a 2-year survival rate of 61.1% was obtained. Although the number of patients suitable for IORT is restricted (23% of patients), IORT is the best treatment modality available at present for glioblastoma.

Acknowledgement. This research was supported in part by a Grant-in-Aid for Cancer Research from the Ministry of Health and Welfare (62–8), and from Tokyo Metropolitan Bureau of Public Health.

References

Burger PC, Dubois PJ, Schold SC Jr, Smith KR Jr, Odom GL, Crafts DC, Giangaspero F (1983) Computerized tomographic and pathologic studies of the untreated, quiescent, and recurrent glioblastoma multiforme. J Neurosurg 58:159–169

Edwards MS, Levin VA, Wilson CB (1980) Brain tumor chemotherapy: an evaluation of agents in current use for phase II and III trials. Cancer Treat Rep 64:1179–1205

Gutin PH, Leibel SA, Wara WM, Choucair A, Levin VA, Philips TL, Silver P, Da Silva V, Edwards MB, Davis RL, Weaver KA, Lamb S (1987) Recurrent malignant gliomas: survival following interstitial brachytherapy with high-activity iodine-125 sources. J Neurosurg 67:864–873

Hochberg FH, Pruitt A (1980) Assumption in the radiotherapy of glioblastoma. Neurology 30:907–911

Matsutani M (1989) Intraoperative radiation therapy for malignant brain tumors. In: Dobelbower RR, Abe M (eds) Intraoperative radiation therapy. CRC, Boca Rotan

Matsutani M, Kohno T, Matsuda T, Seto T (1985) Histological evaluation of radiation therapy for glioblastoma multiforme (in Japanese). Rad System Res 2:63–69

Matsutani M, Matsuda T, Kohno T, Asai A, Fujimaki T (1986) Intraoperative radiation therapy for glioblastoma multiforme. In: Walker MD, Thomas DGT (eds) Biology of brain tumor. Nijhoff, Boston, pp 269–275

Takakura K, Abe H, Tanaka R, Kitamura K, Miwa T, Takeuchi K, Yamamoto S, Kageyama N, Handa H, Mogami H, Nishimoto A, Uozumi T, Matsutani M, Nomura K (1986) Effects of ACNU and radiotherapy on malignant glioma. J Neurosurg 64:53–57

Salazar OM, Rubin P, Feldstein ML, Pizzutiello R (1979) High dose radiation therapy in the treatment of malignant gliomas: final report. Int J Radiat Oncol Biol Phys 5:1733–1740

Walker MD, Alexander E Jr, Hunt WE, MacCarty CS, Mahaley MS Jr, Mealey J Jr, Norrell HA, Owens G, Ransohoff J, Wilson CB, Gehan EA, Strike TA (1978) Evaluation of BCNU and/or radiotherapy in the treatment of anaplastic gliomas. A cooperative clinical trial. J Neurosurg 49:333–343

Walker MD, Strike TA, Sheline GE (1979) An analysis of dose-effect relationship in the radiotherapy of malignant gliomas. Int J Radiat Oncol Biol Phys 5:1725–1731

Summary of Discussion: Session 2

G. van Kaick

The starting point for the discussion was the question of the high costs of neutron and proton installations.

When discussing the cost of these new installations (Dr. Wambersie said), we have to distinguish between the neutron programs and the proton programs. As regards neutrons, the price of a treatment is about three times that of a photon treatment at the present time. We made this assessment for the neutron therapy project in Nice, France, assuming a fixed energy cyclotron specially designed for therapy and made best possible use of. Actually, our impression may be falsely slanted, because in many neutron treatment centers the cyclotrons were not primarily designed for therapy and are often sophisticated machines with very high running costs.

Proton beam therapy needs a higher energy range: 200–250 MeV for deep-seated tumors. This implies, of course, an increase in machine costs. However, if one optimizes all parameters, even contemplating using the machine 24 h a day, it is possible to keep running costs within acceptable limits. This is expected for the proton therapy program planned in Loma-Linda in California, where about 1000 treatments a year are foreseen.

The possible combination of proton therapy with sensitizers and/or hyperthermia was commented on by Dr. Wambersie as a radiological problem which is not different for protons than for conventional X-rays. Like photons, proton beams are low lineal energy transfer radiations. Biologically speaking, these beams are very similar; for instance, the difference in relative biological effectiveness (RBE) is only 10%. The benefit expected of proton beams is only improved physical selectivity.

The question was raised whether specific tumor types respond better to neutrons than to photons.

Considering the poor penetration of the d(16)+B neutron beam, the colleagues at Hammersmith hospital selected salivary gland tumors, especially locally extended inoperable tumors, as they are located rather superficially. The results were excellent and there is now general agreement that neutrons are superior to photons for this category of tumor. More generally, the systematic study of Battermann in Amsterdam indicates a correlation between tumor doubling time and therapeutic gain from fast neutrons. Briefly, if the tumor doubling time is longer than 100 days, the RBE of neutrons is higher in the tumor than in normal tissue: the therapeutic gain exceeds 1. This is probably the case for salivary gland tumors, which are often well differentiated. By contrast, in rapidly growing tumors, the RBE in the tumor is less than the RBE in normal tissue: fast neutrons should not be used.

The problem of tumor cell repopulation was the first discussed after Dr. Trott's presentation. The question was raised whether the repopulation could be due to the excretion of certain growth factors. Dr. Trott thought it was due either to some sort of chalones or to growth factors which also act in normal tissues where the number of functioning cells is decreased below a certain level. He added that there is no reason to assume that tumors do not have the same control mechanism to keep up some sort of equilibrium.

The question was asked whether the labelling index is an index for the repopulation rate and whether it could be possible to follow the labelling index during therapy. In his answer Dr. Trott said: The labelling index was suggested by us some time ago. It may be related to repopulation but it does not indicate repopulation and has in principle nothing to do with repopulation. We merely suggested that, since the repopulation rate of squamous cell carcinomas gave a doubling time of 4 days, and the mean potential doubling time (T_{pot}) was 4 days for the same tumors, we may obtain some useful information from the labelling index. So far it has become extremely popular, and many people already take it for granted that repopulation is related to T_{pot}. This is very unlikely to be so – at any rate it has to be tested. The European study which is going on may give us some information but it will take another 2 or 3 years before this information is available. Following the labelling index or any other kinetic parameters during radiotherapy does not tell us anything meaningful.

Dr. Trott was asked to comment on the clinical experience of using different fractionation schemes in radiotherapy. He stated that there are various trials under way using several accelerated fractionation schemes. "These trials are ongoing and all make use of a more or less constant fractionation schedule, because we do not know at what time the acceleration starts. The existing knowledge is that for some tumors, especially squamous cell carcinoma, accelerated fractionation treatment gives very favorable results. The best results at the moment are probably those from Mount Vernon Hospital in England, where the whole treatment is over after 12 days. They give three fractions a day at 6-h intervals, including Saturdays and Sundays. Most radiotherapy departments would say that this is impossible – but of course it is possible! You just have to arrange it! The patient are happier and highly motivated and the outcome seems to be extremely good." Dr. Trott foresees profound changes in the organizational structure of radiotherapy departments in the future, to allow much greater flexibility in the treatment of individual patients.

The discussion on computer-assisted planning in radiotherapy was begun by the question: Using a scanning collimator, irradiation times will be dramatically increased; do you think that such treatment techniques can nevertheless been put into practice? Dr. Schlegel replied that, of course, when using dynamic treatment techniques we have to take into account that irradiation times will be longer. However, as there are still reserves in the performance of linear accelerators, this problem could at least partially be solved by increasing the dose rate of the primary beam. The experience of other institutions, e.g. the Joint Center of Radiation Therapy in Boston, shows that treatment times will then be reduced to practical limits.

The next question was: What proportion of the patient population would be suitable for treatment with these techniques?

Dr. Schlegel said that the estimates of how many patients could benefit from such elaborate treatment techniques range from 20% and 30%. In particular, recent studies from Japan and the United States show that these are realistic numbers.

Regarding intraoperative radiation therapy (IORT), Dr. Matsutani was asked to comment on the different indications for interstitial radiation therapy and for intraoperative radiation therapy. He replied that these are two different methods for giving very localized high dose radiation therapy. IORT is used for the most malignant tumors like glioblastoma with relatively good results. Interstitial radiotherapy is indicated for very small tumors and not for the large malignant glioblastomas, as the dose calculation is relatively difficult. Another aspect discussed was the long-term toxicity effects of intraoperative irradiation. Dr. Matsutani pointed out that most patients with malignant glioblastomas do not survive more than 1 or 2 years; side effects could not be observed in these patients even in those few who did survive more than 2 years.

SESSION 3

Hyperthermia

Chairman: M. WANNENMACHER

Hyperthermia in Tumor Treatment*

J. Overgaard

Introduction

More than three-quarters of a century have passed since the German C. Müller in 1910 first described the potential of using hyperthermia as an adjuvant to radiotherapy with the aim of increasing radiation response (Müller 1910, 1912). For many years thereafter sporadic reports enthusiastically demonstrated a likely improvement of radiotherapy in various superficial tumors. It was not, however, until approximately 1970 that a scientific effort was focused upon the potential of increasing radiation response by combining it with hyperthermia (Overgaard 1981, 1983, 1987a, 1989). Associated with this were numerous uncontrolled studies which strongly suggested that adjuvant heat treatment increases the probability of complete response and consequently tumor control (Table 1). This subsequently led to the development of better equipment allowing deep-seated tumors to be heated (Arcangeli et al. 1988; Overgaard 1989; Sapozink et al. 1986).

The purpose of the present paper is to outline the indications for hyperthermia in current radiotherapeutic practice.

Biological Rationale

The biological basis for combining hyperthermia and radiation has been described elsewhere (Overgaard 1980, 1983, 1987a; Overgaard et al. 1987). In principle, it consists of two different mechanisms, namely hyperthermic radiosensitization and direct hyperthermic cytotoxicity.

Hyperthermic radiosensitization is expressed as increased damage from radiation when hyperthermia and radiation are applied concomitantly. This effect does not qualitatively alter the radiation response, but only gives a quantitative enhancement. This hyperthermic radiosensitization occurs to an equal extent in normal tissues and in tumors and is most pronounced by far when the two treatment modalities are applied truly simultaneously.

Hyperthermic cytotoxicity is seen as direct heat killing of cells in a deprived micro-environment, characterized by insufficient blood supply with subsequent poor nutrition and increased acidity due to anaerobic metabolism and accumulation of lactic acid and other waste products. Cells situated in such an area are highly sensitive to hyperthermia and can be destroyed by heat treatment which does not cause

* Supported by the Danish Cancer Society and Legatstiftelsen Pedersholm

Table 1. Effect of adjuvant hyperthermia on the radiation response: complete response after treatment with irradiation given either alone or combined with hyperthermia. Data from Overgaard (1989)

Reference	Tumors (*n*)	Rad. alone (%)	Rad. and heat (%)	Isodose TER
Arcangeli et al.	163	38	74	1.95
Perez et al.	154	41	69	1.68
Overgaard et al.	101	39	62	1.59
U et al.	14	14	86	6.14
Gonzalez et al.	46	33	50	1.52
Kim et al.	238	39	72	1.85
Valdagni et al.	78	36	73	2.03
Bide et al.	76	0	7	>1
van der Zee et al.	71	5	27	5.40
Corry et al.	34	0	62	$\gg 1$
Scott et al.	62	39	87	2.23
Lindholm et al.	85	25	46	1.84
Li et al.	124	29	54	1.86
Steeves et al.	90	31	65	2.10
Dunlop et al.	86	50	60	1.20
Goldobenko et al.	65	86	100	1.16
Muratkhodzhaev et al.	313	25	63	2.52
Hiraoka et al.	33	25	71	2.84
Bey et al.	45	9	42	4.67
Shidna et al.	185	33	64	1.94
Datta et al.	65	46	66	1.43
Uozumi et al.	16	63	88	1.40
Hornback et al.	66	35	72	2.06
Fuwa et al.	24	63	83	1.32
Morita et al.	46	61	94	1.54

TER, thermal enhancement ratio

significant damage to cells in a "normal" environment. Furthermore, the environmental parameters which enhance the hyperthermic damage are typically those which reduce the radiation response (i.e., hypoxia). Thus, the areas of a tumor which because of insufficient vascularization are resistant to radiation are likely to be those which are sensitive to hyperthermia. On the other hand, the well-vascularized tumor areas (characterized by a normal physiological environment) are sensitive to radiotherapy, but relatively resistant to hyperthermia (Overgaard et al. 1987a).

On that basis we have two strategies for applying hyperthermia as an adjuvant to radiotherapy (Overgaard 1983, 1987a, 1989). One is as a radiosensitizing agent enhancing the effect of ionizing radiation in heated tissues. This strategy is only valid if hyperthermia and radiation are applied simultaneously. The other strategy utilizes the specific cytotoxic effect of heat against radioresistant cells, which results in damage to radioresistant areas of the tumors and is achieved by sequential treatment. Although hyperthermic radiosensitization with simultaneous treatment is able to yield the highest thermal enhancement ratio (TER)[1], the clinical applicability of this protocol is dubious because of technical problems, and it is likely that the dominating effect is due to the hyperthermic cytotoxicity.

The biological rationale has been documented in a few clinical studies comparing the effects of simultaneous and sequential treatments in various superficial tumors and normal tissues (Arcangeli et al. 1982; Overgaard 1981; Overgaard 1989).

Heat treatment of superficial tumors normally results in higher temperatures in the tumor than in the surrounding tissue. This has been associated with hyperthermia in experimental systems, causing a differential response between tumor and normal tissue in regard to the effect on blood flow to the tissues. Whereas in most tumors there is a tendency for the blood vessels to collapse at a relatively low temperature, normal tissue will react to the application of heat by increasing the blood flow, tending to reduce the heating effect (Overgaard et al. 1988; Vaupel and Kallinowski 1987). Thus, the differences in heating between tumors and normal tissues are probably a function of these different vascular reactions, which, in association with active vascular cooling, have made it possible to achieve a relatively higher temperature in tumors (Overgaard et al. 1988). Clinically it has been demonstrated that large tumors are relatively more sensitive to hyperthermia and radiation than small tumors, provided that the large tumors are sufficiently heated (Arcangeli et al. 1985; Datta et al. 1988).

Clinical Hyperthermia

There is a dual indication for hyperthermia in clinical radiotherapy (Arcangeli et al. 1988; Kapp 1986; Overgaard 1983, 1987, 1989). First, hyperthermia has an obvious role in palliative treatment, especially of recurrent tumors in previously irradiated areas. Secondly, hyperthermia may be included in the primary treatment of locally advanced tumors where improved local control is expected to result in a subsequent improved curability and survival. So far, clinical evaluation has almost solely been limited to superficial tumors, because of insufficiency of heat delivery, or to situations where interstitial heating is feasible (Arcangeli et al. 1988; Overgaard 1989). External heating of "deep" seated tumors is still preliminary, and most studies are in phase I–II, with the emphasis on toxicity and feasibility. The initial results are promising with regard to improved tumor control and acceptable toxicity (Arcangeli et al. 1988; Overgaard 1989; Sapozink et al. 1986).

In order to illustrate the potential of hyperthermia in radiotherapy, clinical experience of one (superficial) tumor site will be described, namely advanced head and

---

[1] Definition of thermal enhancement ratio based on either isoeffect or isodose values:

$$\text{TER (isoeffect)} = \frac{\text{radiation dose alone to achieve end point}}{\text{radiation dose with heat to achieve end point}}$$

$$\text{TER (isodose)} = \frac{\text{frequency of response after radiation with heat}}{\text{frequency of response after same radiation alone}}$$

neck carcinoma. A detailed overview of the overall current clinical status and literature is to be found in a recent paper (Overgaard 1989).

Head and Neck Carcinoma

Early studies investigated the use of hyperthermia together with radiation in the treatment of advanced head and neck carcinoma. Neck nodes especially have been the target of such experimental therapy, because of their superficial localization. Table 2 shows an overview of published trials where the combined effect has been compared to radiation alone. As will be seen, all studies show an isodose TER greater than 1. Although most comparisons have been made against historical controls, the result is also confirmed in the few prospective randomized trials conducted so far.

The difference in response represents different radiation dose levels in the various studies, since some involved primary treatment with a full course of radiotherapy while others involved treatment of nodes recurring in previously irradiated areas. This latter appears to be a major indication for hyperthermia. Tumor control is difficult to achieve in recurrent previously irradiated tumors, but the addition of hyperthermia has markedly improved this.

Compiling the data in Table 1 and other results (Arcangeli et al. 1982, 1985; Datta et al., in press; Emami et al. 1988; Goldobenko et al. 1987; Hofman 1987; Kim et al. 1985; Nishikawa et al. 1986; Perez et al. 1981; Scott et al. 1984; Valdagni et al. 1986, 1988), a well-defined dose-response relationship is obtained for both radiation alone and the combined treatment, with a significant improvement in favour of the combined therapy (Fig. 1). The isoeffect TER at the 50% level turns out to be approximately 1.6.

Most published data have used complete response as the end point, but for the neck nodes, although there was a well-defined connection between complete response and persistent disappearance, the longer the observation time, the more persistent disappearance diverged from complete response, giving results in favour of the combined treatment – i.e., there were fewer recurrences after complete response to combined treatment than after complete response to radiation alone.

Table 2. Adjuvant hyperthermia in the treatment of neck node tumors: tumor response after the same radiation dose given either alone or combined with hyperthermia

Reference	Tumors (*n*)	Rad. alone (%)	Rad. and heat (%)	Isodose TER
Arcangeli et al. (1985)	81	42	79	1.88
Scott et al. (1984)	18	22	88	4.00
Valdagni et al. (1988)	36	37	82	2.22
Emami et al. (1988)	160	13	38	2.92
Goldobenko et al. (1987)	65	86	100	1.16
Datta et al. (1988)	49	60	79	1.32

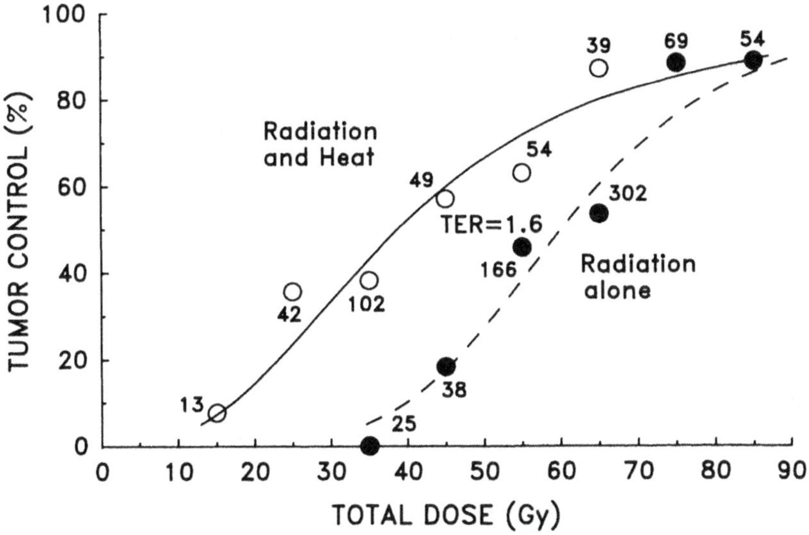

Fig. 1. Dose-response relationship in the neck nodes with squamous cell carcinoma treated with radiation alone or combined radiation and hyperthermia. The total doses were normalized according to Withers et al. (1983) assuming daily fractions of 2 Gy and an α/β ratio of 25 Gy. Data from unpublished observations and literature (Overgaard 1989)

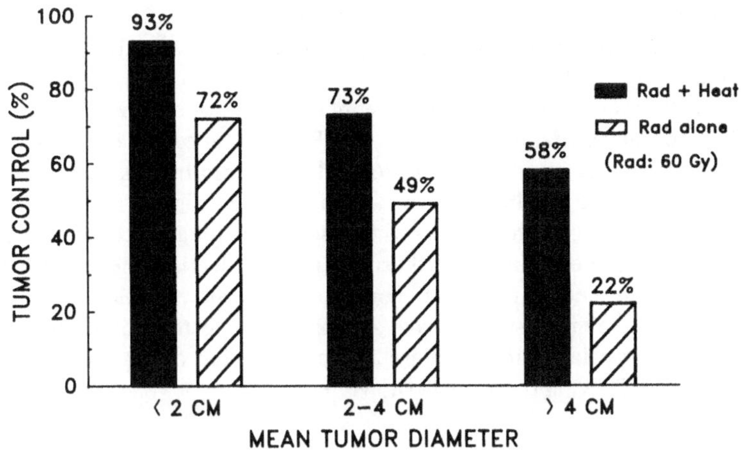

Fig. 2. Relationship between tumor volume and response to radiotherapy given alone or combined with heat. Data from neck node carcinomas described in the literature or from the author's own experience, treated with a total dose of 60 Gy (estimated as described in Fig. 1)

In addition to the radiation dose, several other prognostic parameters may be of importance for the outcome of combined treatment. Those include the quality and amount of heating (Arcangeli et al. 1985; Emami et al. 1988; Overgaard 1989) and tumor volume (Arcangeli et al. 1985; Datta et al. 1988; Emami et al. 1988; Overgaard 1989). There is a tendency towards a relatively better effect of adjuvant heat

Table 3. Adjuvant hyperthermia in the treatment of advanced head and neck tumors: tumor response after the same radiation dose given either alone or combined with hyperthermia. Data from Datta et al. (in press)

Stage and end point (65 patients)	Rad. alone (%)	Rad. and heat (%)	Isodose TER
Local control 2 months			
Stage I–II	88	100	1.14
Stage III–IV	13	46	3.56
All	32	55	1.72
Disease-free surv. 18 months			
Stage I–II	63	80	1.27
Stage III–IV	4	25	6.25
All	19	33	1.74

Radiation: 60–65 Gy/6–7 weeks
Heat: 42–43°C/30–50 min twice weekly before radiation

therapy in larger tumors (providing they can be properly heated), due to a reduced volume dependency of effect when radiation is combined with heat (Fig. 2).

The importance of number of heat fractions has been addressed in a well-conducted study by Valdagni et al. (1988), with results suggesting that only a few heat treatments are needed to achieve optimal effect, probably because of the influence of thermotolerance. However, this is a complex problem which recently has been discussed in detail (Overgaard 1989).

The role of hyperthermia in the primary treatment of the tumor site has also been explored. A small randomized trial by Datta et al. (1988) on advanced head and neck cancer has shown significantly improved local control, with improved survival following in consequence (Table 3). In addition, an on-going European multicenter study (ESHO protocol 4–87) of carcinoma of the base of the tongue, combining a brachytherapy boost with interstitial hyperthermia, is investigating the potential benefit of treating head and neck cancers with combined heat and radiation.

Taken all together, the clinical studies have shown that hyperthermia improves local control of tumors, especially those that are advanced. So far, almost all studies have shown an improved TER, and none has shown the reverse.

Concluding Remarks

The future role of hyperthermia in radiation oncology will depend on the development of better heating equipment. The clinical results so far obtained strongly indicate that there is a place for hyperthermia in general radiotherapy, but the final conclusion must await the outcome of controlled clinical trials (Arcangeli et al. 1988; Overgaard 1987a, b) conducted with a strong emphasis on quality control. Such trials are currently under way, mainly in multi-institutional settings. In Europe most of them are organized by the European Society for Hyperthermic Oncology (Overgaard 1987b), which has activated a number of protocols addressing the role of hyperthermia in primary radiotherapy of advanced tumors (primary advanced breast, base of tongue, and neck nodes, and malignant melanoma). Until such studies have been completed, hyperthermia must still be considered an experimental modality.

References

Arcangeli G, Cividalli A, Creton G, Mauro F, Nervi C (1982) Biological rationale for optimal scheduling of heat and ionizing radiation: clinical results on neck node metastases. NCI Monogr 61:407–409

Arcangeli G, Arcangeli G, Guerra A, Lovisolo GA, Cividalli A, Marino C, Mauro F (1985) Tumour response to heat and radiation: prognostic variables in the treatment of neck node metastases from head and neck cancer. Int J Hyperthermia 1:207–217

Arcangeli G, Overgaard J, Gonzalez Gonzalez D, Shrivastava PN (1988) Hyperthermia trials. Int J Radiat Oncol Biol Phys 14:S93–S109

Datta NR, Bose AK, Kapoor HK, Gupta S (in press) Head and neck cancers: results of thermoradiotherapy versus radiotherapy. Int J Hyperthermia

Emami B, Perez CA, Bignardi M, Leybovich L, Straube W, von Gerichten D, Hederman MA (1988) A retrospective study of irradiation versus combined irradiation plus hyperthermia in recurrent head and neck cancers. Abstract Bg-1, 36th Annual Meeting of the Radiation Research Society, Philadelphia, Pennsylvania, 1988

Goldobenko GV, Durnov LA, Knysh VI, Amiraslanov AT, Kondratieva AP, Matyakin GG, Tkachev SI, Tseitlin GY, Ivanov SM, Kozhushkov AI (1987) Experience in the use of thermoradiotherapy of malignant tumors. (In Russian). Med Radiol (Mosk) 32:36–37

Hofman P (1987) Clinical hyperthermia: medical aspects. Thesis, Utrecht

Kapp DS (1986) Site and disease selection for hyperthermic clinical trials. Int J Hyperthermia 2: 139–156

Kim YH, Ahmad K, Gottlieb CF, Byun YS, Fayos JV (1985) Local hyperthermia and radiation for advanced superficial tumor. Endocurietherapy/Hyperthermia Oncology 1:185–191

Müller C (1910) Eine neue Behandlungsmethode bösartiger Geschwülste. Münch Med Wochenschr 28:1490–1493

Müller C (1912) Therapeutische Erfahrungen an 100 mit Kombination von Röntgenstrahlen und Hochfrequenz, resp Diathermie behandelten bösartigen Neubildungen. Münch Med Wochenschr 28:1546–1549

Nishikawa K, Koga K, Watanabe K (1986) Combined radiation therapy and hyperthermia for advanced head and neck cancer: preliminary reports. In: Onoyama Y (ed) Hyperthermic oncology '86 in Japan. Proceedings of the 3rd Annual Meeting of the Japanese Society of Hyperthermic Oncology, pp 329–330

Overgaard J (1980) Simultaneous and sequential hyperthermia and radiation treatment of an experimental tumor and its surrounding normal tissue in vivo. Int J Radiat Oncol Biol Phys 6:1507–1517

Overgaard J (1981) Fractionated radiation and hyperthermia. Experimental and clinical studies. Cancer 48:1116–1123

Overgaard J (1983) Hyperthermic modification of the radiation response in solid tumors. In: Fletcher GH, Nervi C (eds) Biological bases and clinical implications of tumour radioresistance. Masson, New York, pp 337–352

Overgaard J (1987a) The design of clinical trials in hyperthermic oncology. Physics and technology of hyperthermia. In: Field SB, Franconi C (eds) NATO ASI Series E: Applied Sciences – No 127, pp 598–620

Overgaard J (1987b) Hyperthermia as an adjuvant to radiotherapy. Review of the randomized multicenter studies of the European Society for Hyperthermic Oncology. Strahlenther Onkol 163:453–457

Overgaard J (1989) The current and potential role of hyperthermia in radiotherapy. Int J Radiat Oncol Biol Phys 16:535–549

Overgaard J, Nielsen OS, Lindegaard JC (1987) Biological basis for rational design of clinical treatment with combined hyperthermia and radiation. Physics and technology of hyperthermia. In: Field SB, Franconi C (eds) NATO ASI Series E: Applied Sciences – No 127, pp 54–79

Perez CA, Kopecky W, Rao DV, Baglan R, Mann J (1981) Local microwave hyperthermia and irradiation in cancer therapy: preliminary observations and directions for future clinical trials. Int J Radiat Oncol Biol Phys 7:765–772

Sapozink MD, Gibbs FA, Egger MJ, Stewart JR (1986) Regional hyperthermia for clinically advanced deep-seated pelvic malignancy. Am J Clin Oncol 9:162–169

Scott RS, Johnson RJR, Story KV, Clay L (1984) Local hyperthermia in combination with definitive radiotherapy: Increased tumor clearance, reduced recurrence rate in extended follow-up. Int J Radiat Oncol Biol Phys 10:2119–2123

Valdagni R, Kapp DS, Valdagni C (1986) N_3 (TNM-UICC) metastatic neck nodes managed by combined radiation therapy and hyperthermia: clinical results and analysis of treatment parameters. Int J Hyperthermia 2:189–200

Valdagni R, Amichetti M, Pani G (1988) Radical radiation alone versus radical radiation plus microwave hyperthermia for N3 (TNM-UICC) neck nodes: a prospective randomized clinical trial. Int J Radiat Oncol Biol Phys 15:13–24

Vaupel P, Kallinowski F (1987) Physiological effects of hyperthermia. Recent Results Cancer Res 104:71–109

Withers HR, Thames HD, Peters LJ (1983) A new isoeffect curve for change in dose per fraction. Radiother Oncol 1:187–191

Regional Hyperthermia and Systemic Chemotherapy*

R. D. Issels and K. Krieger

Introduction

Since 1970, profound research in the field of thermobiology has produced a scientific basis for the application of hyperthermia as a new modality of cancer treatment. More recently, hyperthermia in combination with ionizing radiation or chemotherapy is becoming accepted clinically, due to the substantial technical improvements made in achieving selective increase of temperatures in tumor tissues in different anatomic sites. Even the technical problem of heating up more deep-seated solid tumors has been solved principally (for review, see Issels and Wilmanns 1988).

A distinction should be made between whole-body-hyperthermia (WBH) and regional hyperthermia (RHT). The clinical application of heat can be induced by electromagnetic field, ultrasound, or perfusion methods. The latter is essential for the WBH approach, using extracorporeal circulation. At the present time, RHT is most commonly performed using single microwave applicators for superficial hyperthermia and arrays of multiple applicators or multiple interstitial applicators for deep heating. In the annular phased array system (APAS), microwave antennas are arranged cylindrically around the axis of the patient's body to obtain a focus of the electromagnetic field in the center of the antenna by microwave interference. Within the range of frequency used (approx. 60–110 MHz), the focus diameter can be switched from approx. 15 cm at 60 MHz to approx. 8 cm at 100 MHz. Heterogeneity of the electromagnetic field leading to inhomogeneous temperature distribution has been observed frequently at tissue borders (e.g., bone/muscle of fat/muscle). Preferential heating of the tumor region can be achieved by exploiting the lower convection of heat from relatively poorly vasculated tumors compared to their surrounding normal tissues. The measurement of the actual temperature distribution in normal tissue and tumor during hyperthermia treatments is crucially important to the clinical application of RHT. So far, there is a lack of noninvasive methods for temperature measurements in deep-seated tissues. Therefore, thin plastic catheters (outside diameter approx. 1.5 mm) must be implanted either percutaneously or intraoperatively. In general, patients are not handicapped by these flexible catheters, which can remain inserted for as long as 3–6 months. In order to obtain as much information as possible about the temperature distribution, thermal probes (thermistors) are moved automatically back and forward within these catheters ("thermal mapping") during RHT treatments.

* This work is supported by Grants M 12/85 Wi 1, M 41/85 Wi 2, M 10/86 Wi 3, M 41/86 Wi 4, M 10/87 Wi 5, M 39/87 Wi 6 from German Cancer Aid (Deutsche Krebshilfe e.V.)

Thermobiology

Results of thermobiological studies have shown that, dependent on temperature and time of exposure (°C × min), an increase of temperature from 37°C to the range of 42.5°–45°C produces a cytotoxic effect (Westra and Dewey 1971). In contrast, cells exposed to temperatures below 42.5°C (sublethal temperatures) become resistant to continuous heat exposure – which means they become thermotolerant after a certain period of time. Thermotolerance can also be induced by lethal temperatures (> 42.5°C), but its development requires a time interval of about 6–12 h at 37°C before a second heat exposure. The cellular status of thermotolerance is reversible by further incubation and is not detectable about 120 h after the triggering heat dose has been given. Moreover, thermosensitivity itself and the induction of thermotolerance is largely dependent on environmental parameters like pH, partial oxygen pressure, and nutritional supply (Gerweck 1982).

By combining hyperthermia with radiotherapy (thermoradiotherapy), the radiobiological effect upon tumor tissues can be enhanced. Also, cells resistant to radiation can be killed by hyperthermia alone. Due to their environmental parameters (low pH, hypoxia, nutritional deprivation), such cells of poorly vascularized tumors are especially sensitive to hyperthermia.

Combining hyperthermia with chemotherapy (thermochemotherapy), a cooperative effect can be observed dependent on the specific chemotherapeutic agent(s) used (Hahn 1982). In general, cytotoxic drugs showed an enhanced inhibition of clonogenic cell growth in vitro at higher temperatures. Although the mechanisms involved are still unknown at the present time, the modification of the cytotoxic effect of such compounds with increasing temperatures can be classified into four groups: (1) inhibition, (2) independent action, (3) additive effect, and (4) synergistic effect. For example, an inhibition of the cytotoxic action of adriamycin has been shown in thermotolerant cells. Independent action means that the combined effect of heat and drug exposure upon the clonogenic survival of cells is equal to the numerical addition of the effect of each individual treatment alone. Additive and synergistic effects for combined heat and drug treatments have been shown previously for several agents (e.g., cisplatin, bischloronitrosourea (BCNU), cyclophosphamide, mitomycin). These agents should be tested in detail as good candidates for thermochemotherapy (Bull 1984). This latter group also includes "thermosensitizers" which are of interest in preclinical studies because their cytotoxic effects only occur at higher temperatures (e.g., thiol compounds, polyamines).

Pilot Study "Thermochemotherapy" (RHT-86)

Early clinical trials of hyperthermia combined with chemotherapy were mainly confined to isolated extremity/organ perfusion or systemic whole-body hyperthermia. The latter approach admits a systemic dose of cytotoxic drugs at an elevated temperature but is limited, however, with regard to the maximum of the raised temperature (41.8°–42°C) in order to avoid severe systemic side effects (e.g., bone marrow toxicity). Clinical application of RHT for deep-seated tumors in the abdominal or pelvic region combined with systemic chemotherapy has not previously been carried out.

Therefore, based on the rationale outlined above, a pilot study supported by the German Cancer Aid was started in 1986 at the Klinikum Großhadern of the University of Munich to investigate the feasibility and toxicity of this approach, employing an annular phased array applicator system (APAS) in combination with systemic chemotherapy. Only patients with advanced deep-seated tumors in the abdomen, pelvis, or proximal extremities and showing progressive disease under conventional treatment modalities (surgery, radiotherapy and/or chemotherapy) have been selected for this pilot study. Before entering the study the patients had the study design and possible side effects explained to them in detail. Patients with Karnofsky status lower than 40%, earlier myocardial infarction, a cardiac pacemaker, or metallic implants were excluded. At the beginning and end of the study, each patient underwent extensive staging examinations (e.g., X-ray, CT, NMR, bone scan, tumor markers). As described earlier, for patients with refractory sarcomas chemotherapy (ifosfamide 1.5 g/m^2 on days 1–5 and etoposide 80 mg/m^2 on days 1, 3, 5) was given simultaneously with RHT for 1 h on days 1 and 5 in order to avoid thermotolerance for the second heat treatment. Similar repeated cycles of thermochemotherapy were given 4–5 times at intervals of 4 weeks. For patients with progressive colorectal cancer, 5-fluorouracil (500 mg/m^2 on days 1–5) was given combined with RHT in the same order.

Results of the Phase I Study

From July 1986 to June 1988, 209 APAS treatments were performed on 38 patients (209/38) with solid tumors (25 sarcomas, 8 colorectal tumors, 5 others) in the pelvis (171/31), abdomen (26/5) or proximal extremities (12/2; see Tables 1, 2). The ability of the APAS treatments to reach the range of effective temperatures in tumor tissues was found to be dependent on the anatomic site. Although the maximum temperature obtained in pelvic and abdominal tumors was quite similar, the effective tumor dose (expressed as equivalent minutes of 43°C) was essentially higher in pelvic tumors (see Table 2). The compiled data relating to acute side effects are given in Table 3. Partially power-dependent pain has occurred in one-third of RHT treatments. Since such pain can be an early indication of overheated areas in normal tissues ("hot spots"), RHT is performed with patients not anesthesized. Apart from systemic stress (tachycardia in 45% of treatments; drop in central venous pressure in 24%), no severe increase of systemic temperature was observed. Further complica-

Table 1. Data from patients undergoing APAS treatment

No. of patients	38
Sex (F/M)	16/22
Median age (years)	50.5 (7–75)
Mean Karnofsky status	60% (40%–90%)
No. of APAS treatments	209
Mean no. of treatments/patient	5.5 (1–16)
Median tumor volume	785 cm^3 (55–4930 cm^3)

Table 2. APAS treatment data

Tumor site	Pelvis	Abdomen	Proximal extremities
No. of patients	31	5	2
No. of treatments	171	26	12
Tumor volume (cm^3)			
Mean/median	637/250	980/420	2580/2580
Range	55–4930	80–2980	1470–3690
Maximum temperature (°C)			
Mean/median	43.0/42.8	42.5/42.7	44.8/44.8
Range	38.8–52.0	39.5–44.5	43.6–45.6
Maximum tumor dose (min)			
Mean/median	54.8/16.8	19.0/12.0	150.1/150.4
Range	0–2231.9	0–72.2	81.9–266.8

Table 3. Acute side effects after 209 APAS treatments

	Treatments	
	n	%
Pain		
Power-dependent	67	32
Power-independent	75	36
Systemic temperature		
>38°C	30	14
>39°C	5	2
Nausea or vomiting	8	4
Cardiocirculatory symptoms		
Tachycardia (>120/min)	94	45
Arrhythmia	7	3
Stenocardia	1	0.4
Drop in CVP (>3 cm H_2O)	51	24
Neurological symptoms		
Sensory disturbance	5	2
Muscular spasm	1	0.4
Dyspnea	4	2

CVP, central venous pressure

tions consisted of bacteriological infections in the catheters in 11% of all RHT treatments. All other RHT-related complications (e.g., bleeding 1/209, hematuria 1/209, superficial burn 2/209, thrombosis 2/209) were rare events.

The systemic chemotherapy given during RHT treatment was well tolerated by the patients, with no increase of the known acute side effects (e.g., nausea, vomiting); in particular, bone marrow toxicity, measured as the leukocyte nadir, was not affected within the different courses of combined treatments.

Apart from the maximum temperature and heat dose, we also observed heterogeneous temperature distribution in normal and tumor tissues, most likely due to the differences in vascularization and to tissue-specific regulatory mechanisms (Song et al. 1984). RHT seems to be limited by relatively well-perfused areas of the individual tumor or of the surrounding tissue. By analyzing the temperatures measured along the axis of the thermal probes during the course of each RHT treatment, this hypothesis could be confirmed. Despite heating parts of the tumor to greatly elevated temperatures (43°–45°C), the existence of other areas with a temperature range of 40°–42.5°C could be ascribed to the presence of large blood vessels or cavities (e.g., externally cooled bladder). These observations may support the following conclusion in regard to the simultaneous application of RHT and systemic chemotherapy: poorly perfused tumor areas that are hardly reached by chemotherapeutic agents can be heated to a cytotoxic temperature range (> 42.5°C). In addition, due to the external environmental parameters mentioned before, such tumor areas are particularly sensitized to heat. By contrast, well-perfused tumor areas will be reached by the cytotoxic drugs from the blood supply. Despite the lower heating of these areas, a sensitizing effect to chemotherapy should still be expected in a temperature range of 40°–42.5°C.

Tumor Response

At present, tumor response can only be evaluated in 12 patients with sarcomas who have received at least 6 RHT treatments 3 cycles of chemotherapy (duration of observation: 4–23 months; mean: 8.5 months). Four of these patients died from progressive disease despite initial palliative effects (e.g., pain relief). Three patients still show no change, whereas partial remission (> 50% reduction of the tumor mass) was be achieved in two patients. In three patients with nonresectable, chemotherapy-resistant, progressive pelvic tumors, the tumor mass was largely reduced by RHT combined with chemotherapy (IFO/VP-16) followed by complete resection without mutilation. In each case histological examination of the resected material showed tumor cell-free margins and these three patients have no evidence of disease at present.

Future Prospects for the Use of Hyperthermia

Hyperthermia of deep-seated tumors in specific sites could become a promising new therapeutic approach in clinical oncology. After combining systemic chemotherapy with regional hyperthermia, large, nonresectable pelvic tumors may become resectable without mutilation and damage to the surrounding tissue. A further advantage could be the possibility of postoperative radiation with lower target volume. On the basis of these first data, a phase II study including, for example, nonresponders or poor responders to initial chemotherapy of soft tissue sarcomas, Ewing's sarcomas and/or osteogenic sarcomas, should be performed to evaluate the potential of RHT in these patients. At present, it is completely uncertain whether other advanced tumors in the pelvic area (e.g., colorectal, ovarian, bladder, prostate) could be treated by RHT combined with chemotherapy.

Further technical improvements (e.g., enhanced focusing of the tumor target, noninvasive temperature measurement) and efforts in thermobiological research (e.g., development of new thermosensitizing compounds) are essential to enhance the clinical potential of RHT in the treatment of solid tumors.

References

Bull MC (1984) An update on the anticancer effects of a combination of chemotherapy and hyperthermia. Cancer Res [Suppl] 44:4853–4856

Gerweck LE (1982) Effect of microenvironmental factors on the response of cells to single and fractionated heat treatments. NCI Monogr 61:19–26

Hahn GM (1982) Hyperthermia and cancer. In: Hahn GM (ed) Hyperthermia and cancer. Plenum, New York

Issels R, Wilmanns W (1988) Application of hyperthermia in the treatment of cancer. Springer, Berlin Heidelberg New York (Recent results in cancer research, vol 107)

Song CW, Lokshina A, Rhee JG, Patten M, Levitt SH (1984) Implication of blood flow in hyperthermic treatment of tumors. IEEE Trans Biomed Eng 31:9–16

Westra A, Dewey WC (1971) Variation in sensitivity to heat shock during the cell-cycle of chinese hamster cells in vitro. Int J Radiat Biol 19:467–477

Summary of Discussion: Session 3

E. W. HAHN

Hyperthermia in Tumor Treatment

The question was raised as to what experience has there been with the combination of high LET (linear energy transfer) radiation and hyperthermia. It appears that very little work has been done in this area. Dr. Hahn and his colleagues did some work at the Memorial Sloan-Kettering Cancer Center in New York (Hahn et al. 1976, Radiat Res 68:39–56), where they found that heat in combination with fast neutrons offered no significant advantage over treatment with neutrons alone. In this same report they showed that the combination of hyperthermia and photons (300 kV X-rays) gave essentially the same response as neutrons alone. In fact, because of these results, the combination of photons plus hyperthermia was called "the poor man's high LET radiation." This has been the only study reporting this effect, but it was carried out using the Ridgeway osteogenic sarcoma, which is a rapidly proliferating mouse tumor and exquisitely sensitive to radiation. This tumor was used because the neutron beam available had a low flux with a dose rate of about 2 cGy/min and thus only low doses of radiation could be given. There are now ongoing studies, using the KARIN neutron generator (dose rate 10–12 cGy/min) at the German Cancer Research Centre with the Dunning prostate tumor (e.g., R-3327 AT-1 subline) which is syngeneic to the Copenhagen rat, slow growing, and fairly radioresistant.

The dose survival curves presented were very persuasive, but one participant wondered if his impression was correct that the results from practically every clinical trial seemed to be as good as every other. It seemed that, as to the method of heating, it really doesn't matter whether you give good or bad hyperthermia, before or after radiation – the results all seem to lie nicely on the sigmoid-shaped curve. Could this really be so, when there were so many differences in the methods of heating and in the treatment schedules, and was it possible to derive better treatment strategies from these experiences?

It remains unclear how the fractionated combined treatments work. It is very possible that the incidence of good or bad heating of the tumor is the same in most of the clinical studies. In all likelihood, all one needs is one good heating every so often during the treatment schedule. However, there is one heating technique that is superior to all others and that is interstitial hyperthermia. The results for this are very impressive in, for instance, recurrent tumors, and are probably due to the more uniform heating of the tumor. The 60%–70% long-term local tumor control achieved in most clinical trials is therefore probably the minimum result that we are likely to get with the combined treatment.

With respect to the thermal enhancement ratio (TER) and its dependence on the sequence of treatment, two questions were asked. Firstly, if the normal tissues were protected, would the simultaneous application of heat and radiation yield better results, and, secondly, is the situation the same for all tumors? The answer was "yes" to the first and "probably yes" to the second. If one can give simultaneous treatment, for instance, as can be done with interstitial hyperthermia, one is likely to obtain a better response – but one must be able to protect the normal tissues. Dr. Overgaard felt that to protect the normal tissues one could either introduce a time interval between the radiation and heat, or cool the normal tissue. The current philosophy in combined therapy is to use heat as the adjuvant treatment. This in principle means that we should not change the currently accepted fractionation schedule of radiation for a particular tumor type. Therefore by using a routinely used fractionation we can introduce an adjuvant treatment which would then not enhance normal tissue damage. Thus using a time interval or cooling down the normal tissues seems judicious.

It is important to point out that hyperthermia is not in competition with other conventional forms of therapy, with perhaps one exception and that is in the case of malignant melanoma. In this instance, combined heat and radiation therapy may be superior to surgical excision.

A further question was raised concerning whether there might be a diurnal effect of hyperthermia, in other words was hyperthermia more effective when given for instance, during the daytime as opposed to during the nighttime. No clearcut information was available to answer this question. However, it is well-known that one heat treatment induces a subsequent resistance to the next heat treatment. This transient phenomenon is called thermal tolerance. Thus, in essence, if one good heat treatment is given on day 1, a second heat treatment on day 2 will have little biological effect. Thermal tolerance in combination with radiation has not been demonstrated to be of significance in the clinical studies. If one heat treatment out of say five applications is good, the following ones are not likely to have a significant effect unless they are each separated by a few days. This may account for the lack of apparent differences in the clinical studies.

Influence of Hyperthermia on Chemotherapy

As to the power and radio frequency available to the heating equipment, Dr. Issels uses a frequency range between 50 and 80 MHz at 300–400 watts at the beginning of treatment, increasing the power to a maximum of 1500 watts if necessary. A new machine, the BSD 2000, will soon be installed in Munich. This new equipment, which should be easier to use and safer for the patient, will by means of amplitude and phase shifting of the microwave applicators allow more directed heating of extensive tumors within the body.

Some in vitro cell culture data which were presented indicated that hyperthermia may be able to reverse acquired drug resistance. Did this mean that hyperthermia could be used to overcome pleiotropic drug resistance in patients which is considered to be a major problem in cancer chemotherapy today?

The data on cisplatin and methotrexate suggest that acquired resistance to these drugs can indeed be overcome by treatment with hyperthermia. In the case of bleomycin-resistant cells, after heat treatment they become more sensitive to bleomycin than the original, nonresistant cell line. The reason for this is not clear, but there is evidence to indicate that the action of bleomycin may be through causing the formation of highly reactive radicals during hyperthermia. Dr. Issels has some patients who initially did not respond to ifosfamide and VP-16 combination treatment, but did respond later when retreated with these same drugs in combination with hyperthermia. Four patients had a complete response with no evidence of disease 3–24 months after treatment.

There is an interesting parallelism between the decrease in both thermal tolerance and drug resistance, for instance with adriamycin (doxorubicin) – apparently, this phenomenon has been reported only for this drug. These phenomena are not related to an increased cellular uptake of adriamycin but rather there seems to be a difference in the action of the drug within the cell.

Hyperthermia induces a raised action of drugs through several mechanisms. In the case of the antimetabolite 5-fluorouracil, it brings about an increased uptake of the drug – in other words, a change in the transport activity. Another mechanism is to cause the drug to be more readily converted to a more reactive form, as happens, for example, with the alkylating agent. There is no one unified mechanism which explains all the drug effects associated with hyperthermia; rather, there seem to be four or five mechanisms. One of the most interesting phenomena described was the effect of hyperthermia on glutathione concentrations and the resulting increasing ratio of oxidized to reduced glutathione. By decreasing the level of glutathione, increased drug sensitivity to alkylating agents, for instance, is obtained. Thus, introducing chemicals which alter glutathione levels may be an important way of obtaining an increased therapeutic response. BSO (buthionine sulfoxamine) is a specific inhibitor of glutathione biosynthesis and when added to cell culture media leads to enhanced thermosensitivity of a drug. Studies are being conducted on the effects of BSO in animal tumor systems but as of yet there are no controlled phase I clinical studies.

A list separating the interaction between heat and drugs into three different categories gave the impression that with some drugs – cisplatin, for instance, – one always obtained a synergistic effect, while for others one would always obtain an additive effect. However, in studies of drug interactions with ionizing radiation, the results vary considerably depending on the cell line and the details of the experiment. Are the data concerning hyperthermia and drugs really that clean and consistent, or could it be that not enough information is available to make that judgment?

It was concluded that before one can critically evaluate the type of interaction of a particular drug with hyperthermia, data on all points must be available. For instance, it appears that the interaction of heat with cisplatin is synergistic over a range of temperatures; with adriamycin the interaction varies according to the temperature studied and is additive only when a temperature above 42.5° is used.

There appears to be quite a heterogeneity in the tumor temperatures attained in the clinical setting. What is the cause of this variation, and can it be moderated by machine manipulation of power, frequency, and phase shifting?

Apparently there is always a certain heterogeneity of temperature distribution within the deep pelvic tumors, due to the physical limitations of the hyperthermia equipment as well as to anatomical configurations and of course blood flow. At each treatment there is always an engineer present who attempts to optimize the treatment set-up. He measures the electric fields and positions the patient. If the tumor does not heat up, the patient may be repositioned, the frequency changed, and a new evaluation made. One such deep treatment takes a minimum of 4 h.

As an extension of this discussion, the question was raised as to which tumors were suitable and which were unsuitable for combined chemotherapy plus hyperthermia treatment. Tumors in the lower abdomen and pelvic area seem to be most appropriate. These would include bladder cancer, ovarian cancer, colorectal cancer, etc. Because of problems of patient positioning experienced with the present equipment used in Munich, tumors in the thorax (for example, lung tumors) cannot be treated. Further, .tumors with a high blood flow, such as angiomas, cannot be adequately heated with this approach. It was emphasized that while there are many studies to be done, the studies that are done must be well-planned, multi-institutional controlled trials.

It appears, at least with the inductive mode of heating, it is easier to heat larger than smaller tumors. Dr. Issels also had that impression and added that it is easier to implant a temperature measuring probe in a larger tumor.

If a temperature probe could be implanted with the same degree of certainty in a smaller tumor mass one might, by varying the treatment parameters, also be able to heat smaller tumors with the same degree of success as larger ones. The temperature variation in larger tumors appears to be greater than seen with smaller tumors. Larger tumors are more apt to have cold spots.

SESSION 4

Chemotherapy

Chairman: C. G. SCHMIDT

New Trends in Chemotherapy of Tumors

W. Wilmanns, C. Clemm, H. Gerhartz, K. Possinger, and H. Sauer

Introduction

Chemotherapy of tumors is not a new treatment; it is rather an established treatment in which some new trends have appeared during the past 10 years. It must be regarded as a part of an interdisciplinary conducted treatment modality applied in any neoplastic disease.

Approximately 25 years ago, the introduction by De Vita of a multiple drug treatment modality, the MOPP regimen (Mustine-Oncovin (vincristine) – procarbazine – prednisone), into the treatment of Hodgkin's disease resulted in a significantly higher cure rate of this disease, even at advanced stages. Similar results had already been obtained in gestational chorion carcinoma and were in the following years achieved in various pediatric tumors, testicular cancer, acute lymphoblastic leukemia of childhood – most recently in adults, too –, highly malignant non-Hodgkin's lymphoma, and also in limited small cell lung cancer (in a small percentage of patients). Thus, it became almost unjustifiable not to treat any neoplastic disease with multiple cytotoxic drug combinations, which were tested in controlled randomized trials and evaluated primarily according to remission rates. But at last we have learned that in tumors for which curative methods are not available, remission rates do not necessarily correlate with survival, nor – a very important aspect – with quality of life. Therefore, the present trend in tumor chemotherapy is to adapt our treatment strategies to prognostic factors and to ask whether in particular tumor, there is a chance of "long-term disease-free survival" – which may mean cure – or whether treatment modalities should be restricted to palliation, with quality of life as the main aim (Brunner 1987).

Curative Cancer Chemotherapy

In a discussion of curative therapy, the first question that arises is how to define "cure" (see Frei 1985). The exact meaning of "cure" is that a successfully treated patient survives a normal life span. According to this precise definition, the word "cure" cannot yet be employed, as chemotherapy has not been in use for long enough, so some physicians avoid it and prefer instead the expression "long-term disease-free survival". This might be inappropriate, however, if the probability of being cured is high. The quality of life and the compliance of patients are highly improved if they can hope that their treatment will lead to cure. For most tumor categories the cure rate can be defined as the disease-free survival plateau. Breast cancer is the only exception of the application of this definition, as the risk of relapse will remain up to 15 years after primary operation, even though the probability of treatment failure decreases constantly during this time.

In the next part of this paper the results of chemotherapy applied with aim to cure patients suffering from testicular cancer, Hodgkin's and non-Hodgkin's lymphoma, and acute leukemia will be discussed.

Testicular Cancer

In 1981 L. H. Einhorn gave the Richard and Hinda Rosenthal Foundation Award Lecture (published in *Cancer Research*), entitled "Testicular Cancer as a Model for a Curable Neoplasm". This dramatic progress in the treatment of a tumor – even at an advanced stage – which strikes young men (aged between 20 and 30 years at the most), and which formerly had a very poor prognosis, was made possible by inclusion of a new cytotoxic compound, cisplatin, into a polychemotherapeutic regimen containing bleomycin and vinblastine. Recently, because of neurotoxic side effects, vinblastine in the PVB regimen has been replaced by etoposide in the PEB regimen (Einhorn 1987; Schmoll and Weissbach 1988). The main treatment strategy is interdisciplinary and is conducted on the basis of histology and staging: In trophoblastic tumors, polychemotherapy at all stages; in teratocarcinomas, after the staging operation, polychemotherapy at stages IIB (as adjuvant treatment), IIC, III, and IV (Schmoll and Weissbach 1988).

The results of treatment effects in more than 200 patients in our hospital are summarized in Table 1. The complete remission rates of patients in stages IIC–IV are over 70%. At second look operation (thoracotomy, retroperitoneal lymphadenectomy) of 61 patients, undifferentiated tumor was removed in only 10%. Only these patients received further chemotherapy. Forty-three percent showed differentiated teratoma and 47% fibrosis. The overall long-term disease-free survival was 75% (Fig. 1).

Some patients with testicular cancer have a very high tumor load ("bulky tumor") at the time of diagnosis and therefore have a bad prognosis. By adding cyclophosphamide to the PEB combination, however, we achieved long-term survival in 15 of 21 patients (70%), even with advanced testicular cancer. Of course this number of patients is still too small and the follow-up too short for definite conclusions to be drawn (Clemm et al. 1988).

Table 1. Complete remissions in patients with nonseminomatous germ cell tumors

Cancer stage	No. of patients	Complete remissions
I	24/ 24	100%
II	78/ 84	93%
III	20/ 26	77%
IV	73/107	68%
IIC–IV	130/176	74%

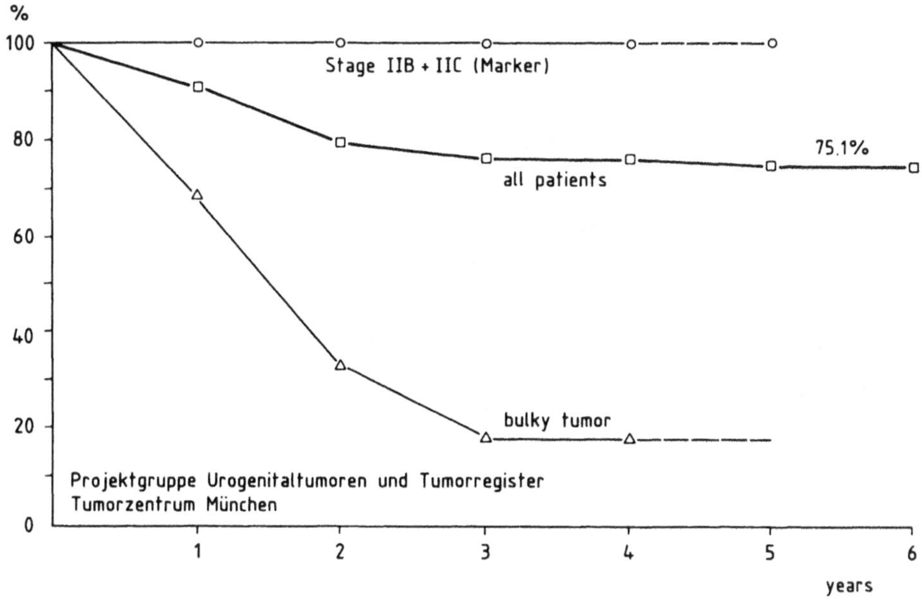

Fig. 1. Nonseminomatous germ cell tumor: survival rate

In advanced seminoma (stages IIC–IV), multiple drug combination chemotherapy also has become the first-line treatment and has replaced radiation. With the VIP regimen (vinblastine/ifosfamide/platin) we achieved complete remissions with long-term disease-free survival in more than 90% of the patients treated. The results were less favorable in cases where prior radiotherapy was performed (Clemm et al. 1986).

Hodgkin's Lymphoma

Hodgkin's lymphoma was the first example of a neoplasm for which the introduction of multiple drug chemotherapy improved the treatment results in terms of cure. A major problem at present is how to adapt treatment strategies to risk factors. This is being investigated in a trial supported by the Bundesministerium für Forschung und Technologie (Loeffler et al. 1988; Pfreundschuh et al. 1986), using a treatment regimen which alternates COPP (cyclophosphamide, vincristine, procarbazine, prednisolone) and ABVD [adriamycin (doxorubicin), bleomycin, vinblastine, dacarbazine] and randomization to different radiotherapeutic treatments after chemotherapy. This treatment regimen is applied to patients with a large mediastinal mass and/or continual involvement of other organs and/or massive splenic involvement. With this regimen even patients with these risk factors have an excellent prognosis, with about 80% long-term disease-free survival. Patients with stage IIIB or IV disease are treated similarly, but with three instead of two cycles of COPP and ABVD in the induction phase. With a long-term disease-free survival of 60%, they have an intermediate prognosis. There is a striking difference between patients with low initial erythrocyte sedimentation rate (ESR) and alkaline phosphatase (AP) and those with

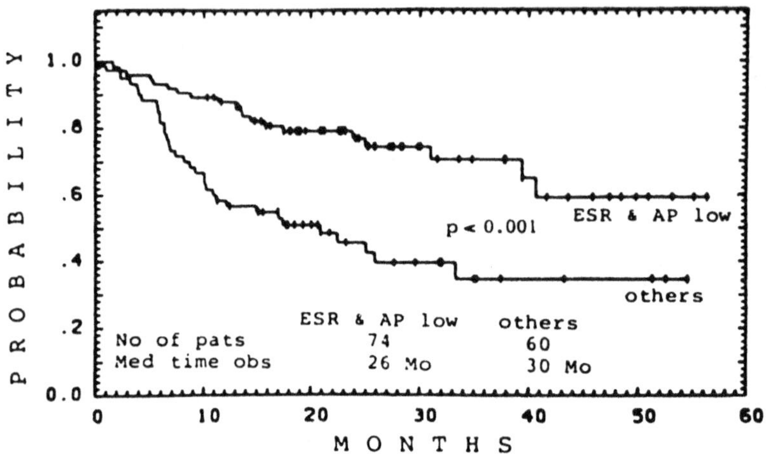

Fig. 2. Hodgkin's lymphoma, advanced stages (IIIB/IV): freedom from treatment failure

high ESR and AP (Fig. 2). The latter have a poor prognosis, with the plateau of freedom from treatment failure at about only 30% of patients treated. These results may have implications on a new definition of B symptoms, and new treatment strategies are urgently needed for this group of patients.

Highly Malignant Non-Hodgkin's Lymphoma

In highly malignant non-Hodgkin's lymphoma, significant improvement of treatment results, in the sense of longer survival and higher cure rates, could be achieved by the introduction of cyclophosphamide, hydroxydaunomycine (adriamycine), oncovine (vincristine), prednisolone (CHOP) and later by COPBLAM (cyclophosphamide, vincristine, prednisolone, bleomycin, adriamycine, methotrexate) and other drug combinations (Pfreundschuh et al. 1986). On the basis of favorable results reported by Gerhartz et al. (1986) in our hospital a prospective trial supported by the Bundesministerium für Forschung und Technologie has been started in West Germany and Austria (Gerhartz et al. 1988). The main characteristics of this trial are the three-cycle-treatment with COPBLAM, which in cases with complete remission is followed by two further cycles of COPBLAM and two cycles of IMVP-16 [ifosfamide, methotrexate, VP-16 (etoposide)] for consolidation. If complete remission is not achieved by the first induction treatment, there is an early switch to IMVP-16. In younger patients below 45 years autologous bone marrow transplantation is discussed. Additional radiation treatment is applied to bulky disease.

Acute Leukemia

As numerous trials have been reported (Champlin and Gale 1987; Gale and Foon 1986; Hoelzer and Gale 1987; Jehn et al. 1988), I restrict myself to standard treatment results, which should be achieved in any hospital involved in the treatment of acute leukemia. These are summarized in Table 2. The remission rate of acute lym-

Table 2. Standard treatment results in acute leukemia

	Remission	Disease-free survival	In remission after 5 years
Children			
ALL	>90%	Cure in 50–75%	
Adults			
ALL/AUL	75–80%		35%
ANLL	60–70%	10–14 months	10–25%

phoblastic leukemia in children is more than 90% with a probability of cure in 50–75%. In adults, the results are less favorable, but even in this population the long-term disease-free survival of patients with acute lymphoblastic leukemia (ALL) has increased to more than 35% and of those with acute nonlymphoblastic leukemia (ANLL) to 10–25%. Many trials are under way in West Germany, the EORTC, and the USA to try to improve results by intensification of induction and consolidation treatment.

The role of maintenance therapy still remains an unsolved question. Treatment results have been improved by bone marrow transplantation during first remission in patients with ANLL and in ALL with high risk factors and during second remission in ALL with low risk factors.

GM-CSF or G-CSF in Neutropenic Patients

Hematological toxicities are the major side effects of many cytotoxic drugs (Brandt et al. 1988; Morstyn et al. 1988). In many tumors the leukocyte and thrombocyte

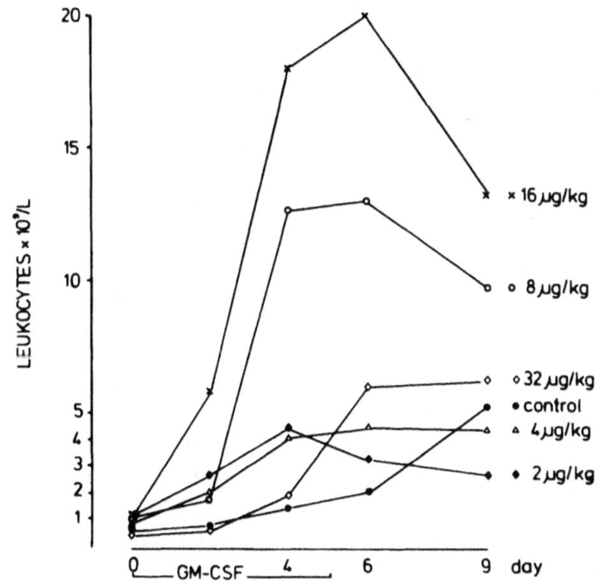

Fig. 3. Effect of 5-day treatment with GM-CSF on leukocyte recovery in chemotherapy-induced leukopenia (mean of three patients in each group; five patients in the control group)

counts after the first treatment course have a significance for dose variation in the subsequent polychemotherapy cycle.

A promising new approach for overcoming the toxicity of myelosuppressive drugs in intensively treated tumor patients is autologous bone marrow transplantation, but this treatment still carries a high risk of morbidity and mortality during the nearly 3-week period required for marrow engraftment and hematopoetic reconstitution. The recent molecular cloning and expression of granulocyte colony stimulating factor (G-CSF) and granulocyte-macrophage colony stimulating factor (GM-CSF) and their ability to accelerate hematopoetic recovery have given new hope for ways of reducing therapy-related toxicity. Results of dose-dependent treatment with GM-CSF given to neutropenic patients after polychemotherapy in our clinic are illustrated in Fig. 3. With the administration of 8 or 16 μg/kg body wt. daily for 5 days, the neutrophiles in the peripheral blood increase dramatically, whereas – interestingly – higher doses (32 μg/kg body wt.) are not that effective. Thus, in the future, the use of colony stimulating factors may allow the development of more intensive and effective chemotherapy schedules for various neoplasms.

Adjuvant Chemotherapy

Experimental studies have indicated that in some tumors treatment which is only partly effective against macroscopic disease is much more effective against microscopic tumors (Frei 1985). On the basis of this assumption, chemotherapy is administered to patients at high risk of disseminating microscopic disease immediately after control of the primary tumor by operation. This treatment is known as adjuvant chemotherapy and has been highly successful in increasing the cure rate in pediatric patients with solid tumors and patients with osteogenic sarcoma and some other tumors, and in prolonging disease-free survival in patients with premenopausal breast cancer with positive lymph nodes (Bonadonna and Valagussa 1987; Kaufmann et al. 1986; Lippmann 1985). It must be stated that, among the last, only a small proportion of patients profit from this kind of treatment. To define the subgroups with breast cancer for whom adjuvant chemotherapy is indicated therefore still remains an important problem in the attempt to avoid unnecessary toxic side effects of cytotoxic drugs in clinically healthy patients (Wilmanns 1989).

Palliative Chemotherapy for Noncurable Tumors: Metastatic Breast Cancer

For the most common tumors – breast cancer, gastrointestinal tumors, non-small-cell lung cancer, ovarian cancer, cancer of the prostate, renal cell cancer, and others – little or no progress in treatment results at the advanced stage has been achieved during the last 10 years (Sauer and Wilmanns 1985). In some of these tumors, we have learned, achievement of remission does not always correlate with longer survival and a better quality of life. In such cases we have to ask whether the palliative effects of cytotoxic treatment outweighs its toxic side effects (Brunner 1987).

Table 3. Advanced breast cancer: prognostic score

Prognostic factors	Points
Site of metastasis	
Skin, soft tissue	1
Bone, effusion	1
Lung: nodular:	
solitary	3
multiple	5
lymphangiosis ca.	6
Liver	6
Bone marrow	4
Receptor status	
Positive	1
Unknown	2
Negative	3
Relapse-free interval	
>2 years	1
≤2 years	3

Favorable prognosis: <7 points
Unfavorable prognosis: ≥7 points

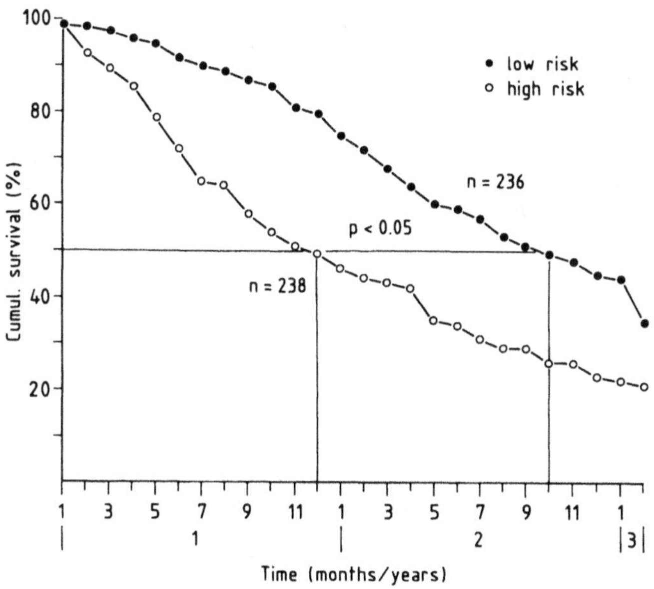

Fig. 4. Advanced breast cancer: survival time measured from the first occurrence of distant metastases

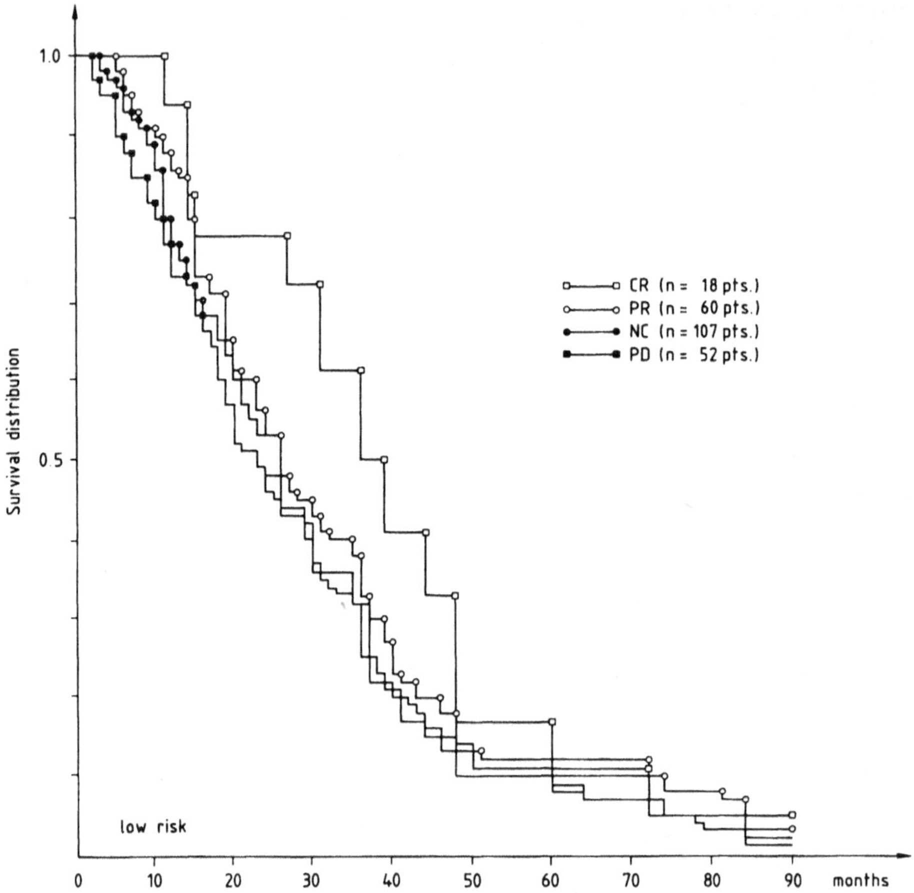

Fig. 5. Advanced breast cancer: survival distribution of patients with favorable prognostic signs (low risk) calculated from the beginning of cytotoxic therapy according to the response to the first cytotoxic therapy. CR, complete remission; PR, partial remission; NC, no change: PD, progressive disease

This problem has been studied intensively in patients with metastasized breast cancer (Possinger et al. 1988). Patients were allocated to a low or a high risk group according to their disease-free interval after operation, number and site of metastases, and hormonal receptor status. For practical reasons prognostic factors were scored by K. Possinger according to Table 3. The therapeutic approach differed between low and high risk patients. Hormones were the first-line treatment for low risk, receptor-positive patients, followed by chemotherapy at relapse. Aggressive polychemotherapy as primary treatment was restricted to patients with high risk factors, especially primary visceral metastases. Of the 501 patients entered the study, data regarding response and survival time are evaluable for 474. Eligibility criteria included histologically proven breast cancer, occurrence of metastases not manageable otherwise (surgery or irradiation), and a prospective survival of more than 2 months.

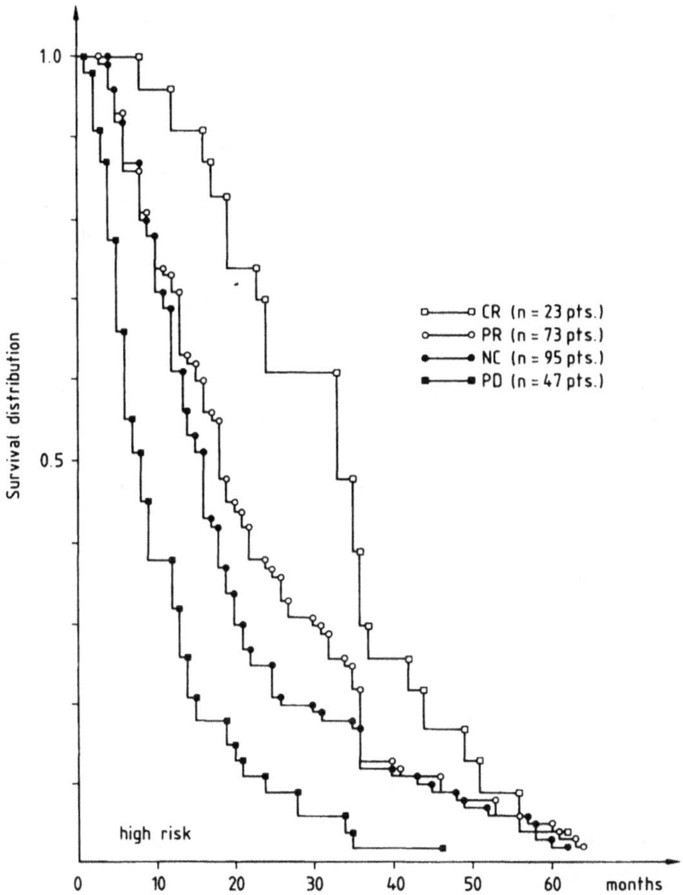

Fig. 6. Advanced breast cancer: survival distribution of patients with unfavorable prognostic signs (high risk) calculated from the beginning of cytotoxic therapy according to the response to the first cytotoxic therapy

The usefulness of the prognostic score was reflected by the survival times of the two patient groups, which were significantly different (Fig. 4). Patients with favorable prognostic signs survived a median of 22 months from the first occurrence of distant metastases, patients with unfavorable signs a median of only 12 months.

Looking at the relation of survival to the response to the first combination chemotherapy, we found considerable differences between the two groups. Patients with favorable prognostic criteria (Fig. 5) had exactly the same survival time, independent of tumor progression, stable disease, or even partial remission. Only patients with complete remission survived longer, but this subgroup (18 of 237 patients) was small. Analyzing these results, it became evident that most patients with favorable prognosis had been overtreated. Only in few patients had polychemotherapy improved the quality of life by reducing tumor-related symptoms; all the other patients had to endure the pronounced toxicity of polychemotherapy for months without any prolongation of survival from this treatment, except for the few who achieved complete remission.

In patients with unfavorable prognosis (high risk), the impact of the therapeutic efficiency of the initial chemotherapy on survival time was completely different (Fig. 6). Patients with primary tumor progression survived for a significantly shorter time than patients with stable disease or partial remission. Those achieving complete remission had the longest survival time. Thus, in contrast to the low risk group, most patients with unfavorable prognostic factors apparently benefited from chemotherapy. In addition, in most of the patients in this group, polychemotherapy induced at least a transient stabilization or an improvement of tumor-induced symptoms.

The conclusion to be drawn from these results, which have been confirmed by evaluation of a large international, prospective, randomized, first-line chemotherapy trial (Possinger et al. 1988), is that chemotherapy for advanced breast cancer must be planned and administered according to the prognostic profile of the individual patient. In palliative treatment therapeutic induction of objective tumor remission does not always correlate with longer survival. One should be careful of overestimating the effects of palliative treatment of advanced breast cancer with favorable prognostic symptoms – and probably other noncurable tumors, too – according to the remission rate, for the following reasons:

1. The definition of remission is variable and the reproducibility poor, especially in a heterogenous tumor disease like breast cancer.
2. Frequently the administration of cytotoxic drugs may cause high toxicity which is not justified when measured against the therapeutic benefit and may thus reduce the quality of life.
3. Thus, overtreatment in order to achieve remission may become treatment failure in noncurable tumors.
4. It has been shown that the remission rate in advanced breast cancer has been overestimated in the past, because there is no correlation between remission rate and longer survival. The situation will probably be similar for other noncurable tumors.

Future Considerations

New methods for evaluation of palliative treatment effects in noncurable tumors – including quality of life – need to be developed. As a consequence that remission rate has been overestimated in the past and does not correlate with longer survival the estimation of the "*T*ime *w*ithout *S*ymptoms and *T*oxicity" (TWJST) and the "*T*ime *to* *P*rogression" (TTP) are factors of much higher value. According to these factors, which can be defined for each noncurable tumor disease within a score (Brunner 1987), the effects, benefits and failures of treatment may be evaluated. This may have implications for our judgement of new treatment modalities, too, such as regional chemotherapy of liver metastases via a catheter to the hepatic artery, and others.

Conclusion

The current trends in chemotherapy of malignant tumors can be summarized as follows:

1. Chemotherapy of tumors has to be integrated into interdisciplinary strategies.
2. In tumor diseases with a chance of cure, better results may be achieved by intensification of induction and consolidation treatment, combined in some tumors with second look operation and radiation.
3. In some tumors a higher cure rate and in others longer survival can be achieved by adjuvant chemotherapy of a microscopic tumor without clinical manifestation.
4. Recombinant colony stimulating factors, at present GM-CSF or G-CSF, are able to reduce toxic side effects of myelosuppressive drugs.
5. The remission rate in merely palliative treatment has been overestimated in the past. More important aspects are quality of life and time to progression.
6. New treatment modalities still at the experimental stage are the application of regional chemotherapy to liver metastases in patients with colorectal cancer, and the combination of chemotherapy with autologous bone marrow transplantation or with local hyperthermia.
7. New treatment modalities should be controlled by pharmacokinetic and biochemical investigations.
8. Most important of course is the development of new drugs ("biological response modifiers"?) with higher efficiency against the malignant tumor and less toxicity to the host.

Acknowledgements. The author acknowledges the help of C. Clemm, H. Gerhartz, K. Possinger, and H. Sauer.

References

Bertino JR (1987) Adjuvant therapy of osteosarcoma. J Clin Oncol 5:831–832
Bonadonna G, Valagussa P (1987) Current status of adjuvant chemotherapy for breast cancer. Semin Oncol 14:8–22
Brandt StJ, Peters WP, Atwater SK, et al (1988) Effect of recombinant human granulocyte-macrophage colony-stimulating factor on hematopoietic reconstitution after high-dose chemotherapy and autologous bone marrow transplantation. N Engl J Med 318:869–876
Brunner KW (1987) Palliative Tumor-Chemotherapie und Lebensqualität: was ist optimal? Schweiz Med Wochenschr 117:688–692
Champlin R, Gale RP (1987) Acute myelogenous leukemia: recent advances in therapy. Blood 69: 1551–1562
Clemm C, Hartenstein R, Willich N, Boening L, Wilmanns W (1986) Vinblastine, ifosfamide, cisplatin treatment of bulky seminoma. Cancer 58:2203–2207
Clemm C, Hartenstein R, Mair W, Wiesel N, Ledderose G (1988) Vierfach-Kombination beim nichtseminomatösen Hodentumor mit ungünstiger Prognose. In: Schmoll HJ, Weißbach L (eds) Diagnostik und Therapie von Hodentumoren. Springer, Berlin Heidelberg New York, pp 212–221
Einhorn LH (1981) Testicular cancer as a model for a curable neoplasm: the Richard and Hinda Rosenthal Foundation Award Lecture. Cancer Res 41:3275–3280
Einhorn LH (1987) Chemotherapy of disseminated germ cell tumors. Cancer 60:570–573
Frei E (1985) Curative cancer chemotherapy. Cancer Res 45:6523–6537

Gale RP, Foon KA (1986) Acute myeloid leukemia: recent advances in therapy. Clin Lab Haematol 15:781–810

Gerhartz HH, Thiel E, Hiller E, Nerl C, Wilmanns W, Huhn D für die Münchner Lymphomgruppe (1986) Vergleich der CHOP- und COP-BLAM-Chemotherapie hochmaligner Non-Hodgkin-Lymphome. Dtsch Med Wochenschr 111:1511–1515

Gerhartz HH, Thiel E, Brittinger G, et al (NHL Study Group) (1988) German-Austrian multicenter trial for aggressive non-Hodgkin lymphomas: COP-BLAM/-IMVP-16 chemotherapy with randomized adjuvant radiotherapy. Blut 56:139–142

Hartenstein R, Clemm C, Jäckel R, Wilmanns W (1988) Prognostische Kriterien beim nicht-seminomatösen Hodenkarzinomen: retrospektive Analyse 1979–1985. In: Schmoll HJ, Weissbach L (eds) Springer, Berlin Heidelberg New York, pp 111–124

Hoelzer D, Gale RP (1987) Acute lymphoblastic leukemia in adults: recent progress, future directions. Semin Hematol 24:27–39

Jehn U, Knüppel W, Wilmanns W (1988) Intensive maintenance treatment in acute myelogenous leukemia (AML): single institution experience of a multicenter randomized trial. Onkologie 11:13–17

Kaufmann M, Jonat W, Maass H (1986) Adjuvante Hormon- und Chemotherapie beim Mammakarzinom. Dtsch Arztebl 83:248–250

Lippman ME (1985) The NIH consensus development conference on adjuvant chemotherapy for breast cancer – a commentary. Breast Cancer Res Treat 6:195–200

Loeffler M, Pfreundschuh M, Hasenclever D, Hiller E, Gerhartz HH, Wilmanns W, et al (1988) Prognostic risk factors in advanced Hodgkin's lymphoma. Report of the German Hodgkin Study Group. Blut 56:273–281

Morstyn G, Souza LM, Keech J, Sheridan W, et al (1988) Effect of granulocyte colony stimulating factor on neutropenia induced by cytotoxic chemotherapy. Lancet 667–671

Pfreundschuh M, Schaadt M, Diehl V (1986) Chemotherapie der Non-Hodgkin-Lymphome. Internist (Berlin) 27:506–524

Pfreundschuh M, Schaadt M, Diehl V, et al (1986) Hodgkin-Lymphoma im Erwachsenenalter. Dtsch Arztebl 83:2538–2540

Possinger K, Sauer H-J, Wilmanns W (1988) Chemotherapie metastasierter Mammakarzinome. Dtsch Med Wochenschr 113:224–231

Sauer H-J, Wilmanns W (1985) Internistische Therapie maligner Erkrankungen, 2nd edn. Urban and Schwarzenberg, Munich

Schmoll HJ, Weissbach L (eds) (1988) Diagnostik und Therapie von Hodentumoren. Springer, Berlin Heidelberg New York

Wilmanns W (1987) Dem Patienten niemals die Hoffnung nehmen! Internistische Behandlung maligner Tumoren unter Berücksichtigung der Lebensqualität. Dtsch Arztbl 84:2261–2263

Wilmanns W (1989) Adjuvante Therapie beim Mammakarzinom. Aktueller Stand der adjuvanten Chemotherapie. In: Bohmert H (ed) Brustkrebs. Organerhaltung und Rekonstruktion. Thieme, Stuttgart, pp 496–502

New Antineoplastic Agents*

D. Schmähl, M. R. Berger, B. K. Keppler, and T. Klenner

Introduction

New antineoplastic agents are being developed predominantly in industrial laboratories and only to a limited extent in university and other research institutes. The results of so-called screening assays, as conducted especially by the National Cancer Institute, have been disappointing in particular since the testing of many hundreds or thousands of substances did not yield any appreciable result. It therefore seems to be important to find a rational basis for research and not to use a shotgun method to detect new antineoplastic agents.

Due to the restricted space, not all approaches can be discussed here. Thus the activities carried out in this field at our institute are presented as representative of similar research projects pursued in other laboratories.

Titanium and Ruthenium Complexes

In cancer therapy, one of the milestones of the past few years has been the development of the metal complex cisplatin. This drug turned testicular cancer, which until then had almost always been fatal in spite of all therapeutic efforts, into a disease that can be cured in most cases. Cisplatin is also active against tumors of the head and neck, bladder tumors, and ovarian tumors. It exhibits only minor activity in a few other tumors such as the small-cell lung carcinoma and is not at all or only insufficiently active in adenoid tumors such as adenocarcinomas of the lung and colon and rectum.

In order to expand the rather narrow spectrum of indication of cisplatin, a large number of direct derivatives have meanwhile been synthesized, but none has shown any major advantages over cisplatin except that they have less severe side effects. The spectrum of curable tumors could not be expanded substantially. Our research has therefore been directed to tumor-inhibiting metal complexes which do not contain platinum as a central metal. In the course of synthesizing and investigating a series of metal complexes we achieved the most significant success with budotitane and two ruthenium compounds (Fig. 1).

Titanium Compounds. Budotitane, diethoxybis(1-phenylbutane-1,3-dionato)titanium(IV), belongs to the class of bis-β-diketonato metal complexes. The antitumor activity of a number of representatives of this class was first described in 1982 (Keller

* This study was financed in part by the Deutsche Krebshilfe

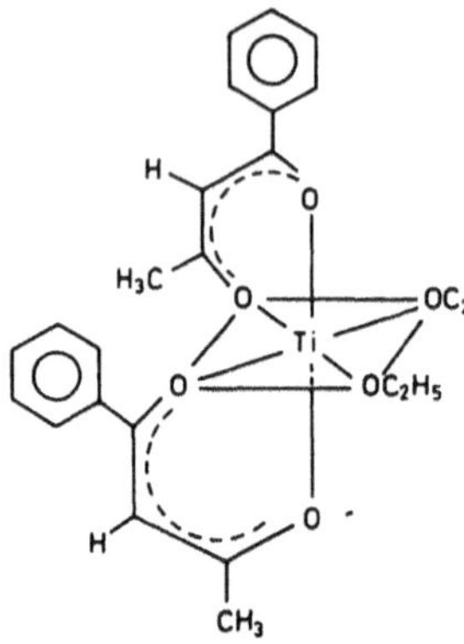

Budotitane (INN),
Diethoxybis (1 - phenylbutane - 1,-
3 - dionato) titanium (IV),
Ti $(bzac)_2(OEt)_2$,
KP 102

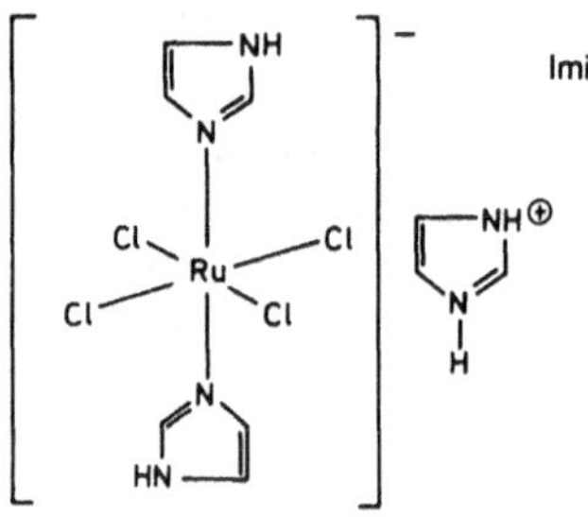

Imidazolium - trans - bisimidazole -
tetrachlororuthenate (III),
ImH $(RuIm_2Cl_4)$, ICR,
KP 418

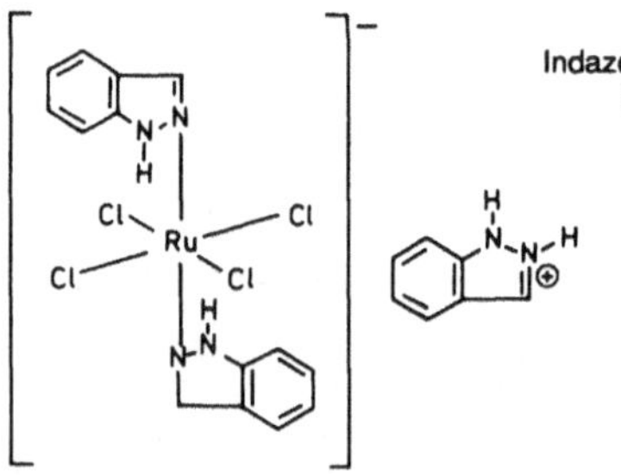

Indazolium - trans - tetrachloro -
bisindazoleruthenate (III),
IndH $(RuInd_2Cl_4)$,
Kp 692

Fig. 1. Chemical structures of budotitane and $ImH(RuIm_2Cl_4)$ and $IndH(RuInd_2Cl_4)$

et al. 1982). They can be synthesized from the corresponding metal tetrahalogenides or alkoxides and the diketonates in an anhydrous organic solvent. The complexes thus obtained are characterized by an octahedral coordinated configuration. Budotitane, the complex with benzoylacetone as a ligand, has by far the best activity (Fig. 1). The antitumor activity of budotitane and its homologs was examined in numerous tumor systems (Table 1) such as the sarcoma 180 tumor model in the ascitic as well as the subcutaneously and intramuscularly transplanted form, the Walker 256 carcinosarcoma, the P388 and L1210 leukemias, the transplantable MAC 15A colon tumor, and the autochthonous acetoxymethylmethylnitrosamine(AMMN)-induced colon tumor (Keppler and Schmähl 1986; Keppler et al. 1988a, b; Bischoff et al. 1987). Budotitane increased the survival times of sarcoma 180 ascitic tumor-bearing mice up to T/C values of 300% after single intraperitoneal administration of about

Table 1. Survey of the results of antitumor activity, which has been obtained with budotitane

Tumor model	Evaluation parameter[a]	Optimum T/C value[b] (%)
Sarcoma 180 ascitic tumor	ST	300[d]
Sarcoma 180 tumor, subcutaneously growing	TW	0[d]
Sarcoma 180 tumor, intramuscularly growing	TW	30
Walker 256 carcinosarcoma	ST	200
L1210 leukemia	ST	130
P388 leukemia	ST	130
Colon ascitic adenocarcinoma MAC 15A	ST	200[d]
Autochthonous AMMN[c]-induced colorectal tumors	ST TW	146 20

[a] ST, survival time; TW, tumor weight
[b] T/C (%), median tumor weight or survival time of treated animals versus control animals × 100
[c] AMMN, acetoxymethylmethylnitrosamine
[d] Fifty percent or more cured

180 mg/kg. The subcutaneously transplanted sarcoma 180 was cured with budotitane by administration of 10 mg/kg twice a week over 4 weeks. The intramuscularly transplanted sarcoma 180 was reduced to 30% when treatment was carried out on days 6, 8, and 10 after tumor transplantation with a dose of 50 mg/kg. Survival time of rats bearing Walker 256 carcinosarcoma was doubled by budotitane therapy. Budotitane was only marginally active in P388 and L1210 leukemias but exhibited excellent activity against MAC 15A colon adenocarcinoma. Here, survival times of about 3 months were achieved, while all the control animals died after 21 days.

Colorectal tumors of the rat induced by AMMN are very similar to those occurring in humans and reflect the activity of clinically established drugs quite well. Cisplatin and other antitumor agents which do not have any effect on these tumors in the clinic also fail in this tumor model. The only compounds to have an effect on colorectal tumors in the clinic are 5-fluorouracil and its derivatives. Comparison of the activities of 5-fluorouracil, cisplatin, and budotitane in the autochthonous colorectal tumors proved budotitane to be significantly more active than 5-fluorouracil, while cisplatin even stimulated the tumor growth (Fig. 2).

The LD_{50} of budotitane in female SD rats is 70–80 mg/kg, administered intravenously as a single dose. The LD_{50} in mice is about twice as high. The main side effect of budotitane is hepatotoxicity. Multiple focal necroses of the liver developed in the range of the LD_{50}. In addition, hyaline thrombi in the kidney glomeruli were found and there was also an increase in the enzymes glutamic oxaloacetic transaminase (GOT), glutamic pyruvic transaminase (GPT), and lactate dehydrogenase (LDH) but no signs of myelosuppression in the peripheral blood.

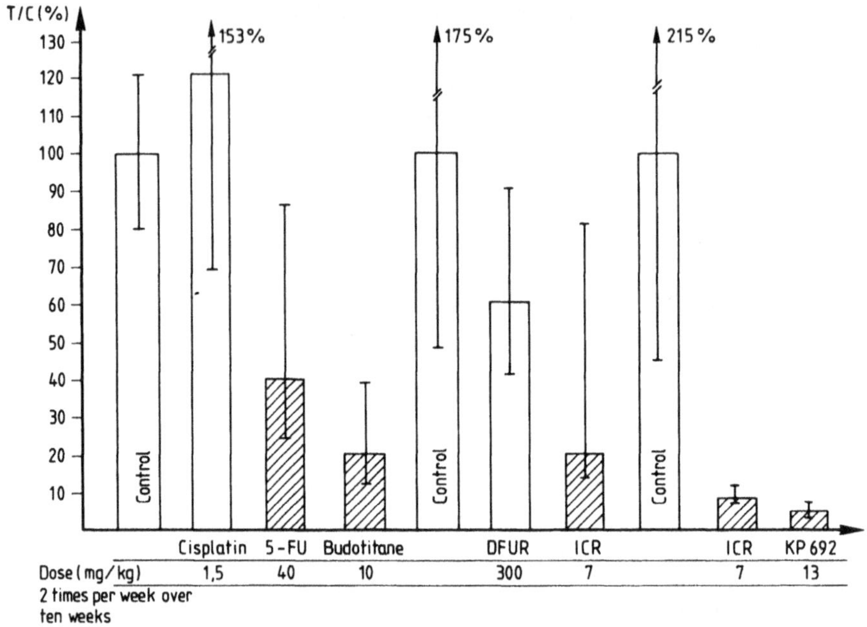

5-FU = 5-Fluorouracil; Budotitane = Diethoxybis (1-phenylbutane-1,3-dionato) titanium (IV), Ti $(bzac)_2(OEt)_2$, DFUR = 5′-Deoxy-5-fluorouridine; ICR = Imidazolium-trans-bisimidazoletetrachlororuthenate (III), ImH$(RuIm_2Cl_4)$; KP692 = Indazolium-trans-tetrachlorobisindazoleruthenate (III), IndH$(RuInd_2Cl_4)$.

Fig. 2. Survey of the test results with budotitane and two ruthenium compounds against autochthonous colorectal tumors compared with cisplatin, 5-fluoro-5′-desoxyuridike (DFUR), and 5-fluorouracil

Chronic administration of budotitane at up to 18 mg/kg twice a week over 12 weeks was tolerated without mortality. This corresponds to a total dose of 432 mg/kg. Here, a significant increase in creatinine and urea was observed.

In a clinical phase I trial started with budotitane in 1986, the first drug-related symptoms of toxicity were observed at a dose of 9 mg/kg, when patients complained about reversible impairment of the sense of taste shortly after budotitane infusion. A moderate increase in liver enzymes and LDH was observed at 14 mg/kg. Two of three patients receiving 21 mg/kg showed increased urea and creatinine and reduced creatinine clearance. This was accompanied by nausea, weakness, and malaise. After 4 weeks, the laboratory parameters of urea, creatinine, and creatinine clearance were almost normal again. There was no local toxicity in contrast to preclinical experience. Myelosuppression did not occur at any dose level tested. Hence, the maximum tolerated dose of budotitane is below 21 mg/kg (800 mg/m^2). The repeated administration scheme (twice a week over 4 weeks) included three different dose levels (100, 120, and 150 mg/m^2). The only toxicity observed was a reversible loss of the sense of taste shortly after budotitane infusion (Keppler et al. 1988a, b).

Ruthenium Complexes. After synthesis of a number of heterocycle coordinated ruthenium complexes, it turned out that anionic complexes characterized by *trans*-standing heterocycles exhibited the best activity against various tumor models. Im-

Table 2. Survey of the test results of ICR in experimental tumor models

Tumor model	Evaluation parameter[a]	Optimum T/C value[b] (%)
P388 leukemia	ST	190
Walker 256 carcinosarcoma	ST	250
B 16 melanoma, s.c. growing	TW	30
Sarcoma 180, i.m. growing	TW	45
AMMN[c]-induced colorectal tumors of the rat	TW	10

[a] ST, survival time; TW, tumor weight
[b] T/C (%), median tumor weight or survival time of treated animals versus control animals × 100
[c] AMMN, acetoxymethylmethylnitrosamine

idazolium-*trans*-bisimidazoletetrachlororuthenate(III) (ICR) and indazolium-*trans*-tetrachlorobisindazoleruthenate(III) ($IndH(RuInd_2Cl_4)$) proved to be most active (Fig. 1). The complexes can be synthesized by reaction of $RuCl_3$ with the organic ligand in a hydrochloric acid solution.

Table 2 summarizes some results obtained with ICR in experimental tumor models. T/C values of about 190% were obtained in P388 leukemia when 70 mg/kg was administered on days 1, 5, and 9 after tumor transplantation. T/C values of 250% were reached in treating the Walker 256 carcinosarcoma on days 1, 2, and 3 at 50 mg/kg. In addition, the intramuscularly transplanted sarcoma 180 was reduced to 45% by administering 80 mg/kg ICR on days 6, 8, and 10 after tumor transplantation (Keppler and Rupp 1986). The subcutaneously growing B 16 melanoma was reduced by up to 30% when 8 mg/kg ICR was administered daily for 12 days (Keppler and Rupp 1986). All solid tumors were treated intravenously.

As previously described, T/C values of 10% were reached with ICR and of 5% with $Ind(RuInd_2Cl_4)$ in AMMN-induced colorectal tumors of the rat, i.e., a tumor growth inhibition of 90% and 95%.

In a single-dose mortality study, the LD_{50} of ICR was determined at about 125 mg/kg. Major histologic findings included tubular necroses in the kidneys and single-cell necroses in the liver. Hematologic findings were erythropenia and increased creatinine and liver enzymes.

In summary, the new titanium and ruthenium complexes exhibited significant antineoplastic activity against a colon tumor model that does not at all respond to cisplatin and has a high predictivity for the clinical situation. Budotitane has been introduced to clinical studies while the two ruthenium compounds presented here have been selected as candidates for clinical trials.

Alkylphosphocholines

Synthetic ether lipids and related substances, originally conceived as analogs of natural lysolecithin, have been characterized as an effective class of antineoplastic

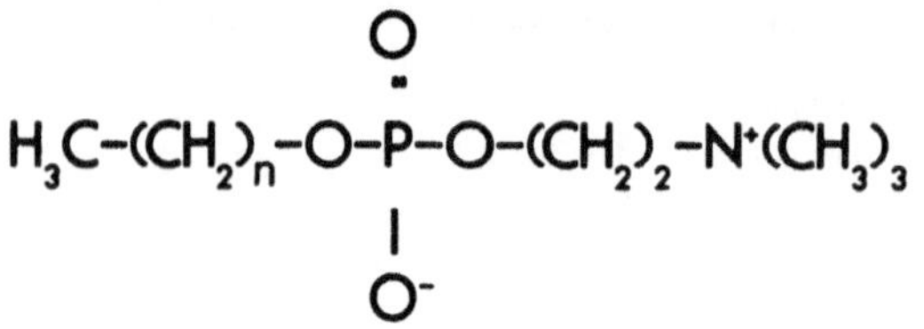

n=13 Tetradecylphosphocholine
n=15 Hexadecylphosphocholine
n=17 Octadecylphosphocholine

Fig. 3. Chemical structures of the alkylphosphocholines

Table 3. Antineoplastic efficacy of tetradecylphosphocholine (TPC), hexadecylphosphocholine (HPC), and octadecylphosphocholine (OPC) in methylnitrosourea-induced mammary carcinomas of SD rats

Group no.	Compound	Dose (μmol/kg)	No. of animals	T/C% [a]	No. of tumors CR [b]	No. of tumors ND [c]	ILS% [d]	% Body weight difference [e]	Mortality [f] N (%)
Ia [g]	Control	–	20	100	0.45	6.21	–	+ 11.8	1 (5)
b [h]	Control	–	20	100	0.06	6.06	–	+ 6.4	5 (25)
IIa [h]	TPC	172	15	42	0.33	4.46	+ 51	± 0	2 (13)
b [g]	TPC	115	15	72	0.33	3.65	+ 5	+ 8.7	2 (13)
c [g]	TPC	77	15	74	0.8	6.16	+ 12	+ 6.5	2 (13)
d [g]	TPC	51	15	92	0.34	5.58	− 5	− 5.4	2 (13)
									3 (20)
IIIa [g]	HPC	115	15	Toxic	2.5	0.14	− 69	Toxic	14 (93)
b [g]	HPC	77	15	2.3	1.99	0.37	+ 26	− 4.4	6 (40)
c [g]	HPC	51	15	13.2	1.62	1.13	+ 23	+ 2.1	0 (0)
d [h]	HPC	34	15	38.6	0.60	2.87	+ 38	+ 7.8	1 (7)
e [h]	HPC	15	10	27.7	0.10	4.37	+ 24	+ 7.5	1 (10)
f [h]	HPC	7	10	74	0.11	5.71	+ 16	+ 2.1	1 (10)
IVa [g]	OPC	115	15	Toxic	Toxic	Toxic	− 76	Toxic	15 (100)
b [g]	OPC	77	15	0.6	4.24	0.1	− 72	− 13.3	12 (80)
c [g]	OPC	51	15	1.8	2.16	0.55	+ 26	− 6.7	5 (33)
d [h]	OPC	34	15	6.0	1.47	1.0	+ 53	± 0	0 (0)
e [h]	OPC	15	15	22.7	0.27	3.47	+ 53	+ 4.3	0 (0)
f [h]	OPC	7	10	74.3	0.40	3.47	+ 2	+ 2.2	2 (20)

[a] Quotient of median tumor volumes of treated and control groups × 100, evaluation at week 6
[b] Mean number of tumors per rat showing complete remission under therapy (weeks 1–6)
[c] Mean number of tumors per rat developing newly under therapy (weeks 1–6)
[d] Percentage increase in life span over untreated controls
[e] Weight difference at the end of treatment in percentage of initial weight
[f] Evaluation at the end of therapy (week 6)
[g] Experiment A
[h] Experiment B

agents (Berdel et al. 1985; Berger et al. 1984; Munder et al. 1981). Several mechanisms of action are being discussed (Berdel et al. 1985) but the smallest common denominator can be presumed in membrane-associated changes in target cells. This type of activity includes changes in membrane properties with regard to uptake and/or release of biologically active materials such as hormones, changes in membrane-bound enzyme reactions, or membrane changes leading to reduced metastasizing capacity of tumor cells or immune system activation. Recently, a subgroup has emerged from this class of agents, the alkylphosphocholines (ALPs), which have a simpler chemical structure to their parent compounds (Fig. 3). These agents were highly active in chemically induced autochthonous mammary carcinoma of the rat (Table 3) (Hilgard et al. 1988; Muschiol et al. 1987) but displayed only marginal antineoplastic efficacy in two transplanted mammary carcinomas of the rat (Scherf et al. 1987) and were inactive in estrogen receptor negative well differentiated ductal (MXT) mammary carcinoma of the mouse (Muschiol et al. 1987).

One agent of this group, hexadecylphosphocholine (HPC), was selected for more intensive preclinical investigation, to be processed to clinical studies. HPC showed borderline activity against benzo(a)pyrene-induced fibrosarcomas of the rat, but no activity in AMMN-induced colorectal cancer of the rat (Berger et al. 1987; Muschiol et al. 1987) and in L5222 leukemia of the rat (unpublished).

Toxicologic examinations revealed the liver and gastrointestinal tract as target organs of HPC-derived toxicity whereas no adverse effects were found in the hematopoietic system (Berger et al. 1987).

First clinical trials (Unger et al. 1988) have demonstrated the anticancer efficacy of topical HPC administration against skin metastases of recurrent breast cancer. The response rate of 25% observed in heavily pretreated patients is encouraging for the ongoing phase I studies with systemic administration (Unger et al. 1988).

In summary, ALPs are a new group of anticancer agents with an unusual spectrum of activity in preclinical tumor models. The toxicity of HPC is obviously different from that of "typical" antineoplastic agents; the low bone marrow toxicity permits its being used in combination chemotherapy. The activity of HPC observed in the clinical phase I study further supports the impression of a highly promising development in anticancer chemotherapy.

Bisphosphonates

Bisphosphonates, especially those which have a P-C-P bond (geminal bisphosphonates), are powerful inhibitors of bone resorption. This was demonstrated in organ culture (Boonekamp et al. 1986) as well as in animals (Reitsma et al. 1983; Marie et al. 1985; Schenk et al. 1986). However, the mechanism of action is still unclear. At present, bisphosphonates have considerable value in the treatment of diseases characterized by abnormal bone destruction, e.g., Paget's disease (Adami et al. 1986; Harinck et al. 1987; Meunier et al. 1987), tumor-induced hypercalcemia (Canfield 1987; Coleman and Rubens 1987), and bone metastasis (Attardo-Parrinello et al. 1987; Scher and Yagoda 1987; van Holten-Verzantvoort et al. 1987). This class of compounds has the ability to adsorb to the bone matrix (Shinoda et al. 1983). For disodium-3-amino-1-hydroxypropylidene-1,1-diphosphonate (APD), a half-time was

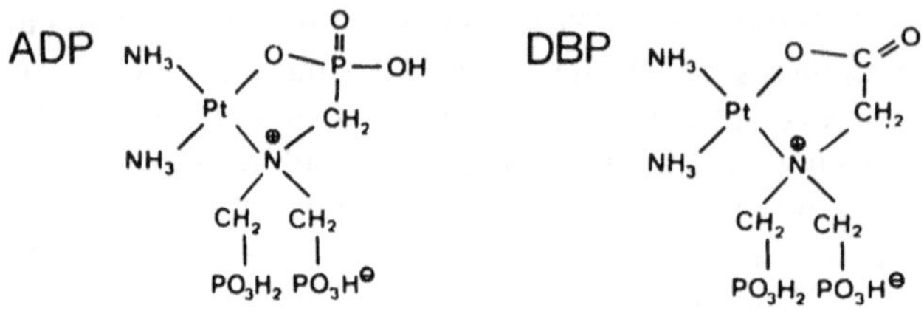

ADP = Aminotris(methylenephosphonato)diamminoplatinum(II)
DBP = Diammino(bis(methylenephosphonato)aminoacetato)platinum(II)

Fig. 4. Chemical structures of cisplatin-linked phosphonates

300 days in an experimental setup with rats (Wingen and Schmähl 1987). This led to the suggestion of using the bisphosphonates in prophylactic treatment to prevent bone metastasis (Wingen et al. 1986a), which was achieved for a period of 8 weeks when using APD (Krempien et al. 1988). Recently, the effect was found to be enhanced when using the dimethyl derivative of APD in the same model. Methyl derivatives of APD were even more effective than APD in vitro (Löwik et al. 1987) and in vivo (Papapoulos et al. 1987).

A new approach in using bisphosphonates has been the introduction of compounds composed of a cytostatic moiety such as melphalan or cisplatin and of a bisphosphonic acid of varying structure. The first compound to be investigated was 4-[4-[bis(2-chloroethyl)amino]phenyl]-1-hydroxybutane-1,1-bisphosphonate (BAD), which is composed of APD and melphalan. The compound proved to maintain the cytotoxic properties of melphalan and at the same time the osteotropic properties of

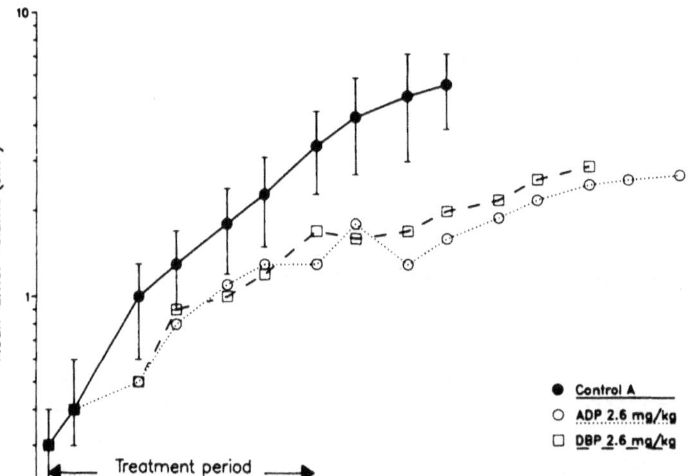

a

Fig. 5a–c. Mean tumor volumes after therapy with ADP and/or DBP. **a** Low-dose ADP and DBP; **b** medium and highest-dose ADP; **c** medium and highest-dose DBP

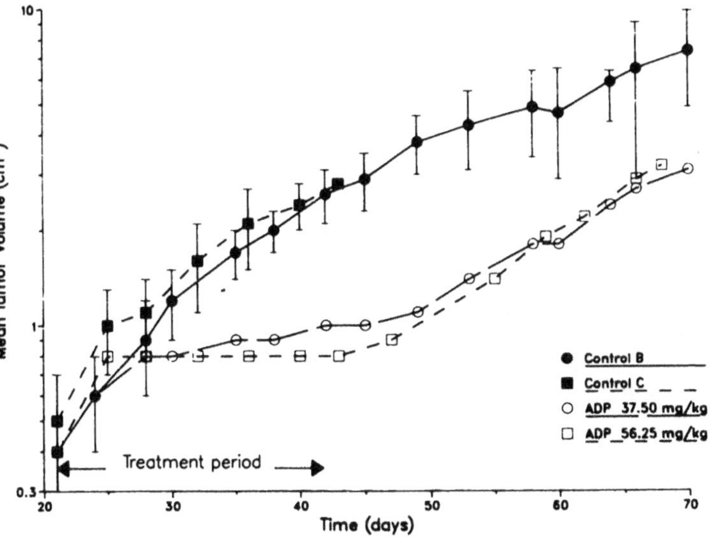

Fig. 5b

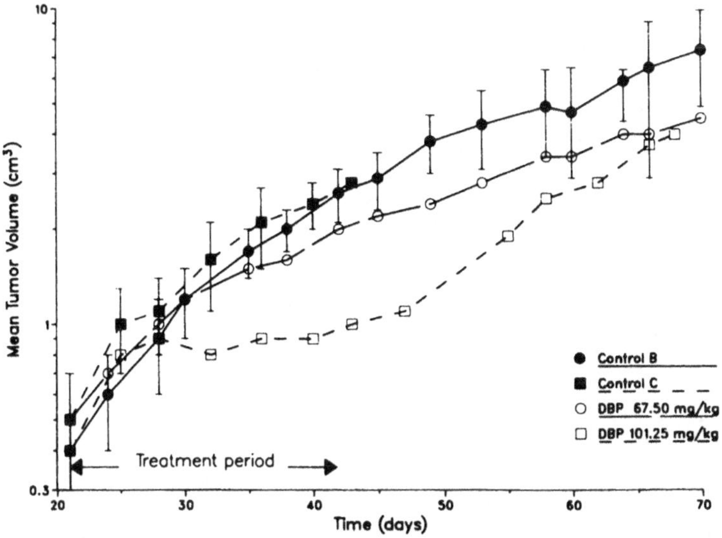

Fig. 5c

the bisphosphonate (Wingen et al. 1986b). In recent studies on other compounds using cisplatin as a cytotoxic moiety and different phosphonates, the antitumor potential of two representatives of this class was investigated in the transplantable osteosarcoma of the rat. This tumor model is characterized by osteoid formation, spontaneous metastatic spread to lungs, kidneys, and lymph nodes, and sensitivity to various cytostatics.

The following compounds were investigated: aminotris(methylenephosphonato)-diamminoplatinum(II) (ADP) and diammino-(bis(methylenephosphonato)amino-

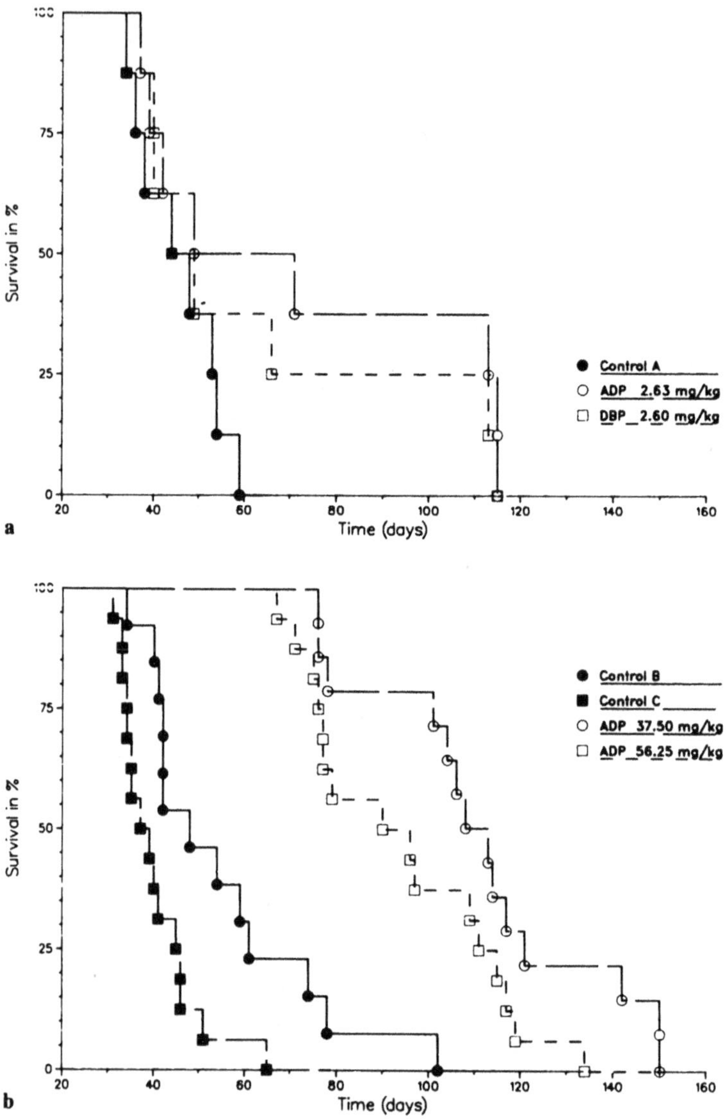

Fig. 6a–c. Survival plot after therapy with ADP and/or DBP. **a** Low-dose ADP and DBP; **b** medium and highest-dose ADP; **c** medium and highest-dose DBP

acetato)platinum(II) (DBP) (Fig. 4). They were synthesized by reaction of amino-tris(methylenephosphonic) acid or bis(methylenephosphonato)amino-acetic acid with $Pt(NH_3)_2(OH)_2$ in H_2O. All compounds were characterized by elemental analysis, IR, ^{3}H-NMR, and ^{31}P-nuclear magnetic resonance (NMR) spectra.

Animals and Tumor Transplantation. Osteosarcoma fragments of approximately 10 mg were transplanted into the tibial bone cavity of 15-day-old SD rats. Therapy of tumor-bearing animals was started from day 21 after transplantation. The com-

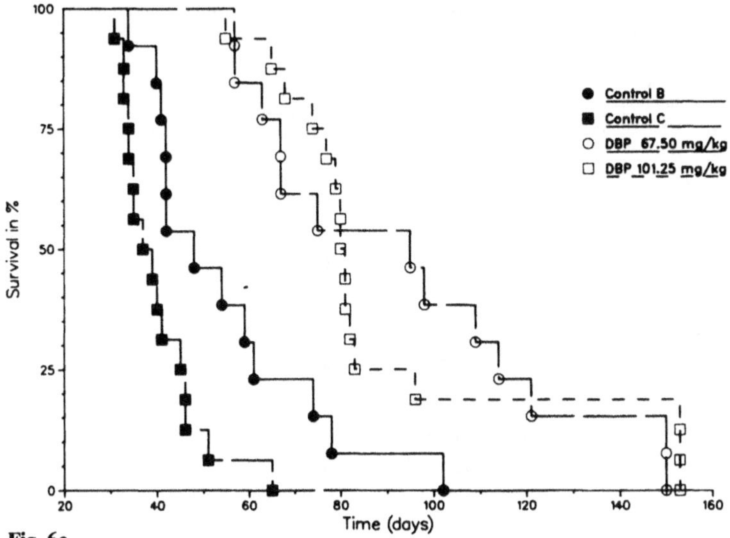

Fig. 6c

pounds were dissolved in 0.9% saline and injected intravenously twice a week over 3 weeks. Tumor volume, body weight, and survival time were recorded. Therapeutic efficacy was evaluated in terms of tumor inhibition in comparison to controls (T/C%).

Treatment with the two compounds resulted in both a significant reduction of tumor volume and an increase in survival time. Comparison of the efficacy of the two cisplatin-linked phosphonates showed a superiority of ADP with respect to tumor inhibition and increase in survival time (Figs. 5, 6). The inhibition of tumor growth by ADP was not enhanced by a dose exceeding 37.5 mg/kg (single dose). Only when looking at T/C% values was a slight increase in antitumor activity seen, since the highest dose effected T/C values below 30% (Table 4). Good antitumor activity was already found at low dose levels, which indicates a broad therapeutic range (Fig. 5). DBP inhibited tumor volume growth only at the highest dosage (Table 3) to an extent comparable to that of ADP at the highest dosage (Fig. 5).

The survival time was significantly increased in comparison to the respective control at a medium dose of ADP and the highest dose of ADP and DBP (Table 4). The main cause of death was multiple lung metastases – as seen at dissection in all control animals. They were also observed in all other animals after prolonged life periods. Whether the increase in survival time is due to an antimetastatic potential of the compounds – as seems possible – has to be verified in further investigations.

The investigated compounds represent a new class of substances which do not have a geminal bisphosphonate moiety (P-C-P bond) but two or three phosphonic acid groups which are linked to nitrogen via a methylen group (P-N-C-N-P bond) and a cisplatin moiety as the cytotoxic property of the molecule. The molar concentration of both compounds used to achieve the same static tumor inhibition was 0.6 mmol/kg ADP and 0.9 mmol/kg DBP (Tables 4, 5). The compounds differ in respect of the number of phosphate groups, ADP having three and DBP having two. We therefore conclude that the amount of phosphate groups which can bind to the bone matrix is at least in part responsible for the activity of the compounds. This must also

Table 4. Design of experiment on new cisplatin-linked bisphosphonates in transplantable osteosarcoma of the rat

Group	Single dose		Total dose (mg/kg)	Number of animals	
	(mmol/kg)	(mg/kg)		Male	Female
Control A	–	–	–	5	3
Control B	–	–	–	7	6
Control C	–	–	–	8	8
ADP a	0.028	2.6	15.6	4	4
b	0.400	37.5	225.0	7	7
c	0.600	56.25	337.5	8	8
DBP a	0.023	2.6	15.6	4	4
b	0.600	67.5	405.0	7	7
c	0.900	101.25	607.5	8	8

Table 5. Results of new cisplatin-linked bisphosphonates in transplantable osteosarcoma of the rat

Group	T/C%		Survival (days) (median + 95%)	P $\alpha = 0.05$
	42nd day PTR	52nd day PTR		
Control A	–	–	46 (34– 59)	
Control B	–	–	48 (41– 74)	
Control C	–	–	38 (34– 46)	
ADP a	38	30	60 (37–115)	NS[a]
b	38	33	111 (78–142)	0.0000
c	29	26	93 (76–104)	0.0000
DBP a	50	36	47 (34–115)	NS[a]
b	77	65	95 (63–121)	0.0009
c	36	36	81 (74– 96)	0.0000

PTR, post-transplant

[a] NS, not significant according to Kaplan-Meier estimates

be verified in further investigations. To sum up, this new class of compounds gives the chance to combine cytostatic and osteotropic agents without loosing the abilities of the unlinked components.

4-Amino-*N*-(2′-aminophenyl)benzamide

4-Amino-*N*-(2′-aminophenyl)benzamide (Dinaline, Fig. 7) was characterized originally as a potentially anticonvulsive agent. In toxicologic investigations, marked inhibition of peripheral blood cells and of spermatogenesis was observed in rats following continuous administration.

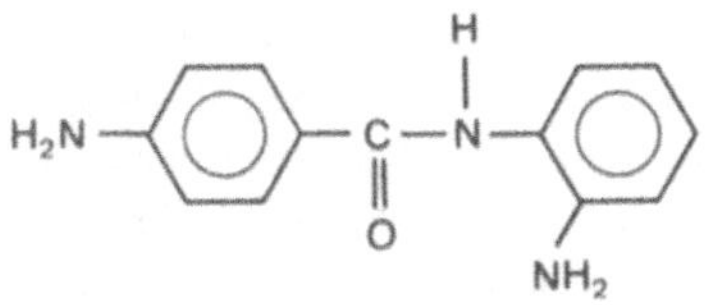

Fig. 7. Chemical structure of 4-amino-*N*-(2′-amino-phenyl)benzamide (GOE 1734)

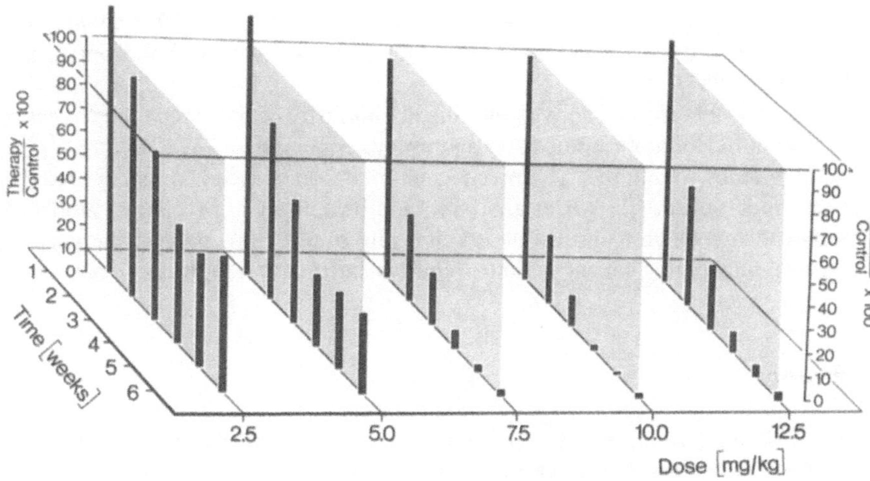

Fig. 8. Dose-response and -time relationship following treatment of methylnitrosourea-induced rat mammary carcinoma with 4-amino-*N*-(2′aminophenyl)benzamide

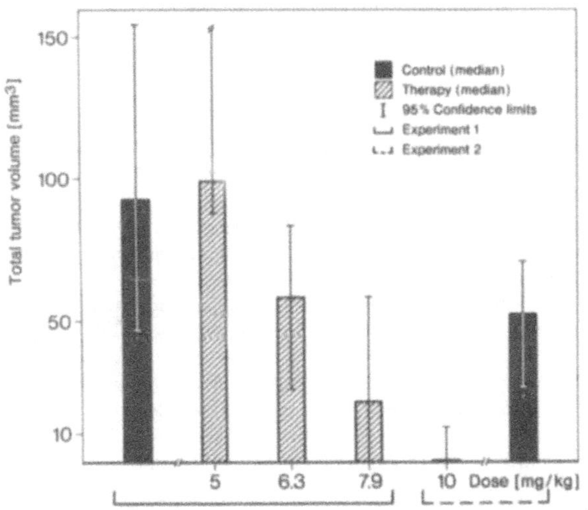

Fig. 9. Antineoplastic efficacy of 4-amino-*N*-(2′-aminophenyl)benzamide against acetoxymethyl-methylnitrosamine-induced colorectal cancer in SD rats

Accordingly, the hematopoietic/lymphatic system, the gonads and, additionally, the gastrointestinal tract and the lung were considered as target organs of toxicity. Investigations on anticancer activity, which had been prompted by these results, showed efficacy against a select but unusual spectrum of rodent tumor models. Although without activity against typical sensitive tumors such as leukemia L5222, Yoshida sarcoma, and Walker 256 carcinosarcoma in rats (Berger et al. 1985) as well as leukemias L1210 and P388 in mice (Leopold et al. 1987), the compound displayed significant activity against chemically induced autochthonous carcinomas of the mammary gland (Fig. 8) and the distal colorectum in rats (Fig. 9) (Berger et al. 1985) as well as in a variety of transplanted, generally less sensitive, solid tumors in mice (Leopold et al. 1987).

This unusual spectrum of activity and the dissimilarity of the mechanism of action to that of all hitherto known anticancer agents make Dinaline a key structure for further systematic investigations. The mechanism of action, which is possibly linked to cell energy metabolism (Berger et al. 1988), and its activity in preclinical models of colorectal cancer, which is insensitive to clinically used drugs, suggest the value of this new drug in treating cancer patients requires clarification in the near future.

Conclusions

Due to the limited space, the present paper does not include all our activities in the development of antineoplastic agents. Further research has been directed, for instance, to linking cytostatic nitrosourea groups with carrier molecules from the class of sex hormones and adrenocortical hormones (Eisenbrand et al. 1988). These investigations aim at finding organotropic antineoplastic agents. Of particular importance in these investigations are the pharmacokinetics (Betsch 1988). Initial preclinical tests have yielded promising results.

References

Adami S, Salvagno G, Guarrera G, Montesanti F, Garavelli S, Rosini S, LoCascio V (1986) Treatment of Paget's disease of bone with intravenous 4-amino-1-hydroxybutylidene-1,1-bisphosphonate. Calcif Tissue Int 39:226–229

Attardo-Parrinello G, Merlini G, Pavesi F, Crema F, Fiorentini ML, Ascari E (1987) Effects of a new aminodiphosphonate (aminohydroxybutylidene diphosphonate) in patients with osteolytic lesions from metastases and myelomatosis. Arch Intern Med 147:1629–1633

Berdel WE, Andreesen R, Munder PG (1985) Synthetic alkylphospholipid analogs: a new class of anticancer agents. In: Kuo JF (ed) Phospholipids and cellular regulation, vol 2. CRC, Boca Raton, pp 41–73

Berger MR, Munder PG, Schmähl D, Westphal O (1984) Influence of the alkyllysophospholipid ET-18-OCH_3 on methylnitrosourea-induced rat mammary carcinomas. Oncology 41:109–113

Berger MR, Bischoff H, Fritschi E, Henne T, Herrmann M, Pool BL, Satzinger G, Schmähl D, Weiershausen U (1985) Synthesis, toxicity, and therapeutic efficacy of 4-amino-*N*-(2′-aminophenyl)benzamide: a new compound preferentially active in slowly growing tumors. Cancer Treat Rep 69:1415–1424

Berger MR, Muschiol C, Schmähl D, Eibl HJ (1987) New cytostatics with experimentally different toxic profiles. Cancer Treat Rev 14:307–317

Betsch B (1988) Pharmakokinetische Studien mit östradiolgekoppelten Nitrosoharnstoffderivaten an Ratten mit chemisch induziertem Mammakarzinom. Dissertation, Heidelberg University

Bischoff H, Berger MR, Keppler BK, Schmähl D (1987) Efficacy of β-diketonato complexes of titanium, zirconium, and hafnium against chemically induced autochthonous colonic tumors in rats. J Cancer Res Clin Oncol 113:446–450

Boonekamp P, van der Wee-Pals LJA, van Wijk-van Lennep MML, Wil Thesing C, Bijvoet OLM (1986) Two modes of action of bisphosphonates on osteoclastic resorption of mineralized matrix. Bone Mineral 1:27–39

Canfield RE (1987) Rationale for diphosphonate therapy in hypercalcemia of malignancy. Am J Med 82(2A):1–5

Coleman RE, Rubens RD (1987) 3(Amino-1,1-hydroxypropylidene)bisphosphonate (APD) for hypercalcemia of breast cancer. Br J Cancer 56:465–469

Eisenbrand G, Berger MR, Fischer J, Schneider MR, Tang W, Zeller WJ (1988) Development of more selective anticancer *N*-nitrosoureas. Anticancer Drug Design 2:351–359

Harinck HIJ, Papapoulos SE, Blanksma HJ, Moolenaar AJ, Vermeij P, Bijvoet OLM (1987) Paget's disease of bone: early and late responses to three different modes of treatment with aminohydroxypropylidene bisphosphonate (APD). Br Med J 295:1301–1305

Hilgard P, Stekar J, Engel J, Schumacher W, Eibl H, Unger C, Berger MR (1988) The antitumor activity of hexadecylphosphocholine (D18506) in DMBA-induced rat mammary carcinomas. Proc Am Assoc Cancer Res 29:362

Keller HJ, Keppler BK, Schmähl D (1982) Antitumor activity of *cis*-dihalogenobis(1-phenyl-1,3-butanedionato)titanium(IV) compounds against Walker 256 carcinosarcoma. Arzneimittelforschung 32:806–807

Keppler BK, Rupp W (1986) Antitumor activity of imidazolium-bisimidazole-tetrachlororuthenate (III). A representative of a new class of inorganic antitumor agents. J Cancer Res Clin Oncol 111:166–168

Keppler BK, Schmähl D (1986) Preclinical evaluation of dichlorobis(1-phenylbutane-1,3-dionato)-titanium(IV) and budotitane. Arzneimittelforschung 36:1822–1828

Keppler BK, Bischoff H, Berger MR, Heim ME, Reznik G, Schmähl D (1988a) Preclinical development and first clinical studies of budotitane. In: Nicolini M (ed) Platinum and other metal coordination compounds in cancer chemotherapy. Martinus Nijhoff Publ, Boston

Keppler BK, Heim ME, Flechtner H, Wingen F, Pool BL (1988b) Assessment of the preclinical activity of budotitane in three different transplantable tumor systems, its lack of mutagenicity, and first results of clinical phase I studies. Arzneimittelforschung (in press)

Krempien B, Wingen F, Eichmann T, Müller M, Schmähl D (1988) Protective effects of a prophylactic treatment with the bisphosphonate 3-amino-1-hydroxypropane-1,1-bisphosphonic acid on the development of tumor osteopathies in the rat: experimental studies with the Walker carcinosarcoma 256. Oncology 45:41–46

Leopold WR, Hook KE, Frey DW (1987) Activity and biochemical properties of GOE 1734 (PD104208), an anticancer agent with a novel mechanism of activity. Proc Am Assoc Cancer Res 28:302

Löwik CWGM, van der Pluijm G, Bijvoet OLM (1987) Migration and phenotypic transformation of osteoclast precursors into mature osteoclasts: the effect of dimethyl-APD (Me_2APD). Calcif Tissue Int [Suppl 2] 41:49

Marie PJ, Hott M, Garba M (1985) Inhibition by aminohydroxypropylidene bisphosphonate (AHPrBP) of 1,25$(OH)_2$ vitamin D_3-induced stimulated bone turnover in the mouse. Calcif Tissue Int 37:268–275

Meunier PJ, Chapuy M, Delmas P, Charhon S, Edouard C, Arlot M (1987) Intravenous disodium etidronate therapy in Paget's disease of bone and hypercalcemia of malignancy. Am J Med 82 (2A):71–78

Munder PG, Modolell M, Bausert W, Öttgen HF, Westphal O (1981) Alkyllysophospholipids in cancer therapy. In: Hersh, et al (eds) Augmenting agents in cancer therapy. Raven, New York, pp 441–458

Muschiol C, Berger MR, Schuler B, Scherf HR, Garzon FT, Zeller WJ, Unger C, Eibl HJ, Schmähl D (1987) Alkylphosphocholines: toxicity and anticancer properties. Lipids 22:930–934

Papapoulos SE, Aleman BMP, Hoekman K, Löwik CWGM, Bijvoet OLM (1987) In vitro assessment of the potency of bisphosphonates can be predictably confirmed in a patient-observer independent clinical model. Calcif Tissue Int [Suppl 2] 41:60

Reitsma HP, Bijvoet OLM, Potokar M, van der Wee-Pals LJA, van Wijk-van Lennep MML (1983) Apposition and resorption of bone during oral treatment with (3-amino-1-hydroxypropylidene)-1,1-bisphosphonate (APD). Calcif Tissue Int 35:357–361

Schenk R, Eggli P, Fleisch H, Rosini S (1986) Quantitative morphometric evaluation of the inhibitory activity of new aminobisphosphonates on bone resorption in the rat. Calcif Tissue Int 38:342–349

Scher HI, Yagoda A (1987) Bone metastasis: pathogenesis, treatment, and rationale for use of resorption inhibitors. Am J Med 82(2A):6–28

Scherf HR, Schuler B, Berger MR, Schmähl D (1987) Therapeutic activity of ET-18-OCH_3 and hexadecylphosphocholine against mammary tumors in BDVI rats. Lipids 22:927–929

Shinoda H, Adamek G, Felix R, Fleisch H, Schenk R, Hagan P (1983) Structure-activity relationship of various bisphosphonates. Calcif Tissue Int 35:87–99

Unger C, Eibl H, von Heyden HW, Nagel GA (1988) Etherlipids in the topical treatment of skin metastases. Proc Am Assoc Cancer Res 29:357

van Holten-Verzantvoort AT, Bijvoet OLM, Hermans J, Harinck HIJ, Elte JWF, Beex LVAM, Cleton FJ, Kroon HM, Vermey P, Neijt JP, Bijlham G (1987) Reduced morbidity from skeletal metastases in breast cancer patients during long-term bisphosphonate (APD) treatment. Lancet 10:983–985

Wingen F, Schmähl D (1987) Pharmacokinetics of the osteotropic diphosphonate 3-amino-1-hydroxypropane-1,1-diphosphonic acid in mammals. Arzneimittelforschung 37:1037–1042

Wingen F, Eichmann T, Manegold C, Krempien B (1986a) Effects of new bisphosphonic acids on tumor-induced bone destruction in the rat. J Cancer Res Clin Oncol 111:35–46

Wingen F, Sterz H, Blum H, Möller H, Pittermann W, Pool BL, Sinn HJ, Spring H, Schmähl D (1986b) Synthesis, antitumor activity, distribution and toxicity of 4-[4-[bis-(2-chloroethyl)amino]-phenyl]-1-hydroxybutane-1,1-bisphosphonate (BAD), a new lost derivative with increased accumulation in rat osteosarcoma. J Cancer Res Clin Oncol 111:209–219

Enzyme-Pattern-Targeted Chemotherapy*

G. Weber

The purpose of this paper is to outline the biochemical and enzymic basis of a novel chemotherapy for refractory acute myelocytic leukemia (AML). The biochemical and clinical rationale will be reported and the results obtained during the 1st year of the study will be discussed. Details of the biochemical and clinical studies will be given elsewhere (Tricot et al. 1989).

Experimental and Clinical Methodology

Biochemical Methods

The activities of inosine monophosphate dehydrogenase (IMP DH) and guanine phosphoribosyltransferase (GPRT), plasma levels of tiazofurin and hypoxanthine, and the concentration of guanosine triphosphate (GTP) were measured and blast cells prepared as previously described (Weber et al. 1988). Tiazofurin was obtained from the National Cancer Institute, Bethesda, MD, and was infused daily in a 1-h period by pump (Tricot et al. 1987). The patients were in end stage AML and the details of these cases have been provided elsewhere (Tricot et al. 1987; Weber et al. 1988), as have the criteria for eligibility of patients for this trial (Tricot et al. 1987). These clinical studies were approved by the Human Studies Committee of Indiana University School of Medicine.

Expression of Biochemical Results

Enzymic activities and concentrations of GTP before and after tiazofurin treatment were calculated in absolute values and were expressed also as percentages of the pretreatment values (Tricot et al. 1987; Weber et al. 1988).

Results and Discussion

Biochemical Imbalance in Purine Metabolism and Increased Capacity for GTP Production

Our earlier work discovered multiple enzymic alterations in purine metabolism in cancer cells which were characterized by an increased capacity for de novo biosyn-

* These studies were supported by Outstanding Investigator Grant CA-42510 awarded to the author

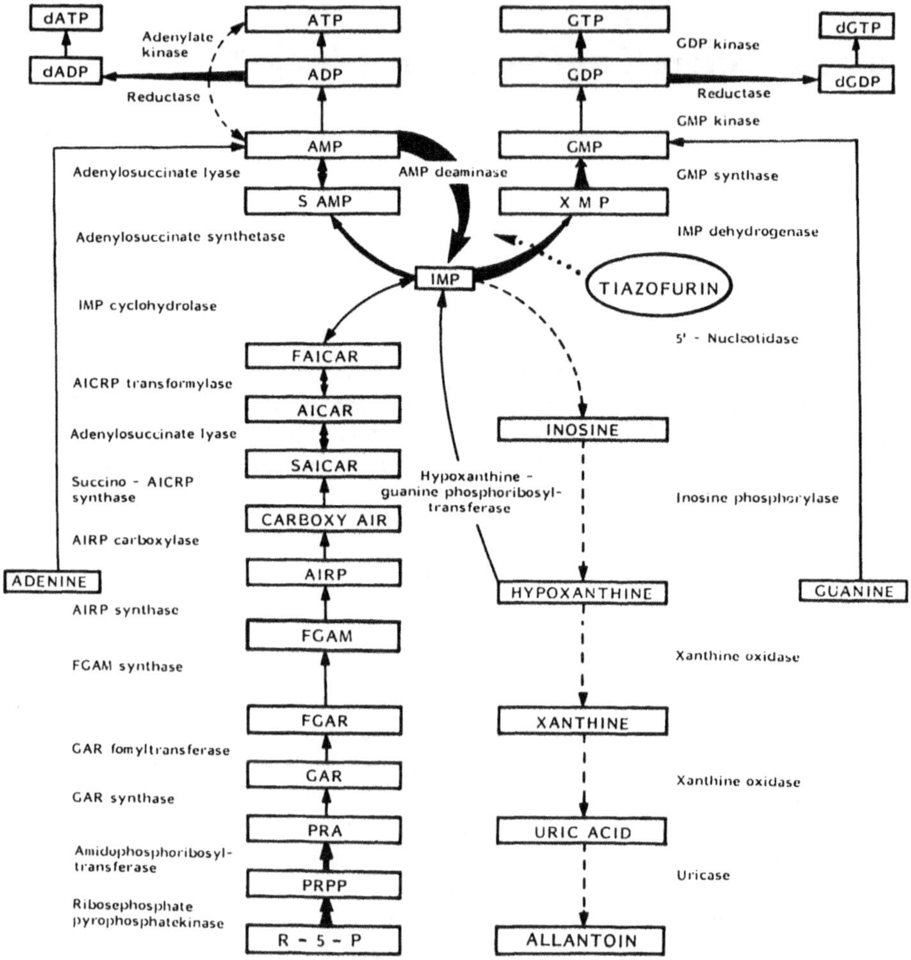

Fig. 1. Biochemical strategy of cancer cells as revealed in the integrated reprogramming of gene expression manifested in the imbalance of the activities of key enzymes of purine de novo and salvage biosynthesis and of the degradative pathway in purine metabolism. SAMP, adenylosuccinate; Ac., acid; FAICAR, formylaminoimidazolecarboximide ribonucleotide; AICRP, aminoimidazolecarboxamide ribose phosphate; AICAR, aminoimidazolecarboximide ribonucleotide; AIR, aminoimidazoleribonucleotide; AIRF, aminoimidazoleribonucleotide-phosphate; FGAM, formylglycinamidine ribonucleotide; FGAR, formylglycine amidoribonucleotide; GAR, glycine aminoribonucleotide; PRA, phosphoribosylamine; R-5-P, ribose 5-phosphate

thesis of purines and a decreased ability to degrade them (Weber 1977, 1983). We interpreted the main biochemical alterations as indicative of an increased capacity for de novo IMP and GTP biosynthesis. The enzymic results indicated that in cancer cells the activity of the rate-limiting enzyme of GTP biosynthesis, IMP DH (EC 1.1.1.205), markedly increased in parallel with the malignancy of the tumors. The specific activity of the salvage enzyme, GPRT, was markedly higher than that of IMP DH and it was maintained at high activity in cancer cells. The original observations

Table 1. Some biological functions of GTP

1.	RNA synthesis (with ATP, CTP, and UTP)
2.	De novo adenylate biosynthesis
3.	Inhibits AMP deaminase activity
4.	mRNA (guanylyltransferase, 5′-"cap" formation)
5.	Protein elongation
6.	Biopterin synthesis
7.	dGTP production
8.	cGMP synthesis; role in cAMP metabolism
9.	Complex glycolipid and glycoprotein synthesis
10.	Krebs cycle
11.	Terminal maturation of myeloid cells
12.	Microtubule polymerization
13.	G-protein function
14.	*ras* oncogene expression
15.	Signal transduction

for purine metabolic imbalance were made in chemically-induced, transplantable rat hepatomas. However, our studies indicated that the biochemical imbalance also applied to other solid tumors (Weber 1977, 1983) (Fig. 1).

The biological significance of GTP and guanylate metabolism is given in Table 1. The brief survey shows that GTP not only plays a role in intermediary metabolism and protein biosynthesis but also in the expression of the *ras* oncogene and in signal transduction. Its role as a precursor of RNA and DNA is of particular significance in chemotherapy targeted against guanylate biosynthesis (Weber et al. 1988).

Chemotherapy Targeted Against IMP DH and GTP Biosynthesis

The main observations and ideas on which the design of anti-IMP DH treatment is based in end stage leukemia are discussed below.

The experimental studies we carried out in human leukemic cells indicated the major differences between normal and leukemic leukocytes that provided a basis for the drug treatment. The activity of IMP DH was markedly higher in leukemic cells than in normal ones. There was also present a high activity of the salvage enzyme, GPRT (Weber et al. 1988). This observation suggested that means must be found not only to inhibit the activity of IMP DH but also that of GPRT, so that the salvage mechanism would not circumvent inhibition of the de novo pathway (Weber et al. 1988). Further evidence was our observation that the active metabolite of tiazofurin, thiazole-4-carboxamide adenine dinucleotide (TAD), markedly accumulated in leukemic cells over that found in normal granulocytes (Jayaram et al. 1986).

Tiazofurin: An Inhibitor of IMP DH Activity

In earlier papers we made the suggestion that IMP DH should be a sensitive target in cancer chemotherapy (Weber 1977, 1983; Weber et al. 1976) and R. K. Robins with the same idea prepared a series of compounds among which tiazofurin was inhibitory to murine leukemias and Lewis lung tumor in mice (Robins 1982). Tiazofurin in sensitive cells is activated by two enzymes to a fraudulent NAD which in turn may be degraded by a phosphodiesterase. The sensitivity or resistance of murine tumors primarily depended on the concentration achieved in the tumor cells of the active metabolite, TAD (Jayaram 1984).

The National Cancer Institute and 10 other centers carried out phase I and II trials with tiazofurin in patients by administering tiazofurin intravenously in a 10-min bolus daily for 5 days or via continuous intravenous infusion for 5 days. Review of the trials indicated that the limiting side effect was neurotoxicity. Plasma tiazofurin content was determined in several trials but there were no reports on TAD concentrations, IMP DH activity, or GTP pools in the tumors of the patients.

Our studies showed a pattern of sequence of activities after tiazofurin administration which included a rapid decline in IMP DH and GTP concentration in animal tumors (Weber 1983). Because of observations in the literature (Becher and Lohr 1979) and our own studies in identifying increased IMP DH activity and high concentration of TAD in leukemic cells (Jayaram et al. 1986; Weber et al. 1988), we decided on a new approach: to avoid or decrease toxicity by intravenous administration of the drug through a 60-min period using the pump for even delivery. The effectiveness of chemotherapy would be monitored by assay of IMP DH activity and GTP concentration in the cancer cells.

Comparison of the Properties of IMP DH from Rat Hepatoma and Human Leukemic Cells

Comparison of the properties of completely purified IMP DH from rat hepatoma and crude extract from blast cells of human patients with AML indicated that constants for ligands and for inhibitory action mechanism by TAD were similar (Weber et al. 1988; Yamada et al. 1988). Therefore, it is assumed that the action of tiazofurin, through TAD, would be similar in rat hepatoma and in human myelocytic leukemia.

Rationale of Enzyme-Pattern-Targeted Chemotherapy in Leukemia

The clinical biochemical study tested the idea that restoration of altered biochemical activities to normal range should have useful chemotherapeutic action and reveal the significance of the enzymic and metabolic alterations for neoplastic growth (Weber 1977, 1983; Weber and Cantero 1957). The reasons for designing an anti-guanylate and anti-IMP DH chemotherapy are as follows: (1) The activity of the rate-limiting enzyme of GTP biosynthesis, IMP DH, is low in normal cells, e.g., liver, but markedly increased in cancer cells, e.g., hepatomas. (2) IMP DH activity increased in all cancer cells in a transformation- and progression-linked fashion. (3) The activity of the subsequent enzyme in GTP biosynthesis, GMP synthase, is markedly increased in cancer cells. (4) The concentration of GMP is increased in hepatomas. (5) The dGTP pool is limiting for DNA biosynthesis in liver and hepatomas. (6) The concentration of dGTP markedly increased in hepatomas of different growth rates. (7) These biochemical alterations confer selective advantages to cancer cells and, therefore, as the molecular correlation concept suggested, the increased IMP DH activity and the elevated capacity for guanylate biosynthesis should provide sensitive targets for anticancer chemotherapy (Weber 1977, 1983; Weber et al. 1976).

In testing this approach for the treatment of human refractory AML with tiazofurin, the following observations provided the rationale. (1) IMP DH activity markedly increased in human leukemic cells. (2) The increased IMP DH activity is transformation- and progression-linked. (3) The activity of GMP synthase is markedly increased in leukemic leukocytes. (4) In patients treated with tiazofurin against various solid tumors, some myelosuppression was observed as a side effect. (5) There is an in vitro predictive test available to determine the sensitivity of leukemic cells to tiazofurin. This is based on the observation that leukemic cells produce over 20-fold higher concentrations of TAD from tiazofurin than normal leukocytes, and as a result in the leukemic leukocytes the GTP pools decreased, whereas there was no change in the normal leukocytes. (6) The biochemical targets, IMP DH activity and GTP concentration in blast cells, make it possible to measure the extent and duration of tiazofurin impact and permit monitoring chemotherapeutic action. (7) The activity of the salvage enzyme, GPRT, is curtailed by the very low concentrations of guanine that are available in the blood. (8) Allopurinol administration increased plasma hypoxanthine concentration which competitively inhibited GPRT activity. (9) Samples of neoplastic and normal cell population are readily available from peripheral blood.

Clinical Response to Chemotherapy and Appearance of In Vivo Differentiation of Leukemic Cells After Tiazofurin Treatment

In patient no. 1 (48-year-old white man) the usual chemotherapeutic means (daunorubicin, cytarabine, 6-deazaguanine and other drugs) were all used but the disease became refractory. Amsacrine, etoposide, and asparaginase were all tried with little success and much toxicity.

The patient was treated with tiazofurin in our first trial and the results were reported (Tricot et al. 1987). This patient and all subsequent patients were given prophylactic allopurinol therapy. Through gradual escalations a dose of 3300 mg/m^2 was reached which resulted in a steady decline in GTP concentrations in the leukemic cells, followed by a decrease in the blast cell count without causing bone marrow hypoplasia or marked neutropenia during a 13-day treatment period and for a few weeks after treatment. The patient had only mild side effects.

Similar results were obtained in the second patient, and by the third patient we were also able to measure plasma tiazofurin and hypoxanthine levels and, most importantly, IMP DH activity (Weber et al. 1988).

Impact of Tiazofurin on Biochemical Parameters and Clinical Course in Long-Term Treatment

Patient no. 3 was a 59-year-old woman with refractory AML. She was treated with 2200 mg/m^2 and after 2 days for an additional 5 days with 3300 mg/m^2 tiazofurin (a total of 7 days), with allopurinol (300 mg) every morning during tiazofurin treatment.

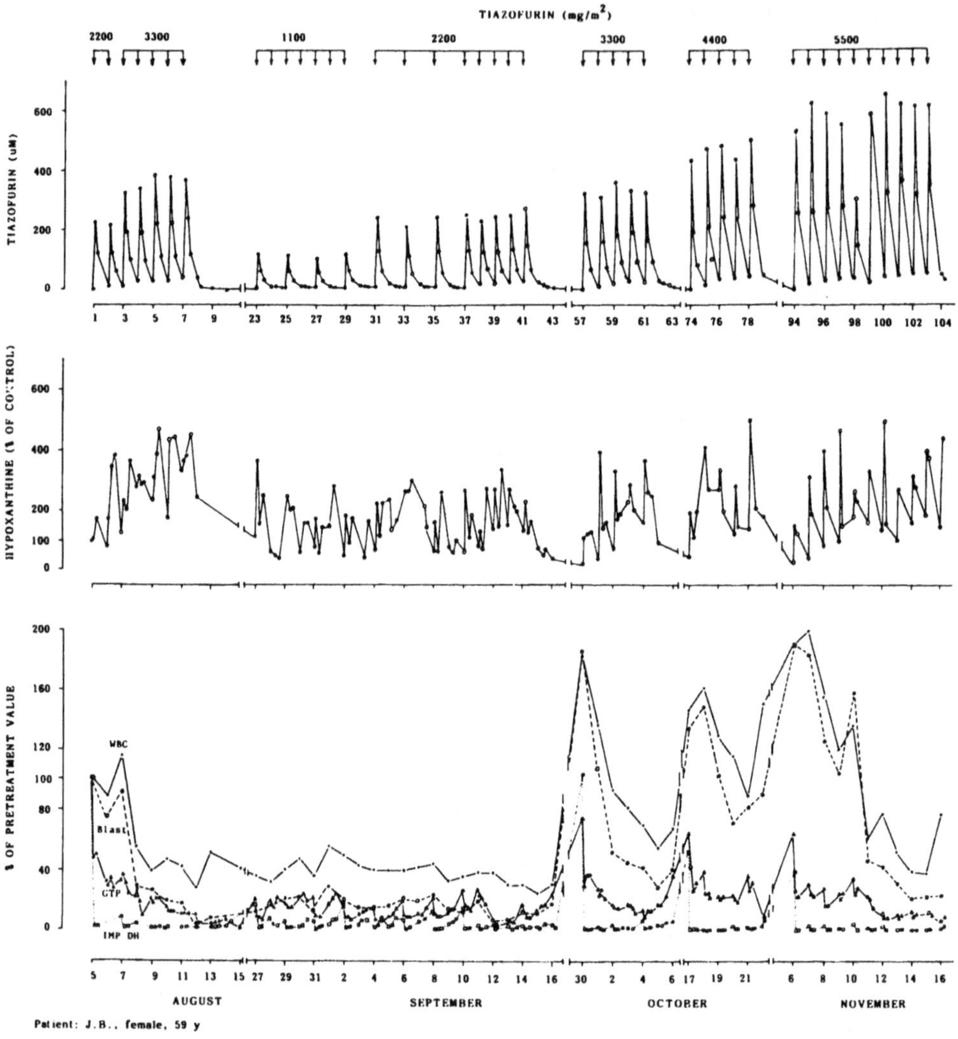

Fig. 2. Impact of infusion of tiazofurin on IMP dehydrogenase activity and GTP concentration in the blast cells of white female patient with end-stage leukemia in myeloid blast crisis. The behavior of blast cell count and white blood cell count and plasma hypoxanthine and tiazofurin concentrations are also shown

After tiazofurin infusion IMP DH activity rapidly declined in the blast cells with a $t_{1/2}$ of 30 min, followed by a decrease in GTP concentration with a $t_{1/2}$ of 2–3 days. These biochemical events were followed by a decline in the blast count, with preservation of the granulocytes and evidence of induced differentiation in the bone marrow. This patient showed some neurotoxicity but cessation of treatment for several days permitted resumption of tiazofurin infusions which the patient then tolerated well. On every relapse the patient received an escalated tiazofurin dose following generally accepted treatment protocol for leukemic patients. The course of the treatment and the behavior of biochemical parameters are shown in Fig. 2. Because the protocol specified a maximum dose of 7600 mg/m^2 tiazofurin, careful analysis of the results was carried out to discover a novel way of treatment which obviated the need for constant escalations on the relapses (Weber et al. 1988).

Combination Chemotherapy Action of Tiazofurin and Allopurinol

The data from patient no. 3 showed that allopurinol given as a single pill (300 mg) in the morning increased plasma hypoxanthine level, but it rapidly decreased by the end of the day. We determined that hypoxanthine can act as a competitive inhibitor of the activity of the salvage enzyme, GPRT, from leukemic blast cells; therefore, it seemed important to sustain a high concentration of hypoxanthine in the plasma (Weber et al. 1988). For this reason we introduced a higher dose of allopurinol given in divided doses every 6 or every 4 h for a total dose of 400 or 800 mg per day. Since our calculation indicated that the high hypoxanthine level should switch off the salvage pathway, we decided to de-escalate the tiazofurin dose for a protocol of 6600 mg/m^2 for induction dose and subsequent 8 or 10 infusions of 2200 mg/m^2. This protocol provided a number of remissions with total treatment lasting for 10 months and was well tolerated by the patient.

Sustained Dose Protocol in the Treatment of Refractory AML

On the basis of results in patient no. 3, several more patients were treated with 2200 or 3300 mg/m^2 on admission and on subsequent relapses. This novel protocol which obviated the need for escalation proved to be helpful in decreasing toxicity and providing good quality of life during treatment and remission.

Tiazofurin-Induced Differentiation in Refractory AML

There have been reports on induced differentiation in vitro in HL-60 tissue culture cells by tiazofurin and other inhibitors of de novo GTP biosynthesis (Lucas et al. 1983; Sokoloski et al. 1986), and this was reviewed (Tricot et al. 1987; Weber et al. 1988). It was also observed that when depletion of GTP concentration was circumvented by providing high concentrations of guanine in the tissue culture system, differentiation did not occur, although IMP DH was inhibited. Thus, in vivo induced differentiation was due to a decrease in GTP concentration (Lucas et al. 1983; Sokoloski et al. 1986).

Our studies are the first ones to demonstrate the production of in vivo differentiation after tiazofurin treatment in patients (Tricot et al. 1987; Weber et al. 1988). Our recent studies on K562 leukemia cells indicated that inhibition of IMP DH activity led to decreased GTP concentration in the cells, resulting in switching off the activity of the GTP-dependent *ras* oncogene (Olah et al. 1988). This was followed by induced differentiation as measured by the new production of hemoglobin in the tiazofurin-treated cells (Olah et al. 1988). Thus, in our patients the tiazofurin-induced decrease in GTP concentration in the leukemic blast cells should achieve chemotherapeutic results by curtailing availability of guanylates (GTP, dGTP) for DNA biosynthesis and replication. The decrease in GTP pool should also curtail the expression of the GTP-dependent oncogene, probably the *ras*, which might be responsible for the observed differentiation of the blast cells in patients. Thus, the induced differentiation might be linked with the tiazofurin-induced down regulation of the C-*ras* oncogene (Olah et al. 1988; Weber et al. 1988).

Major Limitations of Conventional Therapy and Novel Aspects of Tiazofurin Treatment in Leukemia

Some of the major limitations of conventional antileukemia drug treatment are summarized as follows.

1. Current treatment of leukemia is nonselective and profoundly affects normal hematopoietic and other rapidly dividing cells.
2. No rapid predictive in vitro tests are available to assess sensitivity.
3. No methods are available to monitor effect during treatment.
4. In relapsed patients, the effect of antileukemic drugs decreases markedly, but toxicity remains the same.
5. There is 15%–25% mortality due to treatment in newly diagnosed patients and even higher in refractory ones.

Our program with tiazofurin and allopurinol provides combination chemotherapy and yields the following novel aspects for the treatment of leukemia.

1. Rational targeting: IMP DH, GTP.
2. Biochemical monitoring during therapy.
3. Selective action on leukemic cells.
4. Correlation of predictive test with clinical results.
5. Differentiation induced, and neutropenia avoided.
6. Morbidity and mortality of conventional chemotherapy avoided.

The biochemical and clinical details of these studies are being published elsewhere (Tricot et al. 1989).

Summary

The hypothesis was tested that the increased IMP dehydrogenase (IMP DH) activity in human myelocytic leukemic cells might be a sensitive target of chemotherapy by tiazofurin. IMP DH activity in normal leukocytes was 3.1 ± 0.5 nmol h^{-1} mg^{-1} protein and in leukemic cells it was elevated 15- to 40-fold. The activity of the salvage enzyme guanine phosphoribosyltransferase (GPRT) in normal leukocytes was 389 ± 27 nmol h^{-1} mg^{-1} protein and in leukemic cells it increased 3- to 6-fold. Tiazofurin, a C-nucleoside, is metabolized in sensitive cells to thiazole-4-carboxamide adenine dinucleotide (TAD), a strong inhibitor of IMP DH activity, resulting in depression of GTP and dGTP pools and inhibition of cell proliferation in murine tumors. IMP DH of human myelocytic leukemic blast cells was inhibited by TAD ($K_i = 0.1$ μM). The leukemic leukocytes stored 20- to 30-fold higher concentrations of TAD than normal ones.

In a phase I/II trial 16 patients with end stage refractory leukemia were treated with tiazofurin infused daily in a 60-min period with a pump. The trial was directed primarily by the biochemical impact of tiazofurin on IMP dehydrogenase activity and GTP concentration and tiazofurin doses were adjusted accordingly. Allopurinol was given routinely against accumulation of uric acid. Three patients could not be evaluated because of early toxicity and three did not respond. In 10 patients complete or partial remissions were observed, with good quality of life, in some patients for over 6- or 10-month periods with treatment given every 3 to 6 weeks. In the responding patients, tiazofurin decreased IMP DH activity in blast cells with a $t_{1/2}$ of 30–60 min followed by a decline in GTP pools with a $t_{1/2}$ of about 2–3 days and the decline in blast cell count followed with preservation of the granulocytes. Allopurinol, by increasing hypoxanthine concentrations in the plasma, inhibited the activity of GPRT, thus blocking salvage and acting as combination chemotherapy with tiazofurin. Bone marrow aspirates showed a marked shift from immature to more mature cells, suggesting an in vivo induction of differentiation. Tiazofurin given as a 1-h infusion was well tolerated compared to results of other phase I trials using bolus injection or continuous infusion. The preliminary results with tiazofurin are promising and further studies are in progress.

References

Becher HJ, Lohr GW (1979) Inosine 5′-phosphate dehydrogenase in normal and leukemic blood cells. Klin Wochenschr 57:1109–1115

Jayaram HN (1984) Biochemical mechanisms of resistance to tiazofurin. Adv Enzyme Regul 24: 67–89

Jayaram HN, Pillwein K, Nichols CR, Hoffman R, Weber G (1986) Selective sensitivity to tiazofurin of human leukemic cells. Biochem Pharmacol 35:2029–2032

Lucas DL, Robins RK, Knight RD, Wright DG (1983) Induced maturation of the human promyelocytic leukemia cell, HL-60, by 2-β-D-ribofuranosylselenazole-4-carboxamide. Biochem Biophys Res Commun 115:971–980

Olah E, Natsumeda Y, Ikegami T, Kote Z, Horanyi M, Szelenyi J, Paulik E, Kremmer T, Hollan SR, Sugar J, Weber G (1988) Induction of erythroid differentiation and modulation of gene expression by tiazofurin in K562 leukemia cells. Proc Natl Acad Sci USA 85:6533–6537

Robins RK (1982) Nucleoside and nucleotide inhibitors of inosine monophosphate (IMP) dehydrogenase as potential antitumor inhibitors. Nucleosides and Nucleotides 1:35–44

Sokoloski JA, Blair OC, Sartorelli AC (1986) Alterations in glycoprotein synthesis and guanosine triphosphate levels associated with the differentiation of HL-60 leukemia cells produced by inhibitors of inosine 5′-phosphate dehydrogenase. Cancer Res 46:2314–2319

Tricot GJ, Jayaram HN, Nichols CR, Pennington K, Lapis E, Weber G, Hoffman R (1987) Hematological and biochemical action of tiazofurin in a case of refractory acute myeloid leukemia. Cancer Res 47:4988–4991

Tricot GJ, Jayaram HN, Lapis E, Natsumeda Y, Yamada Y, Nichols CR, Kneebone P, Heerema N, Weber G, Hoffman R (1989) Biochemically directed therapy of leukemia with tiazofurin, a selective blocker of inosine 5′-phosphate dehydrogenase activity. Cancer Res 49, July issue

Weber G (1977) Enzymology of cancer cells, parts 1 and 2. N Engl J Med 296:486–493; 541–551

Weber G (1983) Biochemical strategy of cancer cells and the design of chemotherapy. G.H.A. Clowes Memorial Lecture. Cancer Res 43:3466–3492

Weber G, Cantero A (1957) Glucose-6-phosphate utilization in hepatoma, regenerating and newborn rat liver, and in the liver of fed and fasted normal rats. Cancer Res 17:995–1005

Weber G, Prajda N, Jackson RC (1976) Key enzymes of IMP metabolism: transformation- and progression-linked alterations in gene expression. Adv Enzyme Regul 14:3–24

Weber G, Jayaram HN, Lapis E, Natsumeda Y, Yamada Y, Yamaji Y, Tricot GJ, Hoffman R (1988) Enzyme-pattern-targeted chemotherapy with tiazofurin and allopurinol in human leukemia. Adv Enzyme Regul 27:405–433

Yamada Y, Natsumeda Y, Weber G (1988) Action of the active metabolites of tiazofurin and ribavirin on purified IMP dehydrogenase. Biochemistry 27:2193–2196

Nuclear Components and Plasma Membrane as Targets of Chemotherapeutic Agents

H. Grunicke, J. Hofmann, K. Maly, F. Überall, L. Posch, H. Fiebig, Y. Yamada, Y. Natsumeda, W. Helliger, C. Schletterer, H. Talasz, G. Weiss, B. Puschendorf, and G. Weber

Introduction

Autonomous self-stimulation of cellular replication is an intrinsic property of malignant growth. Compounds which inhibit enzymes involved in autonomous growth stimulation should, therefore, be useful agents in tumor chemotherapy. This autonomy is achieved (1) by an autocrine production of growth factors, (2) by modified growth factor receptors which are active even in the absence of the corresponding ligand, or (3) by a constitutive activation of elements of the growth factor signal transduction pathways (Sporn and Todaro 1980; Goustin et al. 1986). Various growth factors cause an activation of phospholipid and Ca^{2+}-dependent protein kinase (protein kinase C); furthermore, this enzyme has been shown to be constitutively activated in some transformed cell lines (Nishizuka 1987; Maly et al. 1988). Therefore, inhibitors of this enzyme seem to be suitable candidates for new antitumor agents. The fact that various isoenzymes have been described for protein kinase C (Coussens et al. 1986; Knopf et al. 1986) may even open up possibilities for tumor-specific effects. We have, therefore, investigated whether inhibitors of protein kinase C inhibit tumor growth and whether these inhibitions are related to a depression of the corresponding enzyme. Furthermore, it seemed of interest to investigate whether combinations of protein kinase C-inhibitors with established antitumor agents can be found in which the antiproliferative activities of the combined drugs exhibit a synergistic or additional behaviour. As protein kinase C (in its active form) is localized in the plasma membrane (Anderson et al. 1985), we have focussed on antitumor agents which are known to interfere with the plasma membrane. Alkylating and platinating agents have been shown to cause a variety of membrane effects at therapeutic concentrations (Grunicke et al. 1971, 1986a; Ihlenfeldt et al. 1981; Baxter et al. 1982; Doppler et al. 1985; Scanlon et al. 1983; Shionoya et al. 1986; Slater et al. 1977; Vassilev et al. 1987); therefore, the combined effects of alkylating or platinating agents with inhibitors of protein kinase C seemed worth investigating.

The mechanisms by which mitogenic signals are transduced to the nucleus are still obscure. Suggestive evidence has been presented, indicating that histone acetyltransferase might be involved in this system (Grunicke et al. 1988). This enzyme was found to be elevated in all hepatomas studied so far and the increased activity seems to represent a progression and transformation-linked phenomenon (Grunicke et al. 1988). Thus, this enzyme may offer an additional interesting target in tumor chemotherapy.

Table 1. Depression of cellular replication and enhancement of the antiproliferative effect of *cis*-platinum by inhibitors of protein kinase C

Inhibitors	Inhibition of			Mode of combined activity
	Protein kinase C	Cell proliferation	Cell proliferation in combination with *cis*-DDP[c]	
	IC_{50} (μM)	IC_{50} (μM)	IC_{50} (μM)	
Quercetin	25	23	3.8	Synergy
Tamoxifen	11.20	12.44	2.24	Synergy
Staurosporine	0.048	0.04	0.004	Synergy
ET-18-OCH_3[a]	24.8	5.8	1.7	Synergy
cis-DDP[b]	>1000	0.23	–	–

[a] 1-0-octadecyl-2-0-methyl-glycero-3-phosphocholine
[b] *cis*-Diaminedichloroplatinum(II)
[c] IC_{50} values of the inhibitors in presence of *cis*-DDP; molar ratios: quercetin/*cis*-DDP 100:1; tamoxifen/*cis*-DDP 10:2; staurosporine/*cis*-DDP 1:100; ET-18-OCH_3/*cis*-DDP 10:1

Protein kinase C was partially purified from Walker cells as described by Kreutter et al. (1985) and the activity determined according to Fabbro et al. (1985). Proliferation of Walker carcinoma cells in culture was determined as described elsewhere (Grunicke et al. 1986). Evaluation of combined drug effects were performed as described by Chou and Talalay (1984)

Protein Kinase C as Target in Chemotherapy

Antitumor Effects of Protein Kinase C Inhibitors

Table 1 shows the effects of various inhibitors of protein kinase C and *cis*-DDP on enzyme activity and cell proliferation of Walker carcinoma cells. As can be seen, all compounds – except *cis*-DDP – inhibit cell proliferation and enzyme activity within the same dose range. In order to investigate whether the drugs affect protein kinase C in intact cells to a similar extent, we studied the phorbol ester stimulated phosphorylation of the ribosomal protein S_6. Phosphorylation of S_6 is catalyzed by a S_6-kinase (Thomas 1986) which is known to be under control of protein kinase C. Thus, the difference in S_6 phosphorylation ± TPA should represent an indirect measure of protein kinase C activity. In all cases it could be demonstrated that those inhibitors listed in Table 1 which depress protein kinase C activity in vitro also reduce S_6-phosphorylation in intact cells (Hofmann et al. 1988). Thus, the data are consistent with the notion that the inhibition of protein kinase C and the depression of cell growth are causally related.

Combination of Protein Kinase C Inhibitors with Alkylating and Platinating Drugs

The compounds listed in Table 1 are relatively nonspecific. This lack of specificity should cause a broad spectrum of unwanted side effects which limits the employment of these drugs, especially for single-drug treatment. We have investigated, therefore,

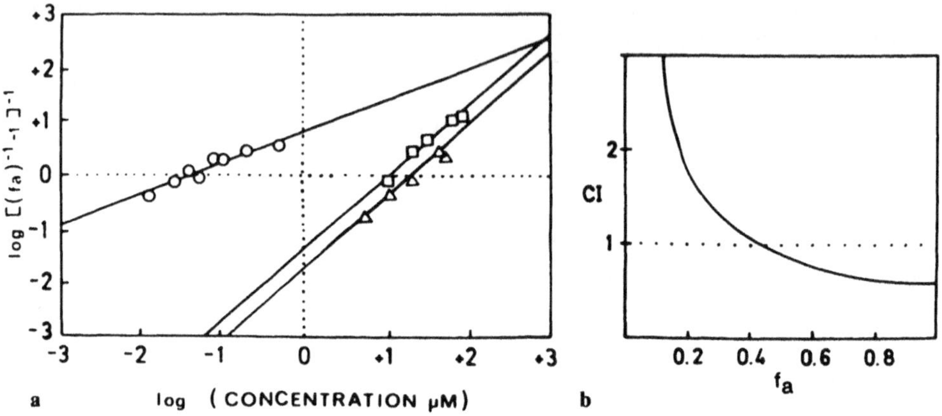

Fig. 1. a Inhibition of cell proliferation by nitrogen mustard (HN2), quercetin, and an HN2/quercetin combination (molar ratio, 1:200). Inhibition of cell multiplication is expressed as fraction affected (f_a) according to Chou and Talalay (1984). △, quercetin; ○, HN2; □, quercetin + HN2. **b** Computer-generated plot of the combination index *CI* with respect to the inhibition of cellular replication by a combination of nitrogen mustard and quercetin. Computation was performed as described by Chou and Talalay (1984) employing the data from Fig. 1a

whether inhibitors of protein kinase C are useful in drug combinations. As the active form of protein kinase C is a membrane-bound enzyme (Anderson et al. 1985), we focussed our interest on established antitumor agents for which an interference with the plasma membrane at therapeutic concentrations had been demonstrated. Alkylating agents and *cis*-platinum complexes have been shown to affect plasma membrane functions and evidence has been presented that these membrane effects contribute to the cytotoxic effect of these drugs (Grunicke et al. 1971, 1986a; Ihlenfeldt et al. 1981; Baxter et al. 1982; Doppler et al. 1985; Scanlon et al. 1983; Shionoya et al. 1986; Slater et al. 1977; Vassilev et al. 1987).

The effects of drug combinations were evaluated by employing the procedure described by Chou and Talalay (1984). In this universally applicable technique, a combination index (CI) is calculated which yields values of CI = 1 in case of summation, CI > 1 in case of antagonistic effects, and CI < 1 if synergy is indicated. Figure 1 demonstrates CI values of quercetin/nitrogen mustard (HN2) combinations as a function of fractional inhibition of cell growth. As can be seen, quercetin synergistically enhances the antiproliferative effect of HN2. The results obtained in combination with *cis*-platinum are summarized in Table 1. All compounds which proved to inhibit protein kinase C cause a synergistic enhancement of the antiproliferative activity of *cis*-DDP.

The results described so far were obtained in tissue culture. It seemed necessary, therefore, to investigate whether these effects can also be observed under in vivo conditions with tumor-bearing animals. The human large cell lung cancer LXFG 529/11 was transplanted s.c. to nude mice and the animals treated with quercetin, *cis*-DDP, or a quercetin/*cis*-DDP combination. Figure 2 demonstrates that 20 mg/kg quercetin, which – alone – is without any effect on tumor growth, dramatically enhances the effect of 5 mg/kg *cis*-DDP. It should be noted that this tumor cannot be

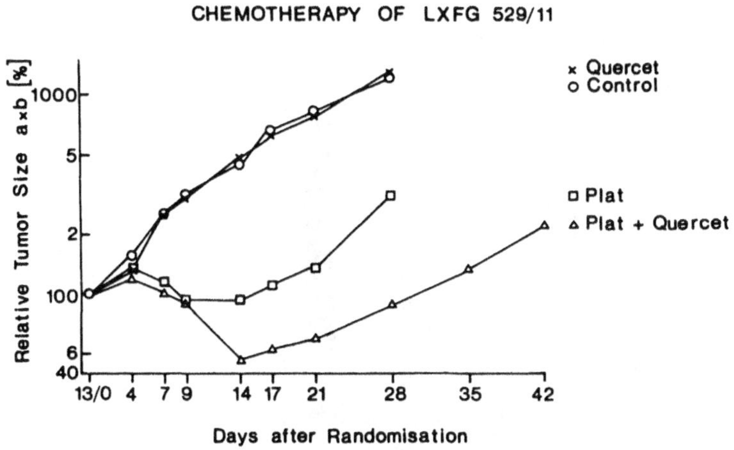

Fig. 2. Enhancement of the antitumor effect of *cis*-diamminedichloroplatinum(II) by quercetin against the human tumor xenograft LXFG in athymic mice. Large-cell lung carcinoma LXFG 529 was transplanted s.c. to athymic mice. Tumor-bearing animals received either 5 mg/kg *cis*-platinum i.p. at days 1, 4, 5 (□), 20 mg quercetin i.p. at days 1, 2, 4, 5, 7, and 8 (×), or *cis*-platinum 5 mg/kg at days 1, 4, and 7 and quercetin 20 mg/kg at days 1, 2, 4, 5, 7, and 8 (△)

cured by *cis*-DDP; therefore, the tumors will resume normal proliferation rates after termination of chemotherapy.

The data indicate that the synergistic enhancement of the antitumor activity of the platinum complexes by inhibitors of protein kinase C should be exploitable in tumor chemotherapy.

Histone Acetyltransferase as a Target in Tumor Chemotherapy

Possible Role of Histone Acetyltransferase in Signal Transduction

The mechanism by which mitogenic signals are transduced to the nucleus is still obscure. Recent data from our laboratory suggest that growth stimulation by serum growth factors (Schletterer et al. 1987), by hepatectomy (Weiss and Puschendorf 1987), or after expression of transforming oncogenes (Schletterer et al. 1987) lead to a transitory increase in histone acetylation which precedes DNA replication. In regenerating liver this replication-associated type of histone acetylation occurs 2–3 h before the onset of DNA synthesis and is well beyond the first maximum of RNA synthesis which is observed 6–8 h after hepatectomy (Grunicke et al. 1988). An acetylation of histones which is in close temporal relation with DNA replication has also been observed in *Physarum polycephalum*, where an acetylation of preexisting histones immediately precedes the entry into S-phase and is followed by an acetylation of newly synthesized histones (Loidl and Gröbner 1987). All these data strongly suggest the existence of a replication-associated type of histone acetylation, which exhibits features of a signaling mechanism. The biological function of the post-translational acetylation of histones is still obscure. It is tempting, however, to speculate

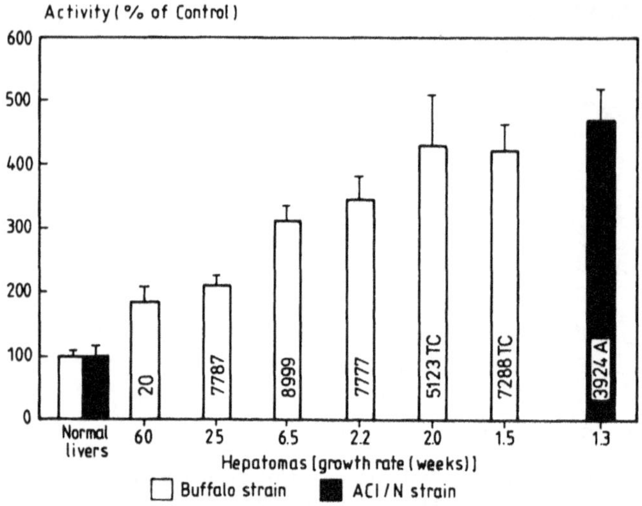

Fig. 3. Histone acetyltransferase activity in nuclei of rat heptomas and corresponding normal livers. ACI/N normal liver is the control of hepatoma 3924A and Buffalo is the control of all the others. *Vertical bars* indicate SEM of three or more experiments in each group. All differences between normal livers and tumors are statistically significant ($P<0.01$). Histone acetyltransferase activity was determined according to Garcea and Alberts (1980). Specific activities were determined as picomoles acetate per hour per milligram protein. One hundred percent corresponds to 208 ± 14 (Buffalo) or 225 ± 32 ACI/N respectively

that histone acetylation leads to a labilization of the nucleosomal structure which in turn facilitates the unfolding of the nucleosome during replication.

Histone Acetyltransferase in Tumors

Increased rates or elevated extents of histone acetylation have been described in experimental tumors (Horiushi et al. 1981; Grunicke et al. 1986b). It remained unclear, however, whether these alterations represent coincidental phenomena or whether changes in histone acetylation are progression- and/or transformation-linked processes. In order to address these questions, histone acetyltransferase activity has been determined in a spectrum of rat hepatomas of low, intermediate, and fast growth rates and the results were compared with the activities obtained from normal rat liver of the same strain, sex, and weight. The results, which are summarized in Fig. 3, demonstrate that the enzyme is increased in all hepatomas and that the rise is proportional to the growth rates of the tumors. The enzyme is significantly elevated even in the slowest-growing hepatoma, which indicates that the increase in histone acetyltransferase is not only a progression (growth related) but possibly also a transformation-linked phenomenon. Thus, this enzyme should represent a particularly interesting target for tumor chemotherapy.

Inhibition of Histone Acetylation by Alkylating Agents

Unfortunately, specific inhibitors for histone acetyltransferase are not yet available. Studies with alkylating agents revealed, however, that these drugs – at therapeutic

Table 2. Effect of nitrogen mustard (HN2) on histone acetyltransferase in nuclei of AS30D rat hepatomas, Ehrlich ascites tumor cells, and the corresponding host livers

	Histone acetyltransferase activity as percentage of untreated controls
Rat liver (host)	92.8 ± 3.2[a]
AS30D hepatoma	50.25 ± 8.3
Mouse liver (host)	94.25 ± 13.1
Ehrlich cells	68.3 ± 5

[a] Mean ± SD

Tumor-bearing animals were injected i.p. with 2.5×20^{-5} mol/kg nitrogen mustard in Tris-buffered saline. After 4 h, the animals were killed, livers and tumors excised, and histone acetyltransferase activity determined in isolated nuclei as described elsewhere (Grunicke et al. 1986b)

concentrations – cause a depression of histone acetylation (Grunicke et al. 1986b; Zwierzina et al. 1984). This inhibition of post-translational histone acetylation is seen at all concentrations of alkylating drugs which depress cellular replication. The antitumor effect of bifunctional alkylating agents is generally ascribed to the formation of DNA-interstrand cross-links, although definite proof that these are the essential lesions after exposure to alkylating drugs is still lacking. Studies with nitrogen mustard-resistant and -sensitive Walker carcinoma cells revealed, however, that neither formation nor repair of DNA-interstrand cross-links are different in resistant versus sensitive cells after exposure to nitrogen mustard (Roberts et al. 1984; Grunicke et al. 1986a). This is in contrast to the inhibition of histone acetylation, which proved to be much less affected in the resistant cells compared with the sensitive counterparts (Grunicke et al. 1986b). These data indicate that the depression of histone acetylation via alkylating agents is perhaps even more closely related to the sensitivity against these drugs than formation or repair of DNA cross-links. The significance of the inhibition of histone acetylation by alkylating agents is further emphasized by the observation that these drugs depress histone acetylation in tumors although not in the host liver (Table 2). The reason for this apparent tumor specificity is most likely the predominance of a replication-associated type of histone acetylation in tumors which – in contrast to histone acetylation in nongrowing tissues – exhibits a particular sensitivity to alkylating agents. That the depression of histone acetylation by alkylating drugs is indeed caused by a depression of the acetyltransferase and not due to an elevated rate of deacetylation as has been shown previously (Grunicke et al. 1986b). In conclusion: histone acetyltransferase is an interesting target of tumor chemotherapy. The observation indicating a particular sensitivity of this enzyme against alkylating drugs should encourage the synthesis of alkylating agents with a higher protein affinity especially to histone acetyltransferase.

Summary

Protein kinase C is an exploitable target in tumor chemotherapy. Inhibitors of this enzyme are especially useful in combination with platinating agents due to their synergistic enhancement of the antiproliferative activity of *cis*-platinum. Histone acetyltransferase seems to be another interesting new target. This enzyme has been shown to be elevated in all tumors studied so far and an increase in the specific activity of histone acetyltransferase seems to represent a progression- and transformation-linked phenomenen. Evidence is presented that alkylating agents inhibit this enzyme and that the depression of histone acetyltransferase is correlated with the antitumor effect of alkylating drugs. These results call for the synthesis of more specific inhibitors of histone acetyltransferase.

Acknowledgment. These studies were supported in part by the Drug Development Program of the Bundesministerium für Forschung und Technologie, FRG, and by the Austrian Science Fund, Project No. P5097.

References

Anderson WB, Estival A, Tabiovaara H, Gopalakrishna R (1985) Altered subcellular distribution of protein kinase C (phorbol ester receptor). Possible role in tumor promotion and the regulation of cell growth. Relationship to changes in adenylate cyclase activity. In: Cooper DMF, Seamon KB (eds) Advances in cyclic nucleotide and protein phosphorylation research, vol 19. Raven, New York, pp 287–306

Baxter JA, Chahavala SB, Hickman JA, Spurgin GE (1982) The effect of N-mustard (HN2) on activities of the plasma membrane of PC6A mouse plasma cytoma cells. Biochem Pharmacol 31: 1773–1778

Chou TC, Talalay B (1984) Quantitative analysis of dose effect relationships: the combined effects of multiple drugs or enzyme inhibitors. Adv Enzyme Regul 22:27–54

Coussens L, Parker PJ, Rhee L, Yang-Feng TL, Chen E, Waterfield M, Francke U, Ullrich A (1986) Multiple, distinct forms of bovine and human protein kinase C suggest diversity in cellular signalling pathways. Science 233:859–866

Doppler W, Hofmann J, Oberhuber H, Maly K, Grunicke H (1985) Nitrogen-mustard interference with potassium transport systems in Ehrlich ascites tumor cells. J Cancer Res Clin Oncol 110: 35–41

Fabbro D, Jungmann RA, Eppenberger U (1985) Subcellular distribution of protein kinase C of GH3-cells. Quantitation and characterization by polyacrylamide gel electrophoresis. Arch Biochem Biophys 239:102–111

Garcea RL, Alberts BM (1980) Comparative studies of histone acetylation in nucleosomes, nuclei and intact cells. J Biol Chem 255:11454–11463

Goustin AS, Leof EB, Shipley GD, Moses HL (1986) Growth factors and cancer. Cancer Res 46: 1015–1029

Grunicke H, Hirsch E, Wolf H, Bauer U, Kiefer G (1975) Selective inhibition of thymidine transport at low doses of the alkylating agent trisethyleneiminobenzoquinone (Trenimon) Exp Cell Res 90:357–364

Grunicke H, Doppler W, Hofmann J, Lindner H, Maly K, Oberhuber H, Ringsdorf H, Roberts JJ (1986a) Plasma membrane as target of alkylating agents. Adv Enzyme Regul 24:247–261

Grunicke H, Helliger W, Hermann BJ, Höck W, Hofmann J, Puschendorf B (1986b) Alkylating antitumor agents reduce histone acetyltransferase activity. Adv Enzyme Regul 25:87–97

Grunicke H, Yamada Y, Natsumeda Y, Helliger W, Schletterer C, Talasz H, Weiss G, Puschendorf B, Weber G (1989) Imbalance of histone metabolism in hepatocellular carcinoma: histone acetylation in normal rat liver and hepatomas. In: Bannasch P, Keppler D, Weber G (eds) Liver cell carcinoma. Kluver Academic Publishers, Dordrecht Boston London, pp 401–410

Hofmann J, Doppler W, Jakob A, Maly K, Posch L, Überall F, Grunicke HH (1988) Enhancement of the antiproliferative effect of *cis*-diamminedichloroplatinum(II) and nitrogen mustard by inhibitors of protein kinase C. Int J Cancer (in press)

Horiuchi K, Fujimoto D, Fukushima M, Kanai K (1981) Increased acetylation and deacetylation in rat ascites hepatoma cells. Cancer Res 41:1488–1491

Ihlenfeldt M, Gantner G, Harrer M, Puschendorf B, Putzer H, Grunicke H (1981) Interaction of the alkylating antitumor agent 2,3,5-tris(ethyleneimino)-benzoquinone with the plasma membrane of Ehrlich ascites tumor cells. Cancer Res. 41:289–293

Knopf JL, Lee M-H, Sultzman LA, Kriz RW, Loomis CR, Hewick RM, Bell RM (1986) Cloning and expression of multiple protein kinase C cDNAs. Cell 46:491–502

Kreutter D, Caldwell A, Morin MJ (1985) Dissociation of protein kinase C activation from phorbol ester induced maturation of HL-60 leukemia cells. J Biol Chem 260:5979–5984

Loidl P, Gröbner P (1987) Postsynthetic acetylation of histones during the cell cycle. A general function for the displacement of histones during chromatin rearrangements. Nucleic Acids Res 15: 8351–8366

Maly K, Oberhuber H, Doppler W, Hoflacher J, Jaggi R, Groner B, Grunicke H (1988) Effect of H-*ras* on phosphatidylinositol metabolism, Na^+/H^+-antiporter and mobilization of intracellular calcium. Adv Enzyme Regul 27:121–131

Nishizuka Y (1987) Protein kinases in signal transduction. In: Bradshaw RA, Prentis ST (eds) Oncogenes and growth factors. Elsevier Science, Amsterdam, pp 248–254

Roberts JJ, Rawlings CJ, Friedlos F (1984) DNA-repair characteristics of Walker rat carcinoma cells sensitive and resistant to *cis*-diamminedichloroplatinum(II) (*cis*-platin) and difunctional alkylating agents. In: Harrap KR, Davies W, Calvert AH (eds) Cancer chemotherapy and selective drug development. Nijhoff, Boston

Scanlon KJ, Safirstein RL, Thies H, Gross RB, Waxman S, Guttenplan JB (1983) Inhibition of aminoacid transport by *cis*-diamminedichloroplatinum(II) derivatives in L1210 murine leukemia cells. Cancer Res 43:4211–4215

Schletterer C, Talasz H, Puschendorf B (1987) Histonacetylierung nach Induktion von c-*myc* and H-*ras* in NIH3T3 Fibroblasten. Proc Annu Meeting Austrian Biochem Soc, Graz 1987

Shionoya S, Ly A, Scanlon KJ (1986) Properties of aminoacid transport systems in K562 cells sensitive and resistant to *cis*-diamminedichloroplatinum(II). Cancer Res 46:3445–3448

Slater TE, Ahmed M, Ibrahim SA (1977) Studies on the nephrotoxicity of *cis*-dichlorodiamine-platinum 2^+ and related substances. J Clin Hepatol Oncol 7:543–546

Sporn M, Todaro GJ (1980) Autocrine secretion and malignant transformation of cells. N Engl J Med 303:878–880

Thomas G (1986) Epidermal growth-factor mediation of S6 phosphorylation during the mitogenic response: a novel S6 kinase. In: Kahn P, Graf T (eds) Oncogenes and growth control. Springer, Berlin Heidelberg New York, pp 177–183

Vassilev PM, Kanazirska MP, Charamella LJ, Dimitrov NV, Tien HT (1987) Changes in calcium channel activity in membranes from *cis*-diamminedichloroplatinum(II)-resistant and -sensitive L1210 cells. Cancer Res. 47:519–522

Weiss G, Puschendorf B (1987) Maximum der Histonacetyltransferase-Aktivität von der DNA-Synthese in regenerierender Rattenleber. Proc Annu Meeting Austrian Biochem Soc, Graz 1987

Zwierzina H, Loidl A, Fuith LC, Helliger W, Puschendorf B, Grunicke H (1984) Depression of histone acetylation by alkylating antitumor agents in murine cells. Cancer Res 44:3336–3339

Drug Resistant Cells as Targets for Chemotherapeutic Agents*

J. R. Bertino, A. Romanini, and J. P. O'Brien

Introduction

During the past decade, as a consequence of developments in molecular biology, there has been a rapid increase in our understanding of the genetic basis of drug resistance. Following the pioneer work of Schimke and his associates, who first reported that amplification of the dehydrofolate reductase (DHFR) gene was the genetic basis of overexpression of this enzyme in methotrexate-resistant cells (Alt et al. 1978), an increasing understanding of drug resistance has occurred. It is now time to use this technology to detect drug resistance in neoplastic cells of patients, and to begin to develop new strategies to avoid, overcome, or selectively eradicate drug resistant cells – the major obstacle to drug cure of tumors.

In this review, we will discuss our current work with methotrexate (MTX) resistance and multidrug resistance (MDR), both in experimental models and in patients, and indicate how this information might guide new drug development and new strategies for drug use.

Resistance to MTX

MTX has been an excellent model drug for the study of resistant mechanisms. Its mechanism of uptake, retention, and binding to the target enzyme DHFR have been extensively investigated. Studies of drug resistance have shown, as for most drugs studied, that resistance may occur by one or more mechanisms; uptake, activation (in the case of MTX, polyglutamate formation, which results in retention of this drug), an increase in the level of the target enzyme, or an alteration of the target enzyme, leading to decreased binding of the drug to the target (Table 1).

In mammalian tumor cells, propagated in vitro or in vivo in rodents, exposure to low dose or conventional dose regimens leads to emergence of a drug-resistant population that is unable to accumulate MTX, or has an increased level of DHFR as a consequence of gene amplification. Less commonly, in these experimental systems, the drug-resistant cells contain a DHFR enzyme with a decreased affinity for MTX. Since MTX is often used clinically in high-dose pulses given weekly or biweekly rather than low-dose continuous administration, we tested MTX-resistant cells emerging after a high-dose schedule of the drug (Pizzorno et al. 1988). The two cell lines obtained in this manner were both markedly impaired in their ability to form

---

* Supported by USPHS Grant CA08010 and The Brookdale Foundation

Table 1. Mechanisms of acquired resistance to methotrexate in mammalian cells

Phenotype expression	Genetic mechanism
1. Increased DHFR activity	Gene amplification
2. Decreased uptake	?
3. Altered DHFR	Mutation in DHFR gene
4. Decreased polyglutamylation	Mutation in Folyl-poly-glutamate synthase gene

polyglutamates of MTX, especially MTX with three or more glutamates. Impairment of folate polyglutamates occurs, but not to the same degree, so the cell is able to retain sufficient folate coenzymes to survive. The basis of this defect is an alteration in the enzyme folylpolyglutamate synthetase (J.J. McGuire, personal communication) which is responsible for polyglutamylation of folates and MTX.

An important attribute of this mechanism of MTX resistance is that this resistance is schedule-dependent, i.e., the cells are still almost as sensitive to low-dose continuous exposure to MTX as the parent cell line (Pizzorno et al. 1988). Since many patients receive MTX on the high-dose pulse schedule, it is possible that re-treatment with MTX at low-dose continuous exposure might be of benefit.

Alteration of DHFR as a Mechanism of MTX Resistance

Resistance to the antifolate trimethoprim, used to treat bacterial infections, is often associated with alterations in the bacterial or plasmid DHFR. By contrast, such alteration has not been commonly observed in cell lines unless they have been treated with a mutagen, which increases the probability of alteration. Several cell lines with an altered DHFR have been described, and the exact locus of the mutation giving rise to the altered enzyme has now been elucidated in two of these cell lines (Simonson and Levinson 1983; Srimatkandada et al. 1988). A MTX-resistant 3T6 cell line initially was resistant as a consequence of an amplification of a normal DHFR gene; as these lection pressure increased, a mutation presumably occurred in one of the normal DHFR genes, and eventually the mutated DHFR also was amplified, resulting in a highly resistant cell line (Haber et al. 1981). This cell line contains both a normal and an altered DHFR enzyme. Both normal cDNA clones and cDNA clones containing the altered enzyme have been obtained (Simonson and Levinson 1983).

The second example of a known mutation in the DHFR gene is also of interest. This cell line is from a human colon carcinoma, an epithelial cancer believed in man to arise as a consequence of one or more mutations in DNA, presumably leading to oncogene activation due to a point mutation (e.g. K-*ras*), or an amplification event. After low-dose continuous exposure to MTX, and with a stepwise increase in concentration, we obtained a highly resistant cell line, able to grow in $10^{-4} M$ MTX. This cell line was found to have an increase in DHFR and gene copies (ca. 50-fold), and the enzyme had a 5- to 8-fold decreased affinity for MTX compared to the parent line (Srimatkandada et al. 1989). This mutation was found to be due to a single base change T-C resulting in a *ser* residue instead of the normal *phe* at position no. 31. A restriction site for $EcoR_1$, is present in the normal human DHFR gene at this site; as a result of this mutation, the restriction site is absent in the resistant cell line. As in the case of the 3T6 MTX-resistant line, both normal and mutated DHFR genes were present, although the majority of the cDNA clones obtained contained the *phe–ser* mutation. Careful analysis of the wild-type DNA by southern blotting after $EcoR_1$, restriction showed that both alleles were initially present. Therefore, we believe that selective amplification of an allele containing the mutation occurred, resulting in high-level MTX-resistance. Evidence for a similar event has been described by Melera et al. (1980) in a Chinese hamster lung cell line resistant to MTX. Recently another human colon line resistant to high levels of 5-fluorodeoxyuridine (FUDR) was also shown to contain polymorphic thymidylate genes, one of which was amplified (Berger 1988). The amplified enzyme was found to have reduced affinity for FdUMP, the active anabolite of FUDR. This enzyme or cDNA has not been sequenced yet, and the mutation responsible for this alteration has not been pinpointed.

These findings suggest the possibility that carcinogen-derived epithelial tumors may also contain mutations in other genes, such as DHFR, which result in natural or rapidly evolved acquired resistance.

Drug Resistant Cells as Selective Targets

Trimetrexate, a "non-classical" antifolate now in extensive phase II trials (Lin and Bertino 1987), is also a potent inhibitor of DHFR (Jackson et al. 1984; Lin and Bertino 1987) but differs from MTX in two important aspects. Firstly, it is taken up avidly by most mammalian tumor cells, including human leukemia cells (Kamen et al. 1984; Lin and Bertino 1987), by a transport process independent of the MTX and reduced folate carrier system; and, secondly, it is not polyglutamylated but is retained in some cells at high levels by mechanisms which are not clear.

We tested the cytotoxicity of trimetrexate in parental and human leukemia cell lines (CEM) with different mechanisms of MTX resistance (Table 2). Only MTX resistant cells with an altered DHFR were still insensitive to trimetrexate; however, it is possible that a mutated DHFR could be still sensitive to trimetrexate but altered in its binding to MTX. Cells with high-level gene amplification (ca. 18-fold) are partially cross-resistant to trimetrexate, while cells with low levels of DHFR gene amplification are even more sensitive to trimetrexate. This sensitivity may reflect the high

Table 2. Cytotoxic effects of trimetrexate in cell lines resistant to MTX

Cell line	Sensitivity to trimetrexate
Sensitive to MTX	++++
Altered DHFR	–
Increased DHFR	++
Decreased polyglutamylation	++++
Impaired uptake	+++++

intracellular level of trimetrexate that results when cells are exposed to this drug (Kamen et al. 1984).

Cells resistant to MTX due to a polyglutamylation defect are still sensitive to trimetrexate. Of perhaps greater interest is the collateral sensitivity of the transport-defective MTX-resistant cell line to trimetrexate (Mini et al. 1985). We believe that this cell line is more sensitive to trimetrexate than the parent cell line, since it contains less folates (ca. 50% total folate) than does the parent line, and consequently that trimetrexate is a better competitive inhibitor of DHFR than MTX (unpublished observations). The use of carboxypeptidase G_2, a folate-depleting enzyme, in conjunction with trimetrexate causes even more cell kill, and we are examining the potency of this combination in mice bearing transplanted tumors.

Another strategy that we have suggested based on these findings is the sequential use of MTX followed by trimetrexate. If early resistance to MTX is due to either low-level gene amplification, impaired uptake, or defective polyglutamylation, after decimation of the cell population with MTX, the sequential use of trimetrexate may eradicate those surviving drug-resistant mutants and lead a more significant cell kill than can be obtained by either drug alone.

What Are the Mechanisms of MTX Resistance in Patients?

It should be clear from the foregoing discussion that in order to utilize new strategies or to develop new drugs targeted to preventing or eradicating drug resistance, a detailed understanding of resistant mechanisms in tumor cells for patients is necessary.

In our initial efforts we have focused on leukemia cells from patients, since the problems of obtaining tumor cells of high purity and repeatedly is less of a problem than in patients with solid tumors. We have started a program to look at both MTX resistance and multidrug resistance in these patients, and some preliminary data will now be presented.

MTX Resistance in Leukemia Patients

We are studying leukemia patients found to be clinically resistant to MTX using a screening in vitro assay (Rodenhuis et al. 1986). We find that there are multiple mechanisms of resistance to MTX in patients with acute lymphocytic leukemia. Initial sensitivity to MTX may be a result of the ability of lymphoblasts to polyglutamylate MTX effectively, and thus retain the drug. In some patients, a defect in this process has occurred, leading to resistance to MTX (Simonson and Levinson 1983).

Additional work is necessary to characterize further the mechanisms of resistance found, in particular gene amplification, sites of alteration of the DHFR in individual patients, and polyglutamylation defect.

Multidrug Resistance

While MTX is a classic example of how a single drug can meet multiple mechanisms of resistance, multidrug resistance (MDR) involves a single mechanism which can result in resistance to a variety of drugs. Strictly used, the term "multidrug resistance" refers to the observation that tumor cells selected in culture for resistance to a single cytotoxic natural product will simultaneously develop resistance to several structurally and functionally unrelated drugs (Biedler and Riehm 1970). Although multiple phenotype changes are seen as cells become MDR, the most consistent finding has been the overexpression of a high-molecular-weight (170–180 kd) membrane glycoprotein called P-glycoprotein (Pgp) (Juliano and Ling 1976). The *mdr*1 gene which encodes Pgp has been cloned (Chen et al. 1986) and its transfection into drug-sensitive cells has resulted in the broad pattern of cross-resistance characteristic of MDR (Gros et al. 1986). Pgp has been shown to have sequence homology to known membrane transport proteins (Chen et al. 1986), to hydrolyze ATP (Hamada and Tsuruo 1988), and to directly interact with certain cytotoxic natural products (Safa et al. 1986) as well as verapamil (Safa et al. 1987). On the basis of this data, MDR in tissue culture is thought to occur through overexpression of Pgp, which, functioning as an energy-dependent drug efflux pump, results in greatly reduced intracellular drug accumulation. Because of its apparent ability to mediate resistance to such important classes of drugs as anthracyclines, vinca alkaloids and epipodophylotoxins, Pgp is a natural target for therapeutic development.

Approaches to Modulation of P-Glycoprotein Function

A considerable number of compounds have been identified which can restore drug sensitivity in MDR cells (Tsuruo et al. 1982; Zamora et al. 1988). These compounds are believed to function by binding to Pgp and reducing its drug efflux capacity. An alternative approach has been the use of monoclonal antibodies (Mab), which bind to external epitopes of Pgp and in doing so modulate its function (Hamada and Tsuruo 1986). To further pursue this strategy, we measured the effect of the Mab HYB-241 on intracellular drug accumulation and drug sensitivity in MDR cells. This antibody, which recognizes an extracellular epitope on the human *mdr*1 gene product (Dr. C. Cordon-Cardo, personal communication), was developed by Hybritech Inc. (San Diego, Calif.) using the human MDR cell line SY5Y/NCR developed by Dr. June Biedler (Rittman-Grauer et al. 1986).

Using the MDR MC-IXC/VCR cell line as a model system, we have found that preincubation of these cells with HYB-241 (10 μg/ml) prior to drug exposure results in an eight-fold and three-fold increase in intracellular accumulation of actinomycin-D and vincristine respectively (Table 3). A substantial increase in cytotoxicity is seen when HYB-241 (10 μg/ml) is added to growth medium, as indicated by the marked lowering of the ED_{50} values for vincristine and actinomycin-D, although there was no detectable effect on doxorubicin (Table 3). When intracellular drug accumulation of vincristine is measured following exposure to HYB-241 plus verapamil a seven-fold increase is obtained, showing the additive effect of these two agents in combination, compared to the three-fold increase with HYB-241 alone or four-fold increase with verapamil alone.

The most intriguing aspect of these studies has been the observation that HYB-241 alone, in the absence of drug, results in a 40% growth inhibition of the MDR MC-IXC/VCR cells, while having no effect on the growth of the drug-sensitive parent

Table 3. Effect of HYB-241 on cytotoxicity and intracellular drug accumulation in MC-IXC/VCR cells

Drug	ED_{50} (μg/ml) − antibody	ED_{50} (μg/ml)[a] + antibody	Fold increase drug uptake
Vincristine	6	2	3 (7)[b]
Actinomycin-D	0.5	0.08	8
Doxorubicin	0.1	0.1	–

[a] ED_{50} values are corrected for effect of antibody alone
[b] Fold increase in drug uptake in presence of antibody plus verapamil (10 μg/ml)

cell line MC-IXC. The ability to inhibit cell growth by interfering with Pgp function in the absence of a cytotoxic drug identifies a collateral sensitivity which has developed as a direct result of cells becoming drug-resistant. A similar and consistent finding has been the observed sensitivity of MDR cells to the growth inhibitory effects of verapamil or nicardipine alone. This effect directly correlates with the degree of resistance to cytotoxic agents and the level of Pgp expression (Biedler et al. 1988). It therefore appears that in MDR cells, Pgp function, even in the absence of cytotoxic agents, is a vital cellular process.

Clinical Studies of Multidrug Resistance

We are currently examining a variety of solid tumors and hematologic malignancies for evidence of Pgp expression and function. In several patients with relapsed acute lymphocytic leukemia, clinically resistant to anthracyclines and vinca alkaloids, Pgp can be readily detected by flow cytometry (Dr. M. Anoreef, personal communication). Using cells from these patients we have found that the intracellular levels of vincristine can be increased by 30%–100% by exposure of cells in vitro to either verapamil or Mab HYB-241. Thus, at least in the few cases studied, we can identify a functional role for Pgp in regulating intracellular drug levels in these clinically drug-resistant human leukemic cells. Further studies in a larger number of patients will be necessary to determine the possible clinical importance of these observations.

References

Alt FW, Kellems RE, Bertino JR, Schimke RT (1978) Multiplication of dihydrofolate reductase genes in methotrexate resistant variants of cultural murine cells. J Biol Chem 253:1357–1370
Berger S (1988) Mol Pharmacol 34:474
Biedler JL, Riehm H (1970) Cellular resistance to actinomycin-D in Chinese hamster cells: cross-resistance, radioautographic and cytogenetic studies. Cancer Res 30:174
Biedler JL, Meyers MB, Spengler BA (1988) Collateral sensitivity of multidrug-resistant Chinese hamster cells to calcium channel blockers: correlation with P-glycoprotein content. Proc Am Assoc Cancer Res 29:1171

Chen C, Chin JE, Ueda K, Clark DP, Patan I, Gottesman MM, Robinson IB (1986) Internal duplication and homology with bacterial transport proteins in the *mdr*1 (P-glycoprotein) gene from multidrug resistant human cells. Cell 47:381

Gros P, Ben Neriah Y, Croop JM, Housman DE (1986) Isolation and expression of a complimentary DNA that confers multidrug resistance. Nature 223:728

Haber DA, Beverly SM, Kiely ML, Schimke RT (1981) Properties of an altered dihydrofolate reductase encoded by amplified genes in cultures of mouse fibroblasts. J Biol Chem 256:9501–9510

Hamada H, Tsuruo T (1986) Functional role for the 170-180 KDa glycoprotein specific to drug resistant tumor cells as revealed by monoclonal antibodies. Proc Natl Acad Sci USA 83:7785

Hamada H, Tsuruo T (1988) Purification of the P-glycoprotein associated with multidrug resistance. J Biol Chem 256:1454

Jackson RC, Fry DN, Boritzki JF, Besserer JA, Loopolo WR, Sloan BJ, Elslager EF (1984) Biochemical pharmacology of the lipophilic antifolate, trimetrexate. Adv Enzyme Regul 22:187–206

Juliano RL, Ling V (1976) A surface glycoprotein modulating drug permeability in Chinese hamster ovary cell mutants. Biochim Biophys Acta 445:152

Kamen BA, Eibl B, Cashmore AR, Bertino JR (1984) Uptake and efficacy of trimetrexate, a nonclassical antifolate in methotrexate-resistant leukemia cells, in vitro. Biochem Pharmacol 33: 1697–1699

Lin JT, Bertino JR (1987) Trimetrexate: a second generation folate antagonist in clinical trial. J Clin Oncol 5:2032–2040

Melera PW, Lewis JA, Biedler JL, Hession C (1980) Antifolate resistant Chinese hamster cells. Evidence for dihydrofolate reductase gene amplification among independently derived sublines overproducing different dihydrofolate reductase. J Biol Chem 255:7024–7028

Mini E, Moroson BA, Franco CT, Bertino JR (1985) Cytoxic effects of folate antagonists against methotrexate-resistant human leukemia lymphoblastic CCRF-CEM cell lines. Cancer Res 45: 325–330

Pizzorno G, Mini E, Coronello M, McGuire JJ, Moroson BA, Cashmore AA, Dreyer RN, Lin JT, Mazzei T, Periti P, Bertino JR (1988) Impaired polyglutamylation of methotrexate as a cause of resistance in CCRF-CEM cells after short-term, high dose treatment with this drug. Cancer Res 48:2149–2155

Rittman-Grauer L, Wilson B, Leung J, Biedler JL (1986) Monoclonal antibodies to human multidrug resistant cells. Proc Am Assoc Cancer Res 78:1564

Rodenhuis S, McGuire JJ, Narayanan R, Bertino JR (1986) Development of an assay system for the detection and classification of methotrexate resistance in fresh human leukemic cells. Cancer Res 46:6513–6519

Safa AR, Glover CJ, Meyers MB, Biedler JL, Felsted RL (1986) Vinblastine photoaffinity labeling of a high molecular weight membrane glycoprotein specific for multidrug resistant cells. J Biol Chem 261:6137

Safa AR, Glover CJ, Sewell JL, Meyers MB, Biedler JL (1987) Identification of the multidrug resistance-related membrane glycoprotein (gp 150–180) as an acceptor for calcium channel blockers. J Biol Chem 262:7884

Simonson CC, Levinson AD (1983) Isolation and expression of an altered mouse dihydrofolate reductase cDNA. Proc Natl Acad Sci USA 80:2495–2499

Srimatkandada S, Schweitzer BI, Moroson BA, Dube S, Bertino JR (1989) Amplification of a polymorphic dihydrofolate reductase gene with decreased binding to methotroxate, in a human colon carcinoma cell line, HCT8, resistant to this drug. J Biol Chem 264:3524

Tsuruo T, Iida H, Tsukagoshi S, Sakurai Y (1982) Increased accumulation of vincristine and adriamycin in drug resistant P388 tumor cells following incubation with calcium antagonists and calmodulin inhibitors. Cancer Res 42:4730

Whitehead VM, Kalinan TI, Rosenblatt DS (1988) Regulation of methotrexate polyglutamate formation in human leukemia cells. Proc Am Assoc Cancer Res 29:1141 (abstr)

Zamora JM, Pearle HL, Beck WT (1988) Physical-chemical properties shared by compounds that modulate multidrug resistance in human leukemic cells. Mol Pharmacol 23:954

Summary of Discussion: Session 4

P. DRINGS

The main problems for clinicians and for the further development of chemotherapy is the frequent discrepancy between high initial remission rates and the long-term survival of patients. The problem of resistance against chemotherapy is overwhelming. Research is urgently wanted to increase our understanding of the different mechanisms through which resistance is occurring and through which it could possibly be overcome. Our understanding of clinical drug resistance to chemotherapeutic agents is still fragmentary but more information is beginning to emerge. Therefore, clinical resistance was the main point of discussion.

Understanding of pharmacokinetics has an important part to play in the development of antineoplastic chemotherapy, e.g., in reduction of toxicity by modification of the drug administration schedule. For example, it is possible to use regional chemotherapy with 5-fluorouracil to treat liver metastases in patients with colorectal cancer.

There were discussions concerning the comparison of clinical trials. The aim of these discussions was to consider the various cytostatic drugs and their administration schedule, and also the prognostic factors relating to the tumors and the patients. Metastatic breast cancer was discussed as a particularly important example. In many clinical trials a considerable difference is evident between the treatment schedule planned and the actual treatment given. This is especially true in palliative treatment. It is not the treatment alone that is of importance, but also the prognostic factors: aggressive treatment is not indicated in breast cancer patients with a relatively good prognosis. Various methods of treatments have been compared in clinical studies, and it was found that outcome was mainly determined by prognostic factors and not by the type of treatment.

The discussion showed also that the polychemotherapy should be individualized and adapted to the acute toxicity of the respective compounds.

In some tumor types the aggressiveness of chemotherapy can be reduced without loosing efficiency. Thus, in clinical trials of childhood cancer and in Hodgkin's disease, aggressive chemotherapy and X-ray treatment were reduced without loosing efficiency.

It is very important to consider the risk factors in the therapeutic strategy. In chemotherapy of breast cancer, many centers are trying to return to monochemotherapy.

As to the regeneration of the bone marrow after chemotherapy, shorter intervals between the treatment cycles are better than longer ones, so as to avoid tumor cell repopulation.

The mechanism of action of phenylbenzamide was briefly discussed. The mechanism of action of this drug is unclear but it has been speculated that it may be linked to changes in energy metabolism.

As regards the clinical application of the new cytostatics presented, there are various phase-II studies still going on in which lipid ethers are being tested. A clinical phase-I trial testing titanium compounds will be completed this year and the testing of phenylbenzamide will begin in 1989.

The value of animal experiments for the clinical medicine was discussed in detail. At present in the German Cancer Research Center in Heidelberg 12 different autochthonous tumor models in animals are available. Treatment of these relatively resistant tumor types with titan compounds resulted in prolongation of life and reduction of 20% of the tumor weight in comparison to controls.

The question was asked whether only one mechanism or several mechanisms of resistance to methotrexate treatment exist. It also appeared to be of interest whether data exist for trimethotrexate. There are no known mechanisms of methotrexate resistance other than the four mentioned by Dr. Bertino. The toxicity of trimethotrexate for normal organs (liver and kidney) does not differ from that of methotrexate.

With respect to tiazofurin, the question arose whether the compound and/or its metabolites were measured in the blast cells. Metabolic components were measured in plasma but not in the blast cells. The mechanism of action of TAD (tiazofurin adenine dinucleotide) and its therapeutic efficiency in myelodysplasia was discussed. It is not definitely known whether TAD induces an increase in inosine monophosphate dehydrogenase activity and guanisyl triphosphate concentration and whether TAD finally influences the cell differentiation.

Tiazofurin is presently in use in a clinical trial for the therapy of myelodysplasia syndrome; preliminary results are promising.

SESSION 5

Biological Response

Chairman: W. Hunstein

Biological Response Modifiers: Mechanisms of Action

G. A. Nagel, A. Ammon, H. H. Bartsch, K. Krönke, and K. Pfizenmaier

Introduction

After surgery, radiotherapy, and chemotherapy, biological response modifiers (BRMs) have become a fourth category of tumor therapy (Oldham 1982). The basic assumption of the BRM concept is that tumors do not represent an autonomous growth, but are still to some extent under the control of the mechanisms governing cellular, tissue, or organ homeostasis.

The earliest example of the successful application of the BRM concept is endocrine therapy of breast cancer (Becher 1986; Wander 1984). In the last twenty years various other defense mechanisms have been described which have lead to the current concept of tumor cells integrated into environments such as the matrix and the autocrine, paracrine, endocrine and neuroendocrine systems (Fig. 1). In today's clinical practice, therapeutic use is made of the endocrine and paracrine axis only. No other therapeutic indications have resulted, because all other interactions in man are insufficiently understood.

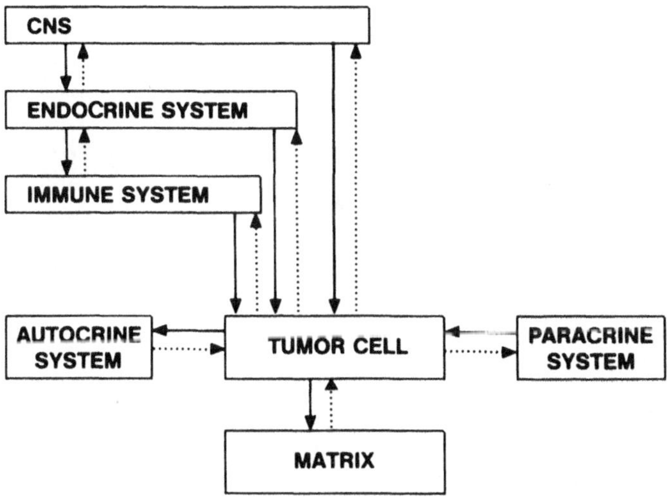

Fig. 1. Host-tumor interactions and possible axes in which use may be made of biological response modifiers. CNS, central nervous system. Effects on tumor cell can be either inhibitory or stimulatory. Tumor cells themselves influence closed response, resulting in, for instance, paraneoplastic syndromes

Two principle mechanisms of BRM action will be discussed: (a) pharmacodynamic effects which interfere with extracellular processes involved in growth control and (b) direct effect of the BRM substance itself in the tumor cell.

Pharmacodynamics of Estrogen Deprivation

Thirty-five percent of all breast carcinomas show estrogen-dependent cell growth activity and can be brought into remission for a certain amount of time by estrogen deprivation (Becher 1986; Wander 1984; Pollow et al. 1988), but they will eventually develop secondary estrogen resistance. The other 65% are primarily estrogen-independent. Before menopause, the female organism synthesizes estrogen in the ovaries under the influence of pituitary gonadotropins. Smaller amounts of estrogens are made independently of gonadotropin influence, mostly in fat and muscle tissue, by peripheral aromatization of androgens secreted by the adrenal cortex (Lipton et al. 1984; Nadjafi 1984). This is then the main source of estrogen in the postmenopausal woman (Lipton et al. 1984). The effects of estrogens in target cells are mediated via estrogen receptors. The cellular synthesis of these receptors is stimulated by estrogens themselves, whereas it is inhibited by gestagens (Lippman et al. 1987; Pollow et al. 1988).

Current concepts of endocrine therapy for breast cancer are entirely based upon principles designed to deprive estrogen-dependent tumor cells of estrogen. These methods are shown in Fig. 2. As of today, there is no clinically available method

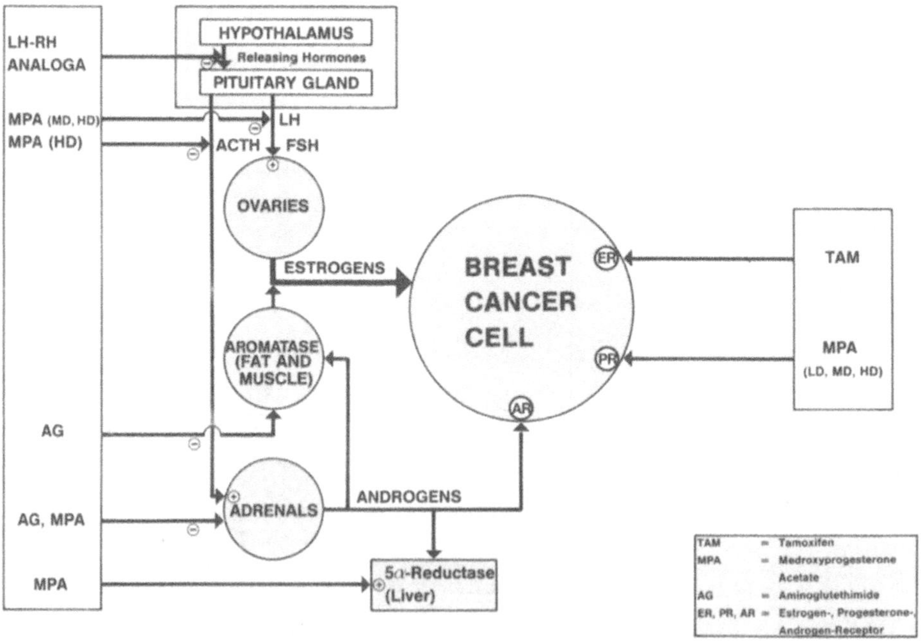

Fig. 2. Endocrine regulation of breast cancer. LD, low dose; MD, medium dose; HD, high dose

of blocking postreceptor events after the estrogen receptor complexes have been formed.

In principle, estrogen deprivation is achieved by:

1. Ablative therapy to interrupt hormone production, i.e., eliminating organs of the endocrine axis which produce estrogens (hypophysectomy, ovarectomy, adrenalectomy; Maass 1985). Since 1985, the development of other effective therapies such as drug-induced hormone deprivation have made endocrine surgery an outdated procedure.
2. Blockage of estrogen synthesis in the ovaries by suppressing stimuli from the hypothalamus and the pituitary gland. There are two major ways to pharmacodynamically interfere with the pituitary-gonadal or pituitary-adrenal axis. The drugs most commonly used are gestagens. As has been shown elsewhere for medroxyprogesterone acetate (MPA), there are three dose-related mechanisms of action of gestagens as antiestrogens (Blossey et al. 1984). At very low doses, gestagens inhibit synthesis of the estrogen receptor without influencing pituitary hormone secretion. An increased dose of MPA suppresses pituitary gonadotropin secretion. At even higher doses, MPA will also block secretion of adrenocorticotropic hormone and stimulate the breakdown of estrogen precursors, namely androgens (Gordon et al. 1971). There is a marked interindividual variation of the doses of MPA needed to reach these effects at the various stages (Wander 1984). The scaled effectiveness of MPA explains why resistance to MPA can be overcome by an increase in dose. The way to block the pituitary–gonadal axis is by luteinizing hormone-releasing hormone (LHRH) analogs (Höffken et al. 1986); this method is still in the clinical phase II trial stage.
3. Inhibition of estrogen synthesis from estrogen precursors by aromatase inhibition. Enzymes of the adrenal cortex, important for the synthesis of androgens as well as microsomal aromatase, which converts androgens to estrogens in peripheral tissue, are specifically inhibited by substances such as aminoglutethimide (Harris et al. 1988; Lipton et al. 1984; Nadjafi 1984; Santen et al. 1982).
4. Prevention of estrogen binding to the receptor by receptor antagonists, antiestrogens, e.g., tamoxifen. These antiestrogens bind at the estrogen receptor without forming an active complex with regard to stimulating the mitotic activity (Noguchi et al. 1988; Pellegrini and Massidda 1982; Wander 1984).

Estrogen/Antiestrogen Resistance

For the development of more effective antiestrogen therapies, it would be important to have a better understanding of the mechanisms of primary and secondary estrogen resistance. Some evidence as to how this resistance develops has emerged only recently. The growth of breast cancer cells from the MCF7 cell line is estrogen-dependent (Albini et al. 1986; Lippman et al. 1987). Transfection with the v-*ras*^{H} oncogene results in estrogen-independent cell growth (Albini et al. 1986; Dickson et al. 1987; Lippman et al. 1987; Roos et al. 1986; Scott Coustin et al. 1986; Stoscheck and King 1986). Like estrogens, the gene product of the v-*ras*^{H} oncogene stimulates the synthesis and secretion of growth factors such as transforming growth factor-α and in-

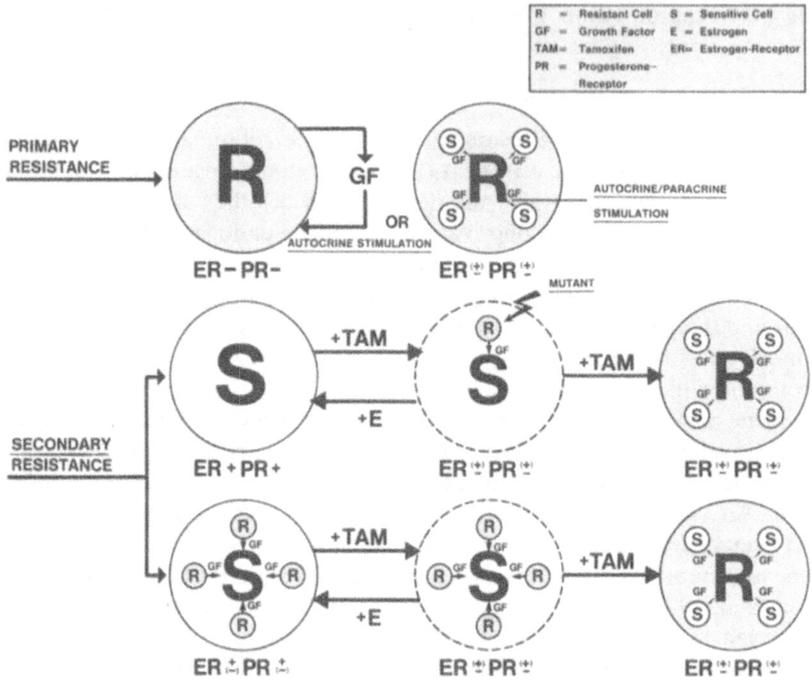

Fig. 3. Primary and secondary resistance of breast cancer to estrogens and antiestrogen therapy

sulin-like growth factor-1 (Albini et al. 1986; Dickson et al. 1987; Lippman et al. 1987; Roos et al. 1986; Scott Coustin et al. 1986; Stoscheck and King 1986). These cells do not lose their estrogen receptors and are still able to bind antiestrogens such as tamoxifen. This binding, however, will not result in arrest of proliferation of the tumor cell (Albini et al. 1986; Dickson et al. 1987; Lippman et al. 1987). From these observations, the following hypothesis about the development of primary and secondary resistance of breast cancer to estrogens evolves (Fig. 3) in the case of primary estrogen resistance, which correlates predominantly with negative estrogen and progesterone receptor status of tumor cells (Wander 1984; Maass 1985), autocrine growth factors maintain self-proliferation. Tumors positive for estrogen and progesterone receptors have shown marked intratumoral heterogeneity as to estrogen receptor expression (Thorpe and Rose 1986). In this case the antiestrogen binds to the estrogen receptor but does not block cell proliferation, because estrogen-independent cell clones within the same tumor would provide paracrine growth factor stimuli. In principle, the same mechanisms are found for secondary resistance. Tumors with positive estrogen and progesterone receptor status sensitive to antiestrogens are considered to contain a high proportion of estrogen-sensitive cell clones without autocrine autonomy. Even if there are some resistant cell clones, a remission would occur if the majority of tumor cells are estrogen-dependent. Following antiestrogen (tamoxifen) therapy, estrogen-independent mutants might occur or overgrow as a result of their growth advantage over estrogen-dependent cell clones; they might also occur in the autocrine and paracrine stages as receptor-positive tumors presenting primary estrogen resistance. Efforts to block such autocrine and paracrine growth factor stimuli are still at the experimental stage (Rochefort et al. 1987).

Tumor Necrosis Factor *α*

Tumor necrosis factor (TNF) was originally identified as a substance in the sera of mice, rats and rabbits, previously treated with Calmette-Guérin bacillus and endotoxin, which caused hemorrhagic necrosis in tumor-bearing mice (Carswell et al. 1975). After the molecular cloning of TNF-*α* cDNA (Pennica et al. 1984), large amounts of the highly purified recombinant cytokine were available for clinical trials and extensive in vitro studies.

Results of first phase I clinical trials with TNF in cancer patients revealed rather modest remission rates (Blick et al. 1987; Creaven et al. 1987; Bartsch et al. 1988). In addition, the definition of the maximal tolerated doses (MTD) for rTNF-*α* revealed a number of side effects. From the oncological perspective, the major questions as to the antitumoral potential of TNF are: how does TNF destroy tumor cells; what determines the responsive state of a tumor target cell; and, how does TNF cause toxic side effects? Clearly, if a rational approach to TNF treatment and therapy of cancer is to be successful, a detailed understanding of the action of TNF in vivo and in vitro is mandatory.

Biological Activities of TNF

The availability of recombinant TNF has sparked extensive laboratory studies. In the past few years, a large body of information has emerged, revealing numerous biological activities of this substance (Old 1985; Beutler and Cerami 1986). Indeed, TNF seems to influence the growth differentiation, function or movement of virtually every cell type investigated (Fig. 4). The complexity of actions makes it difficult to assign a specific role of TNF in vivo. However, TNF is mostly seen as a polypeptide mediator of inflammation and immunological responses. This view is supported by the identity of TNF with cachectin, which has been characterized as an inflammatory substance involved in endotoxin shock and in both acute and chronic infections. The toxic side effects of TNF can be easily explained by its range of inflammatory activities.

Antitumoral Activity of TNF

Its role in inflammation and immunity certainly qualifies TNF as a biological response modifier that eventually contributes to the host's defense against tumors. However, it has been shown that, in addition, TNF is directly cytotoxic for some, but not all tumor cells. The cytolytic activity of TNF seems to be related to its ability to activate phospholipase A2; resulting in the generation of arachidonic acid and release of oxygen radicals (Godfrey et al. 1987). In contrast, the cytostatic action of TNF is associated with its capacity to modulate the expression of genes coding for regulatory proteins (Krönke et al. 1987; Schütze et al. 1988). As shown in Fig. 5a,

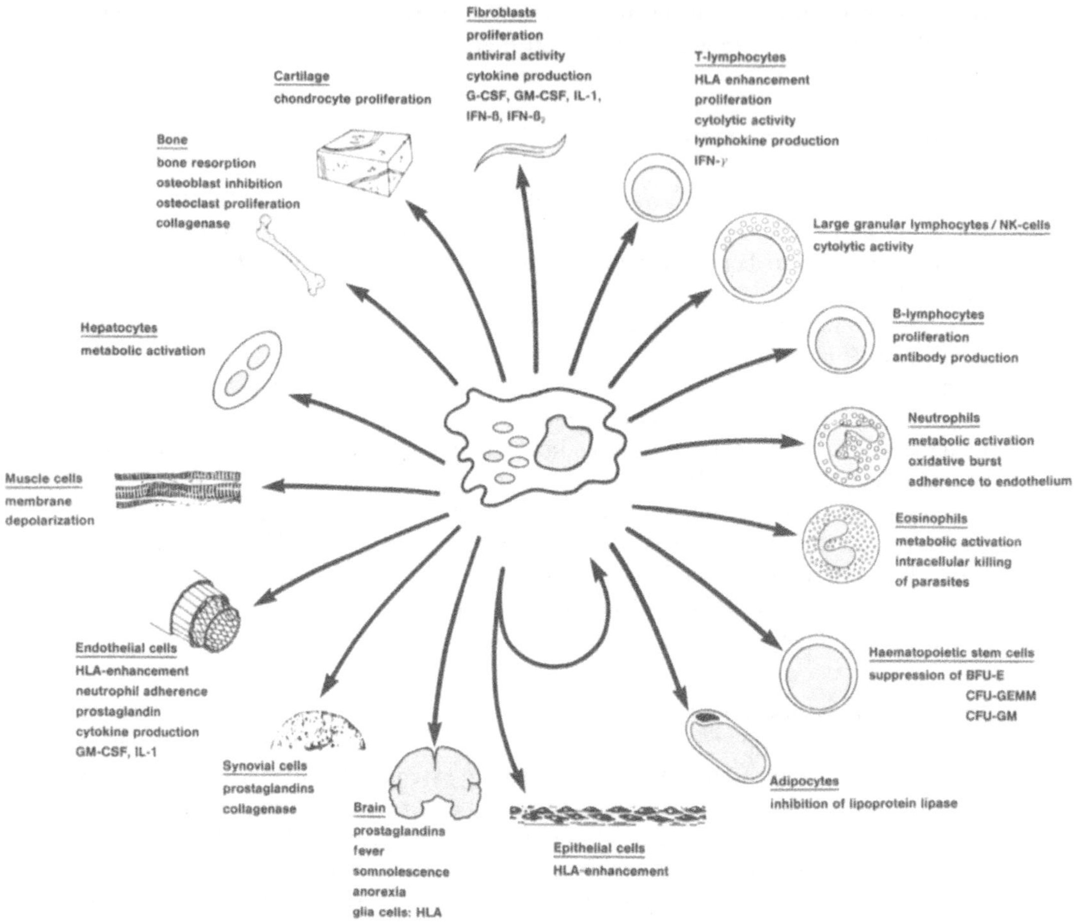

Fig. 4. Actions of TNF-α on normal tissues

TNF reduces the proliferation rate of the human leukemic promyelocytic cell line HL-60. This cytostatic activity of TNF is associated with its ability to decrease mRNA expression in the *myc* oncogene (Fig. 5b), which is highly amplified in HL-60 cells and has been linked to both cell growth and differentiation.

Mechanisms Controlling Resistance to TNF

It is intriguing that TNF is cytotoxic for some, but not all tumor target cells. Little is known about the molecular mechanisms that determine the apparent selectivity of TNF. Deregulated expression of oncogenes has been implicated in the malignant growth of tumor cells. TNF-mediated growth inhibition in general may thus be the result of interference with the expression of one or more oncogenes. As the action of TNF-α requires binding to specific cell surface receptors, TNF sensitivity could be controlled at the level of receptor expression. On the other hand, control at a post-

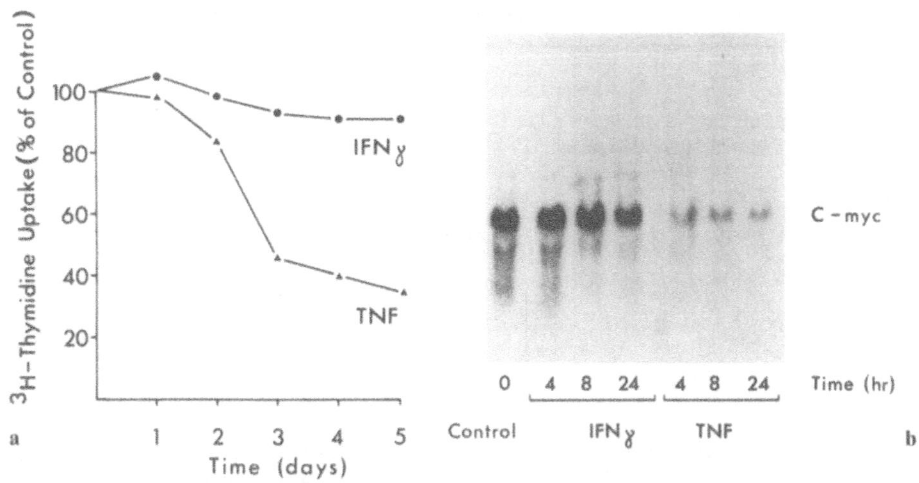

Fig. 5a, b. Cytostatic effects of rTNF-α on HL-60 cells. **a** Cells were treated with either rTNF-α (10 ng/ml) or rIFN-γ (10 ng/ml) and kept a cell density of 105 per milliliter for the times indicated. During the last 6-h cells were incubated with 0.5 Ci [^{3}H]thymidine. Incorporation of [^{3}H]thymidine is expressed in relation to untreated control cells. **b** Inhibitory effects of rTNF-α on *myc* mRNA expression in HL-60 cells. HL-60 cells were untreated *(lane 1)*, treated with rIFN-γ (10 ng/ml; *lanes 2–4*) or rTNF-α (10 ng/ml; *lanes 5–7*) for 4 h *(lanes 2, 5)*, 8 h *(lanes 3, 6)* or 24 h *(lanes 4, 7)*. Twenty micrograms of total cellular RNA was analyzed by RNA gel blotting using a ^{32}P-labeled *myc* (third exon) cDNA probe

receptor level is conceivable. Indeed, recent data suggest that TNF resistance is determined at both levels.

Specific TNF binding sites are apparently constitutively expressed on most, but not all tumor cell lines and primary tumor isolated independent of their tissue origin (Pfizenmaier et al. 1987). While the affinity of binding is within a narrow range (K_d 50–200 pM), a substantial heterogeneity in the quantity of expressed membrane receptors can be found, ranging from 100 to several thousand receptors per cell, depending on the cell line (Kull et al. 1985; Tsujimoto et al. 1985; Scheurich et al. 1986). Initially, this finding raised the question to what extent the number of expressed TNF receptors is directly related to TNF sensitivity. The following observations clarify this question. First, cells lacking specific high-affinity TNF-α binding capacity are resistant to all known actions of TNF. Second, resistance to TNF-α can also be found in cells expressing TNF receptors. From these findings it is apparent that TNF receptor expression is a prerequisite of sensitivity, but itself not sufficient to confer sensitivity. Together, these data indicate that TNF sensitivity of tumor cells must be controlled not only at the level of receptor expression, but also at a post-receptor level.

Development of Resistance to TNF

While some tumors prove to be resistant to TNF, other tumor cells initially sensitive to TNF can develop resistance. With respect to the use of TNF in cancer therapy,

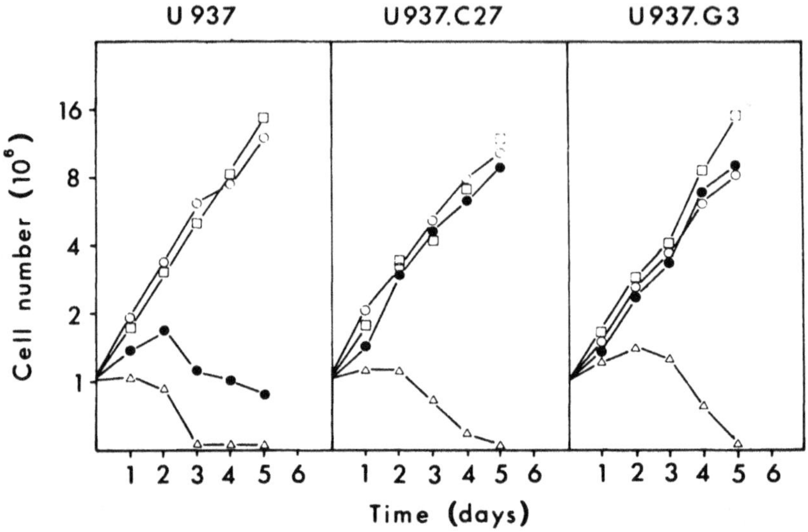

Fig. 6. TNF-α- and IFN-γ-mediated effects on growth of parental U937 cells and their subclones. Cellular proliferation was monitored by microscopic evaluation of aliquots of untreated cultures *(squares)* or cultures treated with 10 ng/ml TNF-α *(open circles)*, 10 ng/ml IFN-γ *(filled circles)*, or a combination of both *(triangles)*. Cells were seeded at a density of 3×10^5 cells/ml (viability 98%) in Click's RMPI 1640 culture medium supplemented with 5% fetal calf serum. Viability was determined by eosin dye exclusion and numbers of viable cells are shown

development of resistance is a serious problem. Some of the processes linked to the development of TNF resistance can be studied in in vitro tumor cell models (Schütze et al. 1988). As shown in Fig. 6, a human histiocytic leukemic cell line, U937, is highly susceptible to the cytostatic action of TNF. A spontaneous variant, C27, obtained by limiting dilution, proved to be TNF-resistant. Such TNF-resistant subclones occur at a frequency of 1/50 and illustrate the heterogeneity of a given tumor. TNF-resistant subclones can be easily selected for by culturing parental U937 cells in the presence of TNF (G3). What distinguishes these subclones from their parental TNF-sensitive U937 cells?

U937, C27, and G3 cells are not distinguishable by morphology or other parameters of monocytic differentiation, such as nonspecific esterase staining, nitroblue tetrazolium reduction, or functional properties like phagocytosis and cell adherence. However, subclones C27 and G3 differ from parental U937 cells by expression of Fc receptors for mouse IgG_1, IgG_2 and IgM (Fig. 7). Also shown in Fig. 7 are the increments of Fc receptor expression induced by TNF and/or interferon-γ. Since Fc receptors are regarded as one marker of monocytic differentiation, these data indicate that (a) C27 and G3 cells may represent discrete higher stages of monocyte differentiation compared to parental U937 cells, and (b) that TNF induces differentiation processes in U937 and C27 cells but not in G3 cells. C27 and G3 cells express a similar number of both high-affinity TNF and interferon-γ receptors when compared to parental U937 cells (not shown), indicating that the different reactivity of the two subclones to TNF is not due to lack of respective receptor expression, but rather must be determined at a postreceptor level. Like many hormone-receptor systems, TNF signal

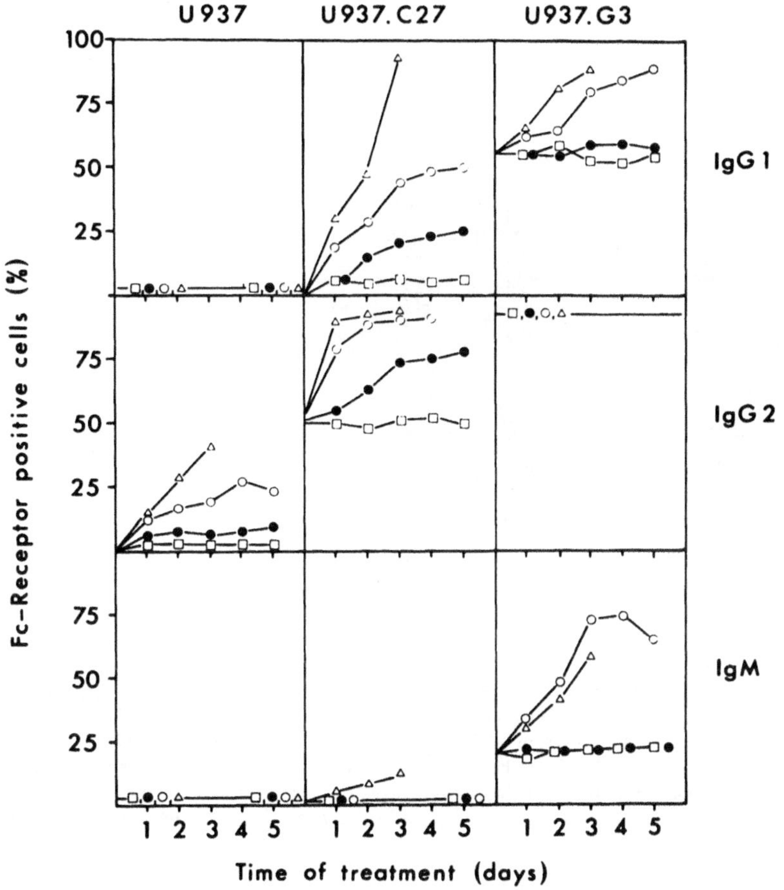

Fig. 7. Expression of Fc receptors by TNF-α- and/or IFN-γ-treated U937 subclones. *Squares,* untreated controls; *open circles,* treatment with 10 ng/ml TNF-α; *filled circles,* 10 ng/ml IFN-γ; *triangles,* a combination of both. The cells were sequentially incubated with murine antibodies of IgG1, IgG2, and IgM subclasses normally used as control antibodies of unknown specificity (Coulter, Krefeld, FRG) followed by incubation with affinity-purified fluorescein isothiocyanate-labeled goat anti-mouse immunoglobulin (Medac, Hamburg, FRG) for 45 min at 0°C. Flow cytometry was performed in an Epics C cytofluorograph. The percentage of positive cells was determined by subtraction of background staining with the goat/antimouse antibody alone and calculated with the Immuno program provided by Coulter

transduction involves protein kinases activating or inactivating enzymes by phosphorylation (Hensel et al. 1987; Schütze et al. 1988). When membrane phosphoprotein patterns of U937 and its two derivatives were compared, clear differences became apparent (Fig. 8), suggesting that altered intracellular signal transduction may account for the differential responsiveness to TNF. Indeed, TNF induces phosphorylation of a cytosolic protein of M_r 26 kDa only in U937 and C27, not in G3 cells (Fig. 9), suggesting that this phosphoprotein may play a role in the TNF signaling pathway linked to differentiation processes rather than to growth control. This model shows a plasticity of the responsive state of three closely related cell lines,

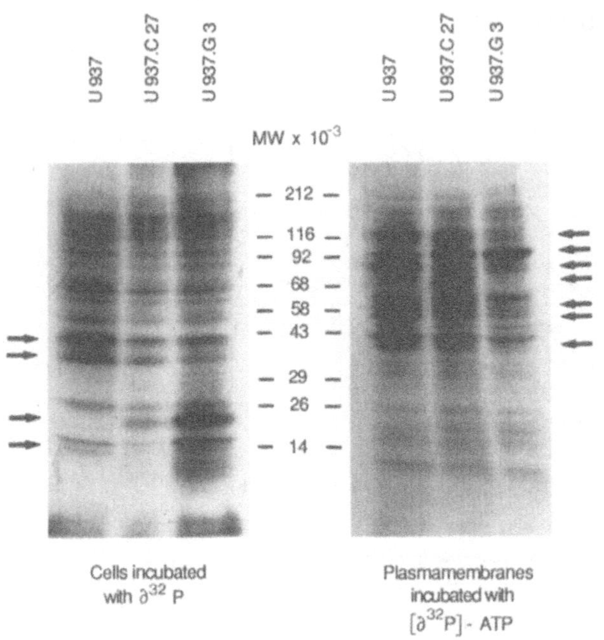

Fig. 8. Constitutive membrane phosphoprotein patterns in U937-subclones. *Left:* Phosphorylation of membrane proteins after labelling of parental U937 *(lane 1)*, U937.C27 *(lane 2)*, and U937.G3 *(lane 3)* cells with [^{32}P] phosphate and subsequent isolation of plasma membranes. *Right:* Phosphorylation of proteins in plasma membranes isolated from U937 *(lane 4)*, U937.C27 *(lane 5)* and U937.G3 *(lane 6)* cells before incubation with [^{32}P] ATP. Phosphoproteins were analyzed on 5%–20% gradient sodium dodecyl sulfate-polyacrylamide gel electrophoresis and autoradiographed with Kodak XAR films at −80°C. Main differences in protein phosphorylation between the subclones are indicated by *arrows*

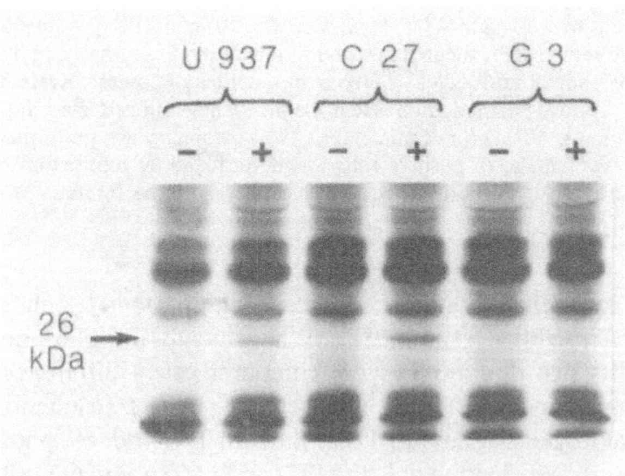

Fig. 9. TNF-induced phosphorylation of a 26 kDA protein in U937 cells and subclones. Cells were labeled with ^{32}P and treated with 20 ng/ml TNF for 10 min at 37°C (+) or left untreated as control (−). Phosphoproteins were analyzed by 7.5% sodium dodecyl sulfate-polyacrylamide electrophoresis

probably due to altered signal transduction pathways. Moreover, the changes in the manner of assimilation of TNF in turn seem to depend – at least in part – on the differentiation status. Since TNF itself is able to induce U937 cell differentiation, there might be only a narrow "window" during monocytic differentiation for the cytostatic action of TNF.

References

Albini A, Graf J, Kitten GT, Kleinmann HK, Martin GR, Veillette A, Lippman ME (1986) 17β-Estradiol regulates and v-Ha-*ras* transfection constitutively enhances MCF7 breast cancer cell interactions with basement membrane. Proc Natl Acad Sci USA 83:8182–8186

Bartsch HH, Nagel GA, Flener R, Mull R, Pfizenmaier K (1988) Phase I trial of recombinant tumor necrosis factor-alpha in patients with advanced malignancies. Mol Biother 1:21–29

Becher R (1986) Der Stellenwert der Hormontherapie im Gesamtkonzept der Behandlung des Mammakarzinoms. In: Höffken K (ed) Aktuelle Aspekte der Hormontherapie des Mammakarzinoms. Enke, Stuttgart, pp 14–24

Beutler B, Cerami A (1986) Cachectin and tumour necrosis factor as two-sides of the same biological coin. Nature 320:584–588

Blick A, Sherwin DA, Rosenblum M, Guttermann J (1987) Phase I study of recombinant tumor necrosis factor in cancer patients. Cancer Res 47:2986–2989

Blossey HC, Wander HE, Koebberling J, Nagel GA (1984) Pharmacokinetic and pharmacodynamic basis for the treatment of metastatic breast cancer with high doses of medroxyprogesterone acetate. Cancer 54:1208–1215

Carswell EA, Old LJ, Kassel RL, Green S, Firoe N, Williamson TS (1975) An endotoxin-induced serum factor that causes necrosis of tumors. Proc Natl Acad Sci USA 25:3666–3670

Creaven PF, Plager JE, Dupere S, Huben RP, Takita H, Mittelman A, Proefrock A (1987) Phase I clinical trial of recombinant human tumor necrosis factor. Cancer Chemother Pharmacol 20: 137–144

Dickson RB, Kasid A, Huff KK, Bates SE, Knabbe C, Bronzer HD, Gelmann EP, Lippman ME (1987) Activation of growth factor secretion in tumorigenic states of breast cancer induced by 17β-estradiol or v-Ha-*ras* oncogene. Proc Natl Acad Sci USA 84:837–841

Godfrey RW, Johnson WJ, Hoffstein ST (1987) Recombinant tumor necrosis factor and interleukin-1 both stimulate human synovial cell arachidonic acid release and phospholipid metabolism. Biochem Biophys Res Commun 142:235–243

Gordon GG, Altmann K, Southern AL, Olivo J (1971) Human hepatic testosterone a-ring reductase activity; effect of medroxyprogesterone acetate. J Clin Endocrin Metab 32(4):457–461

Harris AL, Dowsett M, Jeffocate SL, McKinna JR, Morgan M, Smith IE (1980) Endocrine and therapeutic effects of aminoglutethimide in premenopausal patients with breast cancer. J Clin Endocrin Metab 55(4):718–722

Hensel G, Männel D, Pfizenmaier K, Krönke M (1987) Autocrine stimulation of TNF-alpha-mRNA expression in HL60 cells. Lymphokine Res 6:119–125

Höffken K, Miller AA, Miller B, Becher R, Schmidt CG (1986) Neue Substanzen in der Hormontherapie des Mammakarzinoms. In: Höffken K (ed) Aktuelle Aspekte der Hormontherapie des Mammakarzinoms. Enke, Stuttgart, pp 1–13

Krönke M, Schlüter C, Pfizenmaier K (1987) Tumor necrosis factor inhibits MYC expression in HL60 cells at the level of mRNA transcription. Proc Natl Acad Sci USA 84:469–473

Kull FC Jr, Jacobs S, Cuatrecasas C (1985) Cellular receptor for ^{125}I-labeled tumor necrosis factor: specific binding, affinity labeling, and relationship to sensitivity. Proc Natl Acad Sci USA 82: 5756–5760

Lippman M, Dickson RB, Gelmann EP, Rosen N, Knabbe C, Bates S, Bronzeit D, Huff K, Kasid A (1987) Growth regulation of human breast carcinoma occurs through regulated growth factor secretion. J Cell Biochem 35:1–16

Lipton A, Santen RJ, Harvey HA (1984) Aminoglutethimid beim metastasierenden Mammakarzinom. In: Nagel GA, et al (eds) Aminoglutethimid: ein Antiöstrogen mit Aromatasehemmung. Zuckschwerdt, Munich, pp 20–34 (Aktuelle Onkologie, vol 9)

Maass H (1985) Gesicherte und neue Trends in der Behandlung des Mammakarzinoms. In: Herfarth C, et al (ed) Das Mammakarzinom. Karger, Basel, pp 91–101 (Beiträge zur Onkologie, vol 22)
Nadjafi C (1984) Aminoglutethimid: Chemie, Pharmakokinetik, Pharmakologie, Wirkungsmechanismus. In: Nagel GA, et al (eds) Aminoglutethimid: ein Antiöstrogen mit Aromatasehemmung. Zuckschwerdt, Munich, pp 1–11 (Aktuelle Onkologie, vol 9)
Noguchi S, Miyanchi K, Nishizawa Y, Koyama H (1988) Induction of progesterone receptor with tamoxifen in human breast cancer with special reference to its behavior over time. Cancer 61: 1345–1349
Old LJ (1985) Tumor necrosis factor (TNF) Science 230:630–632
Oldham RK (1982) Biological response modifiers program. J Biol Response Mod 1:81
Pellegrini A, Massidda B (1982) Endokrine Aspekte bei der Behandlung des Brustkrebses. In: Lanius P, et al (eds) German-Italian Oncology Symposium Milan. Kehrer, Freiburg, pp 25–30
Pennica D, Nedwin GE, Hayflick JS, Seebering PH, Derynek R, Palladino MA, Kohr WJ, Aggarwal BA, Goeddel DV (1984) Human tumor necrosis factor: precursor structure, expression and homology to lymphotoxin. Nature 312:724–729
Pfizenmaier K, Scheurich P, Schlüter C, Krönke M (1987) Tumor necrosis factor enhances HLA-A,B,C and HLA-DR gene expression in human tumor cells. J Immunol 138:975–980
Pollow K, Kreienberg R, Grill HJ (1988) Pharmakokinetische und klinische Untersuchungen zur hochdosierten oralen Medroxyprogesteronacetat (MPA-) Therapie beim fortgeschrittenen metastasierenden Mammakarzinom. Tumor Diagnost Therap 9:7–1334
Rochefort H, Capony H, Garcia M, Cavaillis V, Freiss G, Chambon M, Morisset M, Vignon F (1987) Estrogen-induced lysosomal proteases secreted by breast cancer cells: a role in carcinogenesis? J Cell Biochem 35:17–29
Roos W, Fabbio D, King W, Costa SD, Eppenberger U (1986) Correlation between hormone dependency and the regulation of epidermal growth factor receptor by tumor promoters in human mammary carcinoma cells. Proc Natl Acad Sci USA 83:991–995
Santen RJ, Samojlik E, Wells SA (1982) Resistance of the ovary to blockade of aromatization with aminoglutethimide. J Clin Endocrinol Metab 51,3:473–477
Scheurich P, Ücer U, Krönke M, Pfizenmaier K (1986) Quantification and characterization of high-affinity membrane receptors for tumor necrosis factor on human leukemic cell lines. Int J Cancer 38:975–980
Schütze S, Scheurich P, Schlüter C, Ücer C, Pfizenmaier K, Krönke M (1988) Tumor necrosis factor-induced changes of gene expression of U937 cells: differentiation-dependent plasticity of the responsive state. J Immunol 140:3000–3005
Scott Coustin A, Leof EB, Shipley GD, Moses HL (1986) Growth factors and cancer. Cancer Res 46:1015–1029
Stoscheck CM, King LE Jr (1986) Role of epidermal growth factor in carcinogenesis. Cancer Res 46:1030–1037
Thorpe SM, Rose C (1986) Oestrogen and progesterone receptor determinations in breast cancer: technology and biology, Cancer Surv 5(3):505–525
Tsujimoto M, Yip YK, Vilcek J (1985) Tumor necrosis factor: Specific binding and internalization in sensitive and resistant cells. Proc Natl Acad Sci USA 82:7626–7630
Wander HE (1984) Hormonelle Therapie beim metastasierenden Mammakarzinom. Onkologisches Forum für Chemotherapie 2:1–4

Biological Response Modifiers: Clinical Aspects

N. NIEDERLE

Introduction

Until recently, treatment of disseminated malignant disease was limited to administration of cytostatic drugs. This approach can induce complete remissions and even cures, but it is often limited by lack of drug specificity and development of secondary resistance (Chabner 1986; Dexter and Leith 1986; Schnipper 1986). Major efforts are, therefore, now being directed towards development of new drugs which can directly alter the interactions between tumor and host, such as biological response modifiers.

In recent years, several biological agents including interferons, tumor necrosis factor, interleukins, and colony stimulating factors have been introduced into the systemic treatment of cancer (Table 1; Dinarello and Mier 1987; Fauci et al. 1987). These polypeptides regulate the growth, differentiation, and function of cells involved in immunity, inflammation, and hematopoiesis (Old 1987). Via these pathways, they are thought to influence the biological reactions between host and tumor cells, or they may exert a direct antiproliferative effect on normal and transformed cells. Among these drugs, the interferons, described in 1957 by Isaacs and Lindenmann, may be regarded as prototype substances.

Table 1. Biological response modifiers of probable clinical relevance

Interferon (IFN)	IFN-α
	IFN-β
	IFN-γ
Tumor necrosis factor (TNF)	TNF-α
	TNF-β
Interleukin (IL)	IL 1
	IL-2
	IL-3
	IL-4
	IL-5
	IL-6
Colony stimulating factors (CSF)	G-CSF
	GM-CSF
	M-CSF

Interferons

Types

Today, three types of natural and recombinant interferons are undergoing clinical evaluation (Kirchner 1984; Niederle 1988; Pestka 1986; Smyth et al. 1987; Taylor-Papadimitriou 1984): alpha interferons, which are derived from leukocytes, monocytes and lymphoblastoid cells, beta interferons which are usually derived from fibroblasts; and immune or gamma interferons, which are derived from T lymphocytes (Table 2). The natural interferons each represent a mixture of proteins with a specific activity of $1\text{–}3 \times 10^6$ units per milligram protein. The corresponding recombinant types possess a specific activity of $1\text{–}4 \times 10^8$ units per milligram protein. It is the large-scale industrial production of these recombinant types that has made clinical trials feasible.

Alpha interferons consist of a family of about 20 closely related proteins, beta interferons probably consist of two subtypes, and gamma interferon occurs as a single subtype. All in all, alpha and beta interferons are structurally and functionally closely related, while gamma interferons are almost totally different (Gray and Goeddel 1982; Jung et al. 1987; Kelley et al. 1985; Shows et al. 1982). These differences are shown by the number of genes and their location on different chromosomes, the number of amino acids and their homology, and – clinically very important – the binding to specific membrane receptors, of which there is one class for alpha and beta interferons and another for gamma interferon (Branca and Baglioni 1981).

Table 2. Different types of interferon

	INF-α	INF-β_1	INF-β_2	INF-γ
Chromosome	9p	9p	7	12q
Gene	>20	1	1	1
Amino acids	165–166	166	184	143
Molecular weight (KD)	16–20	19	21	17
Glycosylation				
– natural type	–	+	?	+
– recombinant type	–	–		–
Receptor gene (chromosome)	21	21	?	6
Producing cells	Monocytes B-lymphocytes	Fibroblasts	Fibroblasts Monocytes T-lymphocytes	T-lymphocytes

Mode of Action

Binding to specific receptors triggers as yet undefined second messages which transmit regulatory signals to the nucleus or the cell membrane (Hovanessian et al. 1977). Ultimately, a change in the pattern of cellular ribonucleic acid and protein synthesis occurs, with some proteins being switched off and others strongly induced, resulting in altered cellular function.

Theoretically, interferons are believed to exert their antitumor effects in three ways: via the host immune system, by altering some nonimmune host/tumor cell interactions, or by direct effects on the tumor cells (Vilcek et al. 1980). So far, there is little evidence either in laboratory mice or in patients that interferons act via an enhancement of host antitumor immune response, except in the prophylaxis of experimental murine pulmonary metastases. There is, however, considerable evidence that the host may play a role in the effects of interferons. Data indicate an effect on host interaction with the tumor besides involvement of the host immune system. Interferon therapy may interfere with some vital host nutrient or growth factors, or may limit development of an effective stroma, e.g., by inhibiting angiogenesis.

There is a large body of knowledge on the direct action of interferons on tumor cells. At a molecular level, interferons can decrease some messenger ribonucleic acids, which are induced when cells pass through the G_0/G_1 phase of the cell cycle (Einat et al. 1985). Further direct actions of interferons on tumor cells might be changes in cytoskeleton, alterations of membrane structures, and induction of cell differentiation (Pfeffer et al. 1980; Trinchieri and Perussia 1985).

Clinical Data

In most trials, different natural and recombinant products were administered by different routes and in a variety of schedules. Schedule dependency can be shown by pharmacokinetic studies of intravenous, intramuscular, and subcutaneous administration of interferons (Niederle et al. 1987a).

The most impressive results have been achieved in hairy cell leukemia. Since the first report by Quesada and coworkers (1984), several hundred patients have been treated with interferons. Both natural and recombinant alpha interferons are effective in hairy cell leukemia. The remission rates are in the range of 70%–90%, including 10%–30% complete remissions (Niederle and Kloke 1987). So far, response rates are similar in previously untreated patients, splenectomized patients and patients pretreated with cytostatic drugs, although some investigators have reported a higher incidence of complete remissions in the previously untreated group (Golomb et al. 1987; Quesada et al. 1986). All in all, alpha interferons have a significant impact on the course of disease, but they do not seem to be curative, since responses are not durable and patients tend to relapse within 9–12 months after cessation of treatment (Hofmann and Frey 1988; Kloke et al. 1988b; Quesada et al. 1986; Ratain et al. 1987).

In contrast to the positive results with alpha interferons, there is, as yet, no evidence that gamma interferon has a significant effect in hairy cell leukemia patients (Niederle et al. 1987a). The clinically observed difference in the effects of alpha and

Table 3. Hematologic malignancies: results of interferon treatment

Disease	Objective responses (%)	Complete remissions (%)
Hairy cell leukemia	70–90	10–30
Cutaneous T-cell lymphoma	40–60	10
Chronic lymphatic leukemia	10–20	–
Multiple myeloma	15–25	2
Other lymphomas		
– low malignancy (nodular)	40–50	<10
– high malignancy	10	–
Chronic myelogenous leukemia	50–70	~10

gamma interferons on the proliferation of hairy cells was confirmed by laboratory investigations (Paganelli et al. 1986). The different antiproliferative activities of the two cytokines might be due to the fact that alpha interferon is able to interrupt an autocrine loop created by the synthesis of interleukin 4/6 in hairy cells – especially since in active hairy cell leukemia the production of alpha but not gamma interferon seems to be depressed (Ford et al. 1986; Porzsolt et al. 1986). In any case, the effectiveness of alpha interferon treatment in hairy cell leukemia does not appear to be mediated by natural killer cells (Gastl et al. 1986; Sigaux et al. 1987).

Alpha interferon has been shown to be effective in other hematologic malignancies as well – for instance, cutaneous T-cell lymphoma, where objective remissions were documented in 40%–60% of patients who had failed to respond to one or more standard forms of treatment, including systemic chemotherapy (Bunn et al. 1987; Foon et al. 1987; Leavitt et al. 1987). Median duration of response was 5.5 months. Moreover, clinical trials have confirmed the effectiveness of both natural and recombinant alpha interferons in a large number of patients with multiple myeloma (Ahre et al. 1988; Alexanian et al. 1982; Cooper and Welander 1987; Costanzi et al. 1985). The results can be summarized as follows: Remission rates, usually partial ones, are in the range of 15%–25% (Table 3). Objective response rates seem to be higher among patients relapsing after chemotherapy induced remission than among patients who are primarily refractory to conventional treatment. Further positive prognostic factors might be low tumor mass, no pretreatment, and immunoglobulin A myeloma.

Subsequently, treatment with melphalan/prednisone or the more intensive vincristine/melphalan/cyclophosphamide/prednisolone combination was compared to alpha interferon treatment in two prospective randomized trials (Ahre et al. 1984; Ludwig et al. 1986). In these studies, combination chemotherapy induced significantly more and longer-lasting remissions than the interferon monotherapy. Overall survival, however, was similar in both groups. Prospective randomized studies are now being conducted to compare standard drug regimes with or without alpha interferons (Ludwig et al. 1987; Mandelli et al. 1988; Österborg et al. 1987).

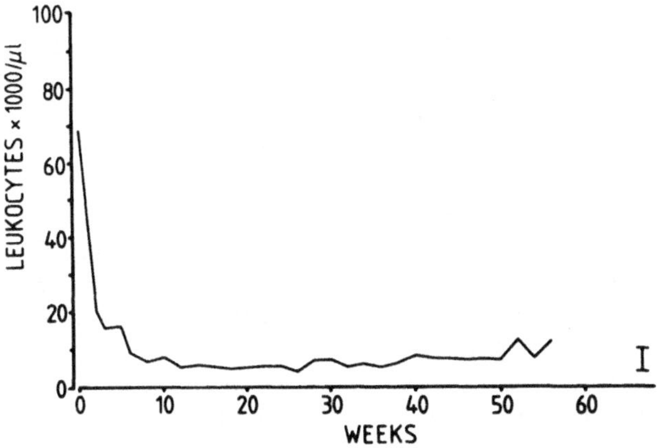

Fig. 1. Chronic myelogenous leukemia: median leukocyte counts in patients who responded to treatment with alpha$_2$ interferon

Interferons have been administered to several hundred pretreated patients with different types of non-Hodgkin's lymphoma who were no longer responding to conventional chemotherapy. In patients with lymphomas of low malignancy, particularly with nodular or follicular histologic patterns, objective response rates between 40%–50% were obtained (Foon et al. 1987; Leavitt et al. 1987). On the other hand, lymphomas of intermediate and high malignancy were relatively resistant to interferon therapy (Table 3). In pretreated chronic lymphocytic leukemia, moreover, alpha interferons seem to have little efficacy (Foon et al. 1985; O'Connell et al. 1986). It was even reported that the comparatively stable or slowly progressing disease of five patients accelerated while they were being treated with interferon (Foon et al. 1985). In untreated disease, however, there might be a place for interferon application (Pangalis and Griva 1988).

Chronic myelogenous leukemia can be palliated but not cured by conventional therapies. Since interferon has been shown to have antiproliferative and differentiation activity in normal and leukemic white cell precursors (McGlave et al. 1987; Neumann and Fauser 1982; Williams et al. 1981), its effect on chronic myeloid leukemia was studied (Alimena et al. 1988; Niederle et al. 1987b; Talpaz et al. 1987). More than 60 patients with chronic myeloid leukemia have been treated in our department during the last 3 years. In chronic phase disease, leukocyte and platelet counts decreased in 70%–80% of patients to normal values after 2–40 (median 6) weeks of therapy (Fig. 1). Serum lactate dehydrogenase levels reflected the changes in leukocyte counts and returned to normal after 3–33 weeks. In some patients, however, a dose-response relationship could be demonstrated. If the interferon dose was reduced too fast from the initial level, or the maintenance dose was too low, all blood counts rose, including leukocytes and platelets as well as hemoglobin and lactate dehydrogenase, and the dosage had to be increased again. During this temporary increase of leukocytes, immature myeloid cells reappeared in the differential counts and the percentage of lymphocytes decreased.

Serial molecular analyses using the Southern blot technique and a 5′ *bcr* probe were performed in 55 patients. During an observation period of 3–24 months, a reduction of the malignant *bcr/abl* band could be shown in three patients. In another two patients, a loss of the marker band was observed. Further investigations using a modified polymerase chain reaction technique for the detection of minimal residual *bcr/abl* transcripts are under way (Lee et al. 1988).

It can be concluded from these data that alpha interferon induces considerable and long-lasting cytoreduction in 50%–70% of patients with chronic phase chronic myelogenous leukemia. In addition, the malignant clone marked with the Philadelphia chromosome or the *bcr/abl* rearrangement may disappear in some patients. However, further follow-up is needed to evaluate whether the substance can slow progression of the disease – especially since it appears to be ineffective when the disease is advanced (Alimena et al. 1988; Niederle et al. 1987b).

In recent years, various alpha interferons have been used in the treatment of a wide range of solid tumors (Goldstein and Laszlo 1986; Kirkwood and Ernstoff 1984; Smyth et al. 1987; Spiegel 1987). Most reports have failed to demonstrate antitumor activity of alpha interferons in colorectal carcinoma, breast cancer, small cell and non-small cell lung cancer, and sarcomas (Table 4). Considerable evidence suggests, however, at least some kind of antitumor activity in malignant melanoma, renal cell carcinoma, epithelial ovarian cancer, and bladder cancer. We and others could achieve convincing palliative effects in midgut carcinoid tumors and cancer of the endocrine pancreas using relatively low doses of alpha interferon (Doberauer et al. 1987; Eriksson et al. 1986; Öberg et al. 1986).

The growth of human tumor cells either in vitro or as xenografts in nude mice is generally inhibited by alpha interferon; however, the same tumor cells fail to respond as solid tumors in humans. The simplest explanation for this is that insufficient interferon reaches the tumor cells in the patient. A second possibility is that growth arrest can not be measured in clinical phase I/II trials. A third explanation is that in the complex host/tumor environment, the growth inhibitory properties of interferons are abrogated by an excess of positive growth signals.

In contrast to the positive responses with alpha interferons, there is no concrete evidence, as yet, for clinical efficacy of gamma interferon (Bonnem and Oldham

Table 4. Solid tumors: objective responses to interferon therapy

Disease	Remission rates (CR) (%)
Colorectal cancer	3
Breast cancer	6
Lung cancer	7
Sarcoma	8
Cervical cancer	11
Malignant melanoma	11 (3)
Renal cell cancer	12 (1)
Ovary cancer (regional)	19 (6)
Bladder cancer (topical)	41
Carcinoid	66
Pancreatic cancer (endocrine)	75

Table 5. Some characteristics of tumor necrosis factor alpha

Producing cells	Macrophages	(BCG, C.p., LPS)
Gene	1	
Chromosome	6	(3 Introns)
Amino acids	157	(No glycosylation)
Molecular weight	17 KD	
Receptors	Specific	
Application	IV, IM, SC, IT	

1987; Ohno 1987). No significant benefit has been seen in lymphoma, chronic myelogenous leukemia, a variety of solid tumors, or even hairy cell leukemia.

All in all, however, clinical testing of gamma interferon lags 2–3 years behind that of alpha interferon. It still seems possible that other alpha interferon-resistant tumors may respond to gamma interferon. Recently, for instance, a beneficial impact of low doses of gamma interferon on the growth of renal cell cancer was demonstrated (Aulitzky et al. 1987).

Tumor Necrosis Factor

Tumor necrosis factor alpha is a protein produced by macrophages after activation with *Corynebacterium parvum* or bacillus Calmette-Guérin and subsequent stimulation with lipopolysaccharides (Carswell et al. 1975). The gene coding for human tumor necrosis factor has been cloned and expressed (Shirai et al. 1985). The recombinant human protein product contains 157 amino acids (Table 5). Like interferons, this polypeptide binds to high-affinity receptors on the surface of target cells (Rubin et al. 1985). The product probably exerts a direct effect on tumor cells (Creasey et al. 1987). Another characteristic is that tumor necrosis factor is not species-specific.

The large-scale industrial production of tumor necrosis factor has made broad preclinical and clinical investigations feasible. In preclinical test systems, the response of human tumor cells has been promising (Munker and Koeffler 1987). In clinical trials, however, almost no beneficial results could be demonstrated in single tumor entities.

Common acute side effects associated with treatment using tumor necrosis factor are fever, chills, headache, nausea and vomiting, fatigue, malaise, myalgia, dry mouth, and hypotension. These adverse reactions generally appear within 1–4 h after the initial dose and usually last for some hours (Niederle et al. 1988). Tachyphylaxis is less marked than after interferon application.

Summary

The number of cloned and sequenced polypeptides regulating cell growth and immune function has grown rapidly in recent years. All these different growth regulators have therapeutic potential individually and in combination. Comprehensive clinical data, however, are available only for alpha interferon. Significant activity of this substance could be demonstrated in a number of hematologic malignancies, especially hairy cell leukemia and chronic myelogenous leukemia. Its efficacy in solid tumors is less impressive.

Experimental studies show that cytokines act best when tumor load is low. It is, therefore, both appropriate and important that future areas for research include effects on minimal tumor burden, for instance, intracavitary application or adjuvant therapy following tumor reduction by surgery or cytostatic chemotherapy (Berek et al. 1986; Mattson 1987; Torti et al. 1988).

An interesting alternative to single agent therapy is to combine cytokines with cytostatic drugs. Data from both in vitro and animal models have shown synergistic or additive interactions between interferons and some cytostatic agents, particularly cisplatin, vinblastine, chlorambucil, cyclophosphamide, and melphalan or other therapeutic modalities (Aapro et al. 1983; Balkwill and Moodie 1984; Bonnem 1987; Creagan et al. 1988; Mattson et al. 1985; Saito et al. 1987; Torrisi et al. 1986; Welander et al. 1985). The molecular basis of these interactions is not understood, however: interferons could interfere with drug metabolism in the tumor, or the enhancing activity may depend on direct interactions during the cell cycle.

On the other hand, recent experimental studies have revealed multiple interactions between the various cytokines (Beran et al. 1988; Fleischmann et al. 1984; Kloke et al. 1988a; Quesada 1988; Williamson et al. 1983). These and other data strongly suggest a potential role for the combined administration of tumor necrosis factor and interferons, or, as we were able to demonstrate earlier in patients with chronic myelogenous leukemia, of alpha and gamma interferon in disorders refractory to alpha interferon alone (Kloke et al. 1987). Therefore, when their mode of action is better understood, cytokines may provide a useful tool in anticancer therapy in addition to the already accepted modalities of surgery, radiotherapy, and chemotherapy.

References

Aapro MS, Alberts DS, Salmon SE (1983) Interactions of human leukocyte interferon with vinca alkaloids and other chemotherapeutic agents against human tumors in clonogenic assay. Cancer Chemother Pharmacol 10:161–166

Ahre A, Björkholm M, Mellstedt H, Brenning G, Engstedt L, Gahrton G, Gyllenhammar H, Holm G, Johansson B, Järnmark M, Karnström L, Killander A, Lerner R, Lockner D, Lönnqvist B, Nilsson B, Simonsson B, Stalfelt A-M, Strander H, Svedmyr E, Wadman B, Wedelin C (1984) Human leukocyte interferon and intermittent high-dose melphalan-prednisone administration in the treatment of multiple myeloma: a randomized clinical trial from the Myeloma Group of Central Sweden. Cancer Treat Rep 68:1331–1338

Ahre A, Björkholm M, Österborg A, Brenning G, Gahrton G, Gyllenhammar H, Holm G, Johansson B, Juliusson G, Järnmark M, Killander A, Lerner R, Lockner D, Nilsson B, Simonsson B, Stalfelt A-M, Strander H, Smedmyr B, Svedmyr E, Uden A-M, Wadman B, Wedelin C, Mellstedt H (1988) High doses of natural interferon (IFN) in the treatment of multiple myeloma – a pilot study from the Myeloma Group of Central Sweden (MGCS) Eur J Haematol 41:123–130

Alexanian R, Gutterman J, Levy H (1982) Interferon treatment for multiple myeloma. Clin Haematol 11:211–220

Alimena G, Morra E, Lazzarino M, Liberati AM, Montefusco E, Inverardi D, Bernasconi P, Mancini M, Donti E, Grignani F, Bernasconi C, Dianzani F, Mandelli F (1988) Interferon alpha-2b as therapy for Ph'-positive chronic myelogenous leukemia: a study of 82 patients treated with intermittent or daily administration. Blood 72:642–647

Aulitzky W, Gastl G, Aulitzky WE, Nachbaur K, Lanske B, Kemmler G, Flener R, Frick J, Huber C (1987) Interferon-γ for the treatment of metastatic renal cancer: dose-dependent stimulation and downregulation of beta-2 microglobulin and neopterin responses. Immunobiology 176:85–95

Balkwill FR, Moodie EM (1984) Positive interactions between human interferon and cyclophosphamide or adriamycin in a human tumor model system. Cancer Res 44:904–908

Beran M, McCredie KB, Keating MJ, Gutterman JU (1988) Antileukemic effect of recombinant tumor necrosis factor alfa in vitro and its modulation by alfa and gamma interferons. Blood 72:728–738

Berek JS, Hacker NF, Lichtenstein A, Jung T, Spina C, Knox RM, Brady J, Greene T, Ettinger LM, Lagasse LD, Bonnem EM, Spiegel RJ, Zighelboim J (1986) Intraperitoneal recombinant alpha-interferon for "salvage" immunotherapy in stage III epithelial ovarian cancer: a Gynecologic Oncology Group Study. Semin Oncol [Suppl 2] 8:61–71

Bonnem EM (1987) Alfa Interferon: combinations with other antineoplastic modalities. Semin Oncol [Suppl 2] 14:48–60

Bonnem EM, Oldham RK (1987) Gamma-interferon: physiology and speculation on its role in medicine. J Biol Response Mod 6:275–301

Branca AA, Baglioni C (1981) Evidence that types I and II interferons have different receptors. Nature 294:768–770

Bunn PA Jr, Ihde DC, Foon KA (1987) Recombinant interferon alpha-2a, an active agent in advanced cutaneous T-cell lymphomas. Int J Cancer [Suppl 1] 40:9–13

Carswell EA, Old LJ, Kassel RL, Green S, Fiore N, Williamson B (1975) An endotoxin-induced serum factor that causes necrosis of tumors. Proc Natl Acad Sci USA 72:3666–3670

Chabner BA (1986) The oncologic end game. J Clin Oncol 4:625–638

Cooper MR, Welander CE (1987) Interferons in the treatment of multiple myeloma. Cancer 59: 594–600

Costanzi JJ, Cooper MR, Scarffe JH, Ozer H, Grubbs SS, Ferraresi RW, Pollard RB, Spiegel RJ (1985) Phase II study of recombinant alpha-2 interferon in resistant multiple myeloma. J Clin Oncol 3:654–659

Creagan ET, Long HJ, Frytak S, Moertel CG (1988) Recombinant leukocyte A interferon with doxorubicin. A phase I study in advanced solid neoplasm and implications for hepatocellular carcinoma. Cancer 61:19–22

Creasey AA, Doyle LV, Reynolds MT, Jung T, Lin LS, Vitt CR (1987) Biological effects of recombinant human tumor necrosis factor and its novel muteins on tumor and normal cell lines. Cancer Res 47:145–149

Dexter DL, Leith JT (1986) Tumor heterogeneity and drug resistance. J Clin Oncol 4:244–257

Dinarello CA, Mier JW (1987) Lymphokines. N Engl J Med 317:940–945

Doberauer C, Niederle N, Kloke O, Kurschel E, Schmidt CG (1987) Zur Behandlung des metastasierten Karzinoids von Ileum und Coecum mit rekombinantem Interferon alpha-2b. Onkologie 10:340–344

Einat M, Resnitzky D, Kimchi A (1985) Close link between reduction of c-*myc* expression by interferon and G0/G1 arrest. Nature 313:597–600

Eriksson B, Öberg K, Alm G, Karlsson A, Lundqvist G, Andersson T, Wilander E, Wide L (1986) Treatment of malignant endocrine pancreatic tumours with human leucocyte interferon. Lancet II:1307–1309

Fauci AS, Rosenberg SA, Sherwin SA, Dinarello CA, Longo DL, Lane HC (1987) Immunomodulators in clinical medicine. Ann Intern Med 106:421–433

Fleischmann WR Jr, Newton RC, Fleischmann CM, Colburn NH, Brysk MM (1984) Discrimination between nonmalignant and malignant cells by combinations of IFN-γ and IFN-α/β. J Biol Response Mod 3:397–405

Foon KA, Bottino GC, Abrams PG, Fer MF, Longo DL, Schoenberger CS, Oldham RK (1985) Phase II trial of recombinant leukocyte A interferon in patients with advanced chronic lymphocytic leukemia. Am J Med 78:216–220

Foon KA, Roth MS, Bunn PA Jr (1987) Interferon therapy of non-Hodgkin's lymphoma. Cancer 59:601–604

Ford RJ, Kwok D, Quesada J, Sahasrabuddhe CG (1986) Production of B cell growth factor(s) by neoplastic B cells from hairy cell leukemia patients. Blood 67:573–577

Gastl G, Aulitzky W, Leiter E, Flener R, Huber C (1986) Alpha-interferon induces remission in hairy cell leukemia without enhancement of natural killing. Blut 52:273–279

Goldstein D, Laszlo J (1986) Interferon therapy in cancer: from imaginon to interferon. Cancer Res 46:4315–4329

Golomb HM, Fefer A, Golde DW, Ozer H, Portlock C, Silber R, Rappeport J, Ratain MJ, Thompson J, Bonnem EM, Spiegel RJ, Tensen L, Burke JS, Vardiman JW (1987) Sequential evaluation of alpha-2b-interferon treatment in 128 patients with hairy cell leukemia. Semin Oncol [Suppl 2] 14:13–17

Gray PW, Goeddel DV (1982) Structure of the human immune interferon gene. Nature 298:859–863

Hofmann V, Frey B (1988) Long-term treatment of hairy cell leukemia with interferon alfa-2b. Cancer Treat Rev [Suppl A] 15:7–13

Hovanessian AG, Brown RE, Kerr IM (1977) Synthesis of low-molecular weight inhibitor of protein synthesis with enzyme from interferon-treated cells. Nature 268:537–539

Isaacs A, Lindenmann J (1957) Virus interference. I. The interferon. Proc R Soc Lond [Biol] 147: 258–267

Jung V, Rashidbaigi A, Jones C, Tischfield JA, Shows TB, Pestka S (1987) Human chromosomes 6 and 21 are required for sensitivity to human interferon gamma. Proc Natl Acad Sci USA 84: 4151–4155

Kelley VE, Fiers W, Strom TB (1985) Cloned human interferon-gamma, but not interferon-beta or -alpha, induces expression of HLA-DR determinants by fetal monocytes and myeloid leukemic cell lines. J Immunol 132:240–245

Kirchner H (1984) Interferons, a group of multiple lymphokines. Springer Semin Immunopathol 7: 347–374

Kirkwood JM, Ernstoff MS (1984) Interferons in the treatment of human cancer. J Clin Oncol 2: 336–352

Kloke O, Becher R, Niederle N (1987) Response to the combined administration of interferons alpha and gamma after failure of single interferon therapy in chronic myelogenous leukaemia. Blut 55:453–458

Kloke O, Kummer G, Matika S, Niederle N, Schmidt CG (1988a) Synergistic effects of tumor necrosis factor and interferons alpha-2b on the proliferation and differentiation of HL-60 cells. Proc Am Assoc Cancer Res 29:415

Kloke O, May D, Niederle N (1988b) Zur Dosierung von Interferon-α in der Induktions- und Erhaltungstherapie der Haarzellenleukämie. Onkologie [Suppl 2] 11:41–45

Leavitt RD, Ratanatharathorn V, Ozer H, Ultmann JE, Portlock C, Myers JW, Kisner D, Norred S, Spiegel RJ, Bonnem EM (1987) Alpha-2b interferon in the treatment of Hodgkin's disease and non-Hodgkin's lymphoma. Semin Oncol [Suppl 2] 14:18–23

Lee MS, Chang KS, Freireich EJ, Kantarjian HM, Talpaz M, Trujillo JM, Stass SA (1988) Detection of minimal residual *bcr/abl* transcripts by a modified polymerase chain reaction. Blood 72: 893–897

Ludwig H, Cortelezzi A, Scheithauer W, van Camp BGK, Kuzmits R, Fillet G, Peetermans M, Polli E, Flener R (1986) Recombinant interferon alpha-2c versus polychemotherapy (VMGP) for treatment of multiple myeloma: a prospective randomized trial. Eur J Cancer Clin Oncol 22: 1111–1116

Ludwig H, Cortelezzi A, Fritz E, Kührer I, Polli E, Scheithauer W, Flener R (1987) Combined interferon-polychemotherapy versus polychemotherapy in multiple myeloma: a phase III study. In: Cantell K, Schellekans H (eds) The biology of interferon system 1986. Nijhoff, Dordrecht

Mandelli F, Tribalto M, Avvisati G, Cantonetti M, Petrucci MT, Boccadoro M, Pileri A, Marmont F, Resegotti L, Lauta V, Dammacco F (1988) Recombinant interferon alpha-2b (INTRON A) as post-induction therapy for responding multiple myeloma patients. M84 protocol. Cancer Treat Rep [Suppl A] 15:43–48

Mattson K (1987) Natural alpha interferon as part of a combined treatment for small cell lung cancer. In: Smyth JF (ed) Interferons in oncology: current status and future directions. Springer, Berlin Heidelberg New York, pp 25–32 (ESO monograph)

Mattson K, Holsti LR, Niiranen A, Kivisaari L, Iivanainen M, Sovijärvi A, Cantell K (1985) Human leukocyte interferon as part of a combined treatment for previously untreated small cell lung cancer. J Biol Response Mod 4:8–17

McGlave P, Mamus S, Vilen B, Dewald G (1987) Effect of recombinant gamma interferon on chronic myelogenous leukemia bone marrow progenitors. Exp Hematol 15:331–335

Munker R, Koeffler PH (1987) Tumor necrosis factor: recent advances. Klin Wochenschr 65:345–352

Neumann HA, Fauser AA (1982) Effect of interferon on pluripotent hemopoietic progenitors (CFU-GEMM) derived from human bone marrow. Exp Hematol 10:587–590

Niederle N (1988) Aspekte und Ergebnisse der Therapie mit Interferonen. Arzneimittelforschung [I] 38:449–453

Niederle N, Kloke O (1987) Interferon in the treatment of hairy cell leukemia and chronic myelogenous leukemia. In: Smyth JF (ed) Interferons in oncology: current status and future directions. Springer, Berlin Heidelberg NewYork, pp 11–24 (ESO monograph)

Niederle N, Doberauer C, Kloke O, Höffken K, Schmidt CG (1987a) Zur Wirksamkeit von IFN-γ und IFN-α bei der Haarzellenleukämie. Klin Wochenschr 65:706–712

Niederle N, Kloke O, Osieka R, Wandl U, Opalka B, Schmidt CG (1987b) Interferon alfa-2b in the treatment of chronic myelogenous leukemia. Semin Oncol [Suppl 2] 14:29–35

Niederle N, Moritz T, Kurschel E, Osieka R, Opalka B, Schlick E, Schmidt CG (1988) Recombinant human tumor necrosis factor alfa (TNF) in the treatment of advanced malignancies: a phase I study. Proc Am Assoc Cancer Res 29:431

Öberg K, Norheim I, Lind E, Ahn G, Lundqvist G, Wide L, Jonsdottir G, Magnusson A, Wilander E (1986) Treatment of malignant carcinoid tumors with human leukocyte interferon: long-term results. Cancer Treat Rep 70:1297–1304

O'Connell MJ, Colgan JP, Oken MM, Ritts RE, Kay NE, Itri LM (1986) Clinical trial of recombinant leukocyte A interferon as initial therapy for favorable histology non-Hodgkin's lymphomas and chronic lymphocytic leukemia. An Eastern Cooperative Oncology Group study. J Clin Oncol 4:128–136

Ohno R (1987) Interferons in the treatment of multiple myeloma. Int J Cancer [Suppl 1] 40:14–20

Old LJ (1987) Polypeptide mediator network. Nature 326:330–331

Österborg A, Björkholm M, Gahrton G, Grimfors G, Gyllenhammar H, Hast R, Holm G, Juliusson G, Järnmark M, Killander A, Kimby E, Lerner R, Paul C, Simonsson B, Smedmyr B, Wedelin C, Ösby E, Mellstedt H (1987) Melphalan/prednisone (MP) therapy vs melphalan/prednisone + human alpha-interferon (MP/IFN) in patients with multiple myeloma, stage II and III. A randomized study from the Myeloma Group of Central Sweden (MGCS). An interimistic report. Abstract, p 169, Ann Meet Swed Med Soc, 2–4 Dec 1987

Paganelli KA, Evans SS, Han T, Ozer H (1986) B cell growth factor-induced proliferation of hairy cell lymphocytes and inhibition by type I interferon in vitro. Blood 67:937–942

Pangalis GA, Griva E (1988) Recombinant alfa-2b-interferon therapy in untreated, stages A and B chronic lymphocytic leukemia. Cancer 61:869–872

Pestka S (1986) Interferon: a decade of accomplishments, foundations of the future in research and therapy. Semin Hematol [Suppl 1] 23: 27–37

Pfeffer LM, Wang E, Tamm E, Tamm I (1980) Interferon effects on microfilament organization, cellular fibronectin distribution, and cell motility in human fibroblasts. J Cell Biol 85:9–17

Porzsolt F, Janik R, Heil G, Brudler O, Raghavachar A, Scholz S, Papendick U, Heimpel H (1986) Deficient IFN alpha production in hairy cell leukemia. Blut 52:185–190

Quesada JR (1988) Biologic response modifiers in the therapy of metastatic renal cell carcinoma. Semin Oncol 15:396–407

Quesada JR, Reuben J, Manning JT, Hersh EM, Gutterman JU (1984) Alpha interferon for induction of remission in hairy-cell leukemia. N Engl J Med 310:15–18

Quesada JR, Hersh EM, Manning J, Reuben J, Keating M, Schnipper E, Itri L, Gutterman JU (1986) Treatment of hairy cell leukemia with recombinant alpha-interferon. Blood 68:493–497

Ratain MJ, Golomb HM, Bardawil RG, Vardiman JW, Westbrook CA, Kaminer LS, Lembersky BC, Bitter MA, Daly K (1987) Durability of response to interferon alfa-2b in advanced hairy cell leukemia. Blood 69:872–877

Rubin BY, Anderson SL, Sullivan SA, Williamson BD, Carswell EA, Old LJ (1985) High affinity binding of ^{125}I-labeled human tumor necrosis factor (LuKII) to specific cell surface receptors. J Exp Med 162:1099–1104

Saito T, Berens ME, Welander CE (1987) Interferon-gamma and cytotoxic agents studied in combination using a soft agarose human tumor clonogenic assay. Cancer Chemother Pharmacol 19: 233–239

Schnipper LE (1986) Clinical implications of tumor-cell heterogeneity. N Engl J Med 314:1423–1431

Shirai T, Yamaguchi H, Ito H, Todd CW, Wallace RB (1985) Cloning and expression in *Escherichia coli* of the gene for human tumour necrosis factor. Nature 313:803–806

Shows TB, Sakaguchi AY, Naylor SL, Goeddel DV, Laen RM (1982) Clusterings of leukocyte and fibroblast interferon clones on human chromosome 9. Science 218:373–376

Sigaux F, Chapuis F, Castaigne S, Degos L, Flandrin G, Gluckman JC (1987) Hairy-cells are not lysed by NK-cells. Blut 54:319–320

Smyth JF, Balkwill FR, Cavalli F, Kimchi A, Mattson K, Niederle NE, Spiegel RJ (1987) Interferons in oncology: current status and future directions. Eur J Cancer Clin Oncol 23:887–889

Spiegel RJ (1987) The alpha interferons: clinical overview. Semin Oncol [Suppl 2] 14:1–12

Talpaz M, Kantarjian HM, McCredie KB, Keating MJ, Trujillo J, Gutterman J (1987) Clinical investigation of human alpha interferon in chronic myelogenous leukemia. Blood 69:1280–1288

Taylor-Papadimitriou J (1984) The interferons. Biochem Soc Symp 49:109–122

Torrisi J, Berg C, Bonnem E, Dritschilo A (1986) The combined use of interferon and radiotherapy in cancer management. Semin Oncol [Suppl 2] 8:78–83

Torti FM, Shortliffe LD, Williams RD, Pitts WC, Kempson RL, Ross JC, Palmer J, Meyers F, Ferrari M, Hannigan J, Spiegel R, McWhirter K, Freiha F (1988) Alpha-interferon in superficial bladder cancer: a Northern California Oncology Group Study. J Clin Oncol 6:476–483

Trinchieri G, Perussia B (1985) Immune interferon: a pleiotropic lymphokine with multiple effects. Immunol Today 6:131–136

Vilcek J, Gresser I, Merigan TC (1980) Regulatory functions of interferons. Ann NY Acad Sci 350: 1129

Welander CE, Morgan TM, Homesley HD, Trotta PP, Spiegel RJ (1985) Combined recombinant human interferon alpha-2 and cytotoxic agents studied in a clonogenic assay. Int J Cancer 35: 721–729

Williams CKO, Svet-Moldavskaya I, Vilcek J, Ohnuma T, Holland JF (1981) Inhibitory effects of human leukocyte and fibroblast interferons on normal and chronic myelogenous leukemic granulocytic progenitor cells. Oncology 38:356–360

Williamson BD, Carswell EA, Rubin BY, Prendergast JS, Old LJ (1983) Human tumor necrosis factor produced by human B-cell lines: synergistic cytotoxic interaction with human interferon. Proc Natl Acad Sci USA 80:5397–5401

Predictive Assays for the Individualization of Tumor Therapy*

C. Streffer

Introduction

It is general clinical experience that the response of human tumors to any given therapeutic modality is very variable, even when the tumors treated are of the same clinical stage and histopathological grade. This is probably due to the intraindividual and to the interindividual heterogeneity of tumors (Sutherland 1988). Heterogeneity has been shown in regard to a number of biological characteristics: the DNA content of tumor cell lines, the number of S-phase cells, and the micromilieu with reference to pH balance, glucose content, and other biological factors can vary tremendously (Sutherland 1988; Barlogie et al. 1980; Tribukait and Gustafson 1980; Streffer et al. 1986). These biological parameters have great relevance to therapeutic response, as radiobiological studies have shown. Determination of such biological parameters is therefore necessary so that tumors can be better characterized as to their individual biological features, and an optimal selection of specific therapy modalities made on an individual basis. Such individualization of tumor therapy could improve the success of treatment.

New therapy modalities are usually tested by randomized studies. The individual heterogeneity of tumors can be a great difficulty in such randomized therapy trials unless factors relevant to therapy are taken into account. Consider the following scenario: Patients with tumors at the same clinical stage and histopathological grade are being treated uniformly, although subpopulations A, B, and C (Fig. 1) could be identified according to differences in tumor vascularization and cell proliferation. Two different therapy modalities are being compared.

In patients of subpopulation B the tumors respond to both therapy modalities to the same degree; therefore, the survival of these patients is the same after both therapy modalities. However, the first therapy modality yields poor survival of patients from subpopulation A, but good survival of patients in subpopulation C (Fig. 1, II). The second therapy modality (Fig. 1, III) yields much better survival in subpopulation A than the first, but patients in subpopulation C have a lower survival rate. Under these conditions, overall survival for subpopulations A, B, and C together will not show any significant difference between the two therapy modalities. However, if it were possible to differentiate between the subpopulations, it is obvious that subpopulation A would profit from the second therapy modality and subpopulation C from the first.

Such an imagined scenario makes evident the necessity of individualized selection of optimal therapy modalities in tumor treatment.

* These studies were supported by the Deutsche Forschungsgemeinschaft, SFB 102

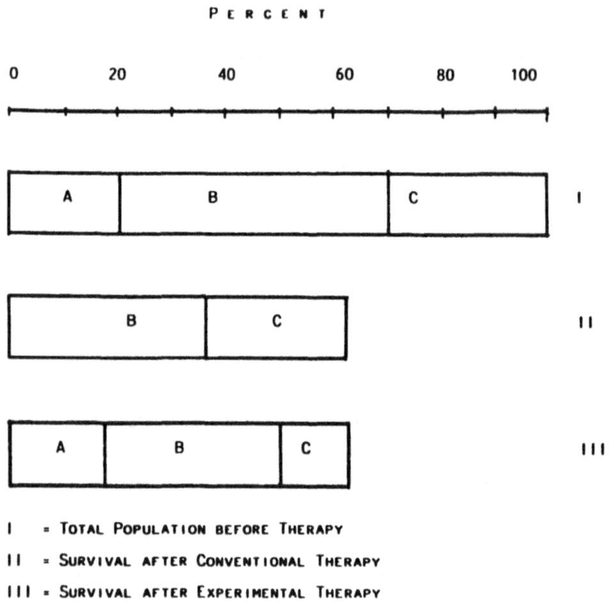

Fig. 1. Imagined clinical trial scenario: subpopulations A, B, and C of patients with tumors of the same type, with identical histopathological grade and clinical stage, before the start of therapy (I); survival of the different subpopulations after therapy with two different modalities (II and III)

Possible Parameters for Predictive Assays

Experimental studies in clinical radiobiology performed with transplantable tumors during recent years have shown the following tumor characteristics to be most important to the therapeutic response (Alper 1979; Hall 1978; Streffer 1987):

1. The intrinsic radiosensitivity of cells, including repair and recovery processes.
2. Cell proliferation kinetics and repopulation.
3. The oxygenation of tumor tissues.

The search for suitable predictive assays must therefore include these characteristics.

The intrinsic radiosensitivity of tumor cells is very important to therapeutic success. The reduction of clonogenic cells by radiation is to a great extent determined by intracellular recovery processes in the dose range of 1–5 Gy, which is the usual dose per fraction in radiotherapy (Fertil and Malaise 1981). Many efforts have been made to determine these processes in tumor cells. The central task is to obtain the relevant data from cells of a primary tumor within a short period, to be used as a basis for selection of the optimal therapy modality for that individual patient. Several authors have shown that the survival rate of cells after a radiation dose of 2 Gy has great predictive relevance to optimization of tumor therapy (Fertil and Malaise 1981). Brock et al. (1985) developed an experimental system by which such data can be obtained within a few days.

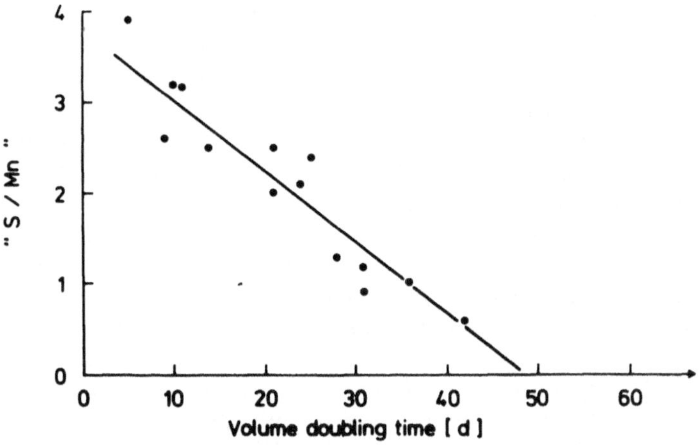

Fig. 2. Tumor volume doubling time of xenograft on nude mice (human melanoma MeWo) in dependence on the ratio of the number of S-phase cells to the number of cells with micronuclei

Cell proliferation can be determined in human tumors by flow cytometry. With this method it is possible to measure the DNA content in single cells. From the DNA histograms the DNA content of the cell line and the distribution of cells in the cell generation cycle can be calculated (Barlogie et al. 1980). Thus it can be seen whether the tumor cell line is diploid or hyperploid. With several tumor entities it has been shown that patients with a diploid tumor cell line have a better prognosis than those with a hyperploid cell line (Tribukait and Gustafson 1980; Streffer et al. 1986). In many tumors only one hyperploid tumor cell line but in some tumors several hyperploid cell lines have been observed. In these cases evaluation becomes complicated.

From the DNA histograms the number of S-phase cells in the tumor can be calculated, which gives an estimate of the rate of cell renewal. However, it has been found that not all cells with a DNA content corresponding to S-phase are DNA-synthesizing cells. Therefore, methods have been developed to label DNA-synthesizing cells by 5-bromodeoxyuridine (BUdR). The incorporation of BUdR into cellular DNA can be shown with monoclonal antibodies which are stained with fluorescent dye (Wilson et al. 1985). Both measurements (cytofluorometric DNA measurements and determination of BUdR incorporation) allow a reasonable analysis of the proliferating activity of tumors. These data have a strong predictive value for tumor radiation therapy, as the expression of radiation response is dependent on cell proliferation (Hall 1978; Streffer 1987).

Tumor growth is dependent on cell renewal and cell loss. So far, it is not possible to determine cell loss directly. Dying cells frequently show cytogenetic damage. It has been demonstrated that cells with micronuclei are potentially lethal cells (Midander and Revesz 1980; van Beuningen et al. 1981). Micronuclei are formed from whole chromosome or from acentric chromosome fragments which are found in the cytoplasm after mitosis (Heddle 1973). These micronuclei are formed spontaneously or after exposure to ionizing radiation and genotoxic chemicals. The incidence of micronuclei is higher in tumors than in normal tissues (Streffer et al. 1986) and can be used as a rough estimate for cell loss. In xenografts on nude mice the number of

S-phase cells as well as the incidence of micronuclei have been measured. Tumor growth has also been determined from caliper measurements, and tumor volume doubling time calculated from the curves of tumor growth. A correlation between tumor volume doubling time and the ratio of the number of S-phase cells to the number of cells with micronuclei has been found (Fig. 2). This ratio thus apparently allows a very rough prediction of tumor growth, although the situation is certainly much more complex in human tumors than in transplanted tumors.

S-phase cells and cells with micronuclei were measured in untreated rectum carcinomas, stage pT_3. A wide variability between individual tumors was seen for both parameters. The number of cells with micronuclei showed a trend to increase when the number of S-phase cells increased. However, a more important finding was that all tumors which developed local recurrence were found to have relatively high numbers of S-phase cells and comparatively few cells with micronuclei (Streffer 1988). Thus, these measurements allow some prediction of the probability of local recurrences. The data from patients who survived longer than 18 months after resection of the tumor appear in the lower part of the diagram with lower numbers of S-phase cells. This observation indicates that cell proliferation is comparatively low in these tumors.

In further studies DNA histograms were measured from biopsies of the rectal mucosa obtained at a distance of 1 cm or 5 cm from the resection border. The measurements show that generally – apart from in one patient – no hyperploid cells were detected in the rectal mucosa, although single hyperploid cells certainly could have been overlooked in these histograms. However, in several patients the number of S-phase cells was remarkably high in the normal-appearing rectal mucosa even at a distance of 5 cm from the resection border (Table 1). In a number of these patients local recurrences were observed within 2 years after the tumor resection. In the one patient in whom hyperploid tumor cells were still found in the normal-appearing rectal mucosa, a local recurrence was seen within a few months after the tumor resection.

Table 1. DNA index and numbers of S-phase cells in rectal carcinomas and nearby rectal mucosa

Patient	Tumor		Mucosa (1 cm away)		Mucosa (5 cm away)	
	DI	S	DI	S	DI	S
1	1.5	21.5	1.0	25.8	1.0	12.5
2	2.6	33.7	2.6	41.2	1.0	11.8
3	1.6	20.2	1.0	26.3	1.0	10.6
4	1.9	32.6	1.0	18.2	1.0	13.7
5	1.5	32.4	1.0	18.3	1.0	17.2
6	1.3	28.8	1.0	11.4	1.0	15.6
7	1.2	27.6	1.0	13.4	1.0	11.7
8	1.7	14.6	1.0	9.3	1.0	7.1
9	1.0	20.1	1.0	23.4	1.0	11.3
10	1.0	26.5	1.0	34.5	1.0	10.7

DI, DNA index; S, S-phase cells. The biopsies of the rectal mucosa were taken at a distance of 1 cm or 5 cm from the border of the tumor resection

Similar data were obtained for squamous cell carcinomas of the head and neck region. Apparently a stimulation of cell proliferation occurs in these individual patients which induced repopulation of tumor cells. This phenomenon could be due to a recruitment of resting cells. A program has therefore been started to measure growth factors and their receptors in tumor patients.

Measurements Before and After Radiotherapy

In several patients with rectal carcinomas or squamous cell carcinomas of the head and neck region, the incidence of micronuclei was measured in single cell suspensions from the tumor biopsies, before and after or during radiotherapy. Rectal tumors were irradiated on 3 consecutive days with 3×2.1 Gy per day (total dose 18.9 Gy); the tumors were resected 1–3 days after the last radiation dose. A good correlation was found between the increase in numbers of micronuclei and the tumor response to radiation. This observation was also made in 10 squamous cell carcinomas. In these tumors a biopsy was studied before radiotherapy and after irradiation of the tumor with 5×2 Gy. Four out of the five patients in whom the incidence of micronuclei increased after radiotherapy had no local recurrence, whereas out of the five patients in whom no increase was seen in the incidence of micronuclei after irradiation, four had local recurrence (Zamboglou and Streffer, unpublished data). Thus, the micronucleus test is apparently a useful assay to determine radiation response early, before tumor regression can be seen.

Prediction of the probability of local recurrence was also possible through determination the proportion of S-phase cells in rectal carcinomas before and after preoperative radiotherapy. The radiation schedule was the same as described before, to a total dose of 18.9 Gy. In 22 out of 43 patients it was observed that the number of S-phase cells was less after radiotherapy than before – an effect to be expected on the basis of radiobiological studies (Hall 1978) –. In this group of 22 patients, 1 local recurrence was observed during the following 2 years. In 9 patients there was no great change in the proportion of S-phase cells, and in this group of patients also 1 local recurrence was seen. In 12 patients, surprisingly, the proportion of S-phase cells increased very shortly after radiotherapy, and 6 of these 12 patients developed local recurrence (Table 2). Thus the probability of a local recurrence was quite high in this latter group. It was suggested that, due to individual factors, the repopulation of tumor cells was extremely high in these patients and induced the local recurrence (Streffer et al. 1986).

Table 2. Change in proportion of S-phase cells in rectal carcinomas before and after preoperative radiotherapy and local recurrences in these patients

	Decrease		No change		Increase	
	n	%	*n*	%	*n*	%
Number of patients	22	51	9	21	12	28
Number of recurrences	1	12.5	1	12.5	6	75

Table 3. Selection of optimal radiotherapy modality for tumors with certain characteristics

Low LET radiation alone	
– Hyperfractionation	Large number of clonogenic cells
– Accelerated fractionation	Rapid repopulation
Low LET radiation combined with	
– Chemotherapeutic drugs	Intrinsic radioresistance
– Hyperthermia	Hypoxia, intrinsic radioresistance
– Hypoxic cell sensitizers	Hypoxia
High LET radiation	Intrinsic radioresistance, hypoxia, poor redistribution

LET, lineal energy transfer

In further studies, radiation response was measured in dependence on the vascular density in rectal carcinomas. The blood vessels were stained through a histochemical method for alkaline phosphatase (Mlynek et al. 1985) and the density of the blood vessels was measured by morphometry. Again, a very wide variation was observed between individual rectal carcinomas (Streffer et al. 1988). The radiation response was especially good in tumors which had a high density of blood vessels.

Conclusions

Studies of human tumors demonstrate that many biological characteristics vary from tumor to tumor considerably. Such characteristics are relevant to tumor therapy, especially radiotherapy. These differences are seen for tumors of the same type, the same histopathological grade, and the same clinical stage. Therefore, to improve individualized selection of optimal tumor therapy modalities, more information is needed about the biology of individual tumors. For these purposes several predictive assays are necessary. A large number of therapy modalities are available today, and experimental radiobiological studies have shown which modality is optimal for tumors with certain characteristics (Table 3).

Some general criteria are necessary for predictive assays:

1. The predictive assay should measure a tumor characteristic which has been shown to correlate to local tumor control.
2. The assay should be independent of the tumor region from which the biopsy was obtained and if possible mirror the intraindividual heterogeneity.
3. The assay should be easy and quick to perform so that the data it yields about a patient can be used for the therapy of that particular patient.
4. The assay should be performed with small biopsies or with harmless in vivo techniques.

Acknowledgments. The studies were performed in cooperation with the Klinik für Strahlentherapie, Klinik für Allgemeine Chirurgie and Klinik für Gesichts- und Kieferchirurgie of the Universitätsklinikum Essen.

References

Alper T (1979) Cellular radiobiology. Cambridge University Press, Cambridge

Barlogie B, Drewinko B, Schumann J, Göhde W, Dosik G, Latreille J, Johnston DA, Freieich EJ (1980) Cellular DNA content as a marker of neoplasia in man. Am J Med 69:196–203

Brock WA, Maor MH, Peters LJ (1985) Predictors of tumor response to radiotherapy. Radiat Res 104:290–296

Fertil B, Malaise EP (1981) Inherent cellular radiosensitivity as a basic concept for human tumor radiotherapy. Int J Radiat Oncol Biol Phys 7:621–629

Hall EJ (1978) Radiobiology for the radiologist. Harper and Row, New York

Heddle JA (1973) A rapid in vivo test for chromosomal damage. Mutat Res 18:187–198

Midander J, Revesz L (1980) The micronucleus (MN) in irradiated cells as a measure of survival. Br J Cancer 41:204

Mlynek ML, van Beuningen D, Leder LD, Streffer C (1985) Measurement of the grade of vascularization in histological tumor tissue sections. Br J Cancer 52:945–948

Streffer C (1987) Biologische Grundlagen der Strahlentherapie. In: Scherer E (ed) Strahlentherapie. Springer, Berlin Heidelberg New York, pp 213–281

Streffer C (1988) Prädiktive Teste zur Verbesserung der Prognose und der Therapie menschlicher Tumoren. Radiobiol Radiother (Berl) 29:377–386

Streffer C, van Beuningen D, Gross E, Schabronath J, Eigler FW, Rebmann A (1986) Predictive assays for the therapy of rectum carcinoma. Radiother Oncol 5:303–310

Streffer C, van Beuningen D, Mylnek ML, Gross E, Eigler FW (1988) Predictive assays for the therapy of rectal carcinoma. Recent Results Cancer Res 110:274–280

Sutherland RM (1988) Cell and environment interactions in tumor microregions: the multicell spheroid model. Science 240:177–184

Tribukait B, Gustafson H (1980) Impulscytophotometrische DNS-Untersuchungen bei Blasenkarzinomen. Onkologie 6:278–288

van Beuningen D, Streffer C, Berthold G (1981) Mikronukleusbildung im Vergleich zur Überlebensrate von menschlichen Melanomzellen nach Röntgen-, Neutronenbestrahlung und Hyperthermie. Strahlentherapie 157:600–606

Wilson GD, McNalla NJ, Dumphy E, Kärcher H, Pfranger R (1985) The labelling index of human and mouse tumours assessed by bromodeoxyuridine staining in vitro and in vivo and flow cytometry. Cytometry 6:641–647

Molecular Genetic Changes as Indicators of Therapeutic Effectiveness

C. R. Bartram

Molecular genetic approaches have considerably increased the current knowledge of various areas in cancer research. Many of these data turned out to be of immediate clinical relevance and established useful diagnostic and prognostic parameters for the classification of human neoplasias as well as for the monitoring of therapeutic effectiveness. The following examples may illustrate this development.

Molecular Genetics of the Philadelphia Translocation – A Paradigm

Chronic myelocytic leukemia (CML) belongs to the first human neoplasias in which the identification of a specific molecular alteration by recombinant DNA techniques showed immediate clinical implications for diagnosis, subclassification, and monitoring of the disease. The cytogenetic hallmark of CML, a reciprocal translocation between chromosome 9 and 22, the Philadelphia (Ph) translocation, is molecularly characterized by a recombination of the *c-abl* and *bcr* genes (Bartram 1988). As a consequence of the *bcr/abl* rearrangement, leukemic cells transcribe a chimeric 8.5-kb RNA species which is translated into a protein, $p210^{bcr\text{-}abl}$, with an associated tyrosine kinase activity that differs from the normal $p145^{abl}$ counterpart (Fig. 1). In contrast to the breakpoints on chromosome 9 which are dispersed over 200 kb of the first *c-abl* intron, the breaks on chromosome 22 also vary individually, but cluster within a limited area, which is therefore called breakpoint cluster region *(bcr)*. Thus Southern blot analyses using appropriate *bcr* probes may be used to diagnose Ph-positive CML, to follow individual leukemia cell clones during the course of the dis-

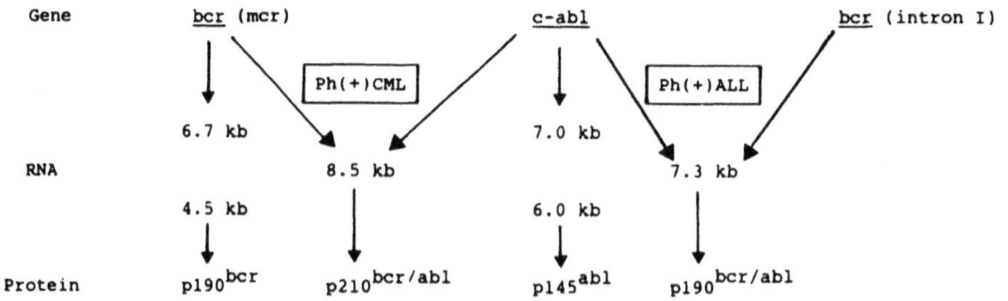

Fig. 1. The Philadelphia translocation in CML and ALL is characterized by a rearrangement of the *c-abl* and *bcr* genes. While in CML the breakpoints are localized within the major cluster region (*mcr*, previously called breakpoint cluster region), and the ALL rearrangements occur within the first intron of the *bcr* gene

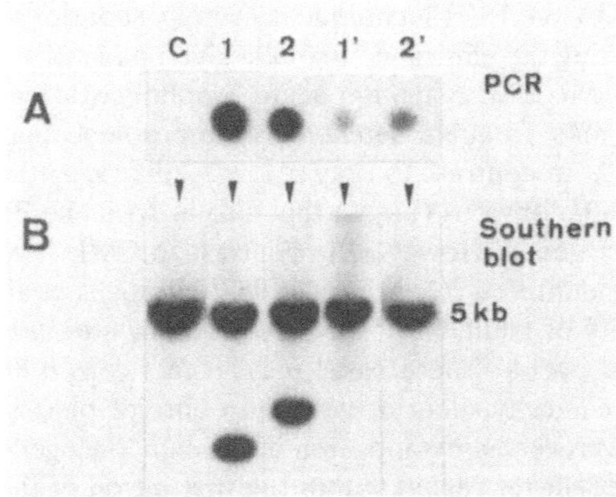

Fig. 2A, B. Comparison of the sensitivities of polymerase chain reaction (PCR) technique and Southern blot analysis in detecting residual leukemic cells in Ph-positive CML following bone marrow transplantation (BMT). In two patients *(lanes 1, 2)* individually rearranged DNA fragments are observed prior to BMT in Southern blots hybridized to 5' *bcr* sequences. After BMT only 5-kb germline bands are visible *(lanes 1', 2')*. Dot blot analysis using the PCR technique, however, demonstrates residual leukemic cells in both patients following BMT. Samples obtained from a healthy control were included *(lanes C)*

ease, and to monitor therapeutic effectiveness of bone marrow transplantation (BMT) or interferon treatment (Bartram et al. 1986; Yoffe et al. 1987). While in general cytogenetic and Southern blot analyses appear to be of comparable sensitivity in detecting residual leukemic cells, 2 out of 14 CML patients treated by allogeneic BMT, who we recently investigated, showed small percentages (5%–10%) of leukemic cells exclusively by the latter technique. Albeit rare, some Ph-positive CML patients exhibit breaks outside the typical region on chromosome 22 and will therefore not be detected by conventional Southern analysis (Bartram et al. 1987; Selleri et al. 1987). These cases can be identified by either cytogenetic studies or pulsed-field gel electrophoresis (Westbrook et al. 1988).

Recently a major breakthrough in the detection of minimal residual disease emerged from the application of a modified polymerase chain reaction (PCR) technique (Saiki et al. 1988). This method is based on the fact that in the vast majority of CML patients, exon 2 or 3 sequences of the breakpoint cluster region are spliced to exon II of the *c-abl* gene (Shtivelman et al. 1986). Thus, despite considerable differences at the genomic level, CML patients are characterized by similar-sized *bcr/abl* transcripts. Respective chimeric cDNAs can be amplified in vitro several hundred thousandfold using *bcr* exon 2 and *c-abl* exon II sequences as primers, and afterwards either directly identified on an agarose gel or by oligomer probes following dot or Southern blotting. This approach allows the detection of less than one leukemic cell in a sample of 10^4 cells. Using this ultrasensitive method, most transplanted CML patients, who previously scored negative by cytogenetic or Southern blot analysis, show residual leukemic cells (Fig. 2). Since occasionally Ph-positive cells may be observed at low frequencies up to several years following BMT without any clinical indications of relapse (Cooperative Study Group 1988), it remains to be elucidated whether monitoring transplanted CML patients by the PCR technique is acutally superior to conventional genetic methods in predicting the clinical course of a given patient.

The *Ph* translocation is not restricted to CML. In adult acute lymphoblastic leukemias (ALL) a Ph chromosome is the most frequent detectable chromosomal aberration, with an incidence of almost 20% in contrast to only 3% of pediatric ALLs showing this hallmark. Recently it became obvious (Fig. 1) that also in ALL the Ph translocation involves the *c-abl* and *bcr* genes. However, in contrast to CML, two molecularly defined subtypes could be identified (Clark et al. 1987; Hermans et al. 1987; Bartram 1988). Thus, the majority of adult Ph-positive ALLs show a *bcr/abl* rearrangement identical to Ph-positive CMLs. These cases may in fact constitute acute phases of CML in the sequel of clinically silent or very short chronic phases. On the other hand, most pediatric ALLs reveal a juxtaposition of the *c-abl* oncogene to sequences 5′ of the CML breakpoint cluster region within the first intron of the *bcr* gene. It should soon become apparent whether both entities, best distinguishable by their respective p210 and p190 *bcr/abl* proteins, are associated with different clinical/biological courses.

Ras Gene Mutations and X-Linked DNA Polymorphism as Clonal Markers in AML and MDS

Two other molecular genetic markers appear to be of clinical value in monitoring therapeutic effectiveness in acute myelocytic leukemia (AML) and myelodysplastic syndromes (MDS). Point mutations leading to the activation of the transforming potential of Ha-*ras*, Ki-*ras*, and N-*ras* have been demonstrated in a variety of different neoplasias. By far the highest incidence (30%–50%) has been reported in colorectal carcinoma and adenocarcinoma of the lung showing Ki-*ras* mutations as well as in AMLs exhibiting a preferential involvement of N-*ras* (Bos et al. 1987). In a recent survey of 78 AML patients, we failed to correlate the presence of mutated *ras* alleles with prognosis, patient's age, or a specific immunological, and cytogenetic subtype. However, *ras* mutations may serve as clonal markers in monitoring leukemic cells through the course of the disease. A limitation of this approach in assessing remission quality is the fact that some AML patients with a *ras* mutation at presentation may relapse with mutation-negative leukemic cells (Farr et al. 1988).

The incidence and clinical significance of *ras* gene mutations in myelodysplastic syndromes is still a matter of controversy. Some authors demonstrated rather high incidences (up to 50%) and, more important, a strong correlation between the presence of mutated *ras* alleles and transition from a preleukemic state into overt AML within the following months (Hirai et al. 1987; Liu et al. 1987). In our own series of some 80 MDS cases we observed *ras* mutations in only 10% of patients, who, moreover, mostly remained in a myelodysplastic state for more than 1 year (Janssen et al. 1987; Lyons et al. 1988). However, as in AML, *ras* mutations are useful markers for clonal analysis in MDS. We were thus able to demonstrate the presence of *ras* mutations in separated granulocyte, monocyte/macrophage, as well as B- and T-lymphocyte cell fractions of different MDS patients (Janssen et al. 1987; Janssen et al. 1989). This result emphasizes that these preleukemic entities originate in a pluripotent stem

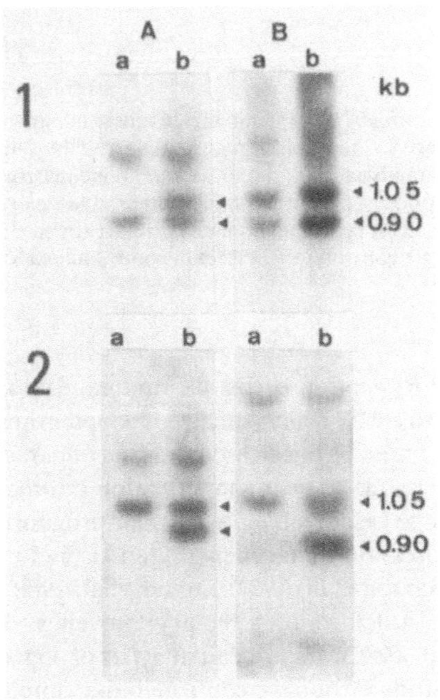

Fig. 3. Clonal composition of blood cell samples from two female AML patients at initial presentation *(A)* and during complete remission *(B)* determined by X-chromosome inactivation analysis. A PGK restriction fragment length polymorphism, characterized by 1.05-kb and 0.9-kb fragments in *Bst*XI/*Pst*I digests, distinguishes the maternal from the paternal allele, and methylation differences as shown by *Hpa*II digestion, distinguish between active and inactive X-chromosomes. DNAs were digested with *Bst*XI and *Pst*I, subsequently divided into two equal aliquots; one was not digested further *(lanes b)*, and the other was digested with *Hpa*II *(lanes a)*. The complete loss of one allele is demonstrated in blood cell samples from both patients prior to therapy after *Hpa*II digestion, indicating a monoclonal cell population *(A)*. Anlaysis of granulocyte fractions in remission *(B)* indicates restoration of a polyclonal pattern in patient 1, but persistence of monoclonality in patient 2

cell. Moreover, the cytotoxic rather than differentiating effect of low-dose cytarabine could be derived from the disappearance of a *ras* gene mutation in MDS patients following treatment with this drug (Layton et al. 1988).

A complementary approach to study clonality in AML and MDS is the use of DNA polymorphism of X-linked genes (Vogelstein et al. 1987). This method is analogous to glucose-6-phosphate dehydrogenase isoenzyme analysis, being based on X-chromosome inactivation. The random nature of X-inactivation renders females mosaic for heterozygous loci. In monoclonal cell populations, however, the same X chromosome will be active in all cells. In the strategy pioneered by Vogelstein and coworkers, active and inactive alleles are differentiated by a methylation-sensitive restriction enzyme. Using this approach persistence of a single dominant hemopoietic clone can be demonstrated in a proportion of AML patients, who are otherwise in complete clinical and hematological remission (Fearon et al. 1986; Fig. 3). This result indicates that in some patients leukemic cells may differentiate to mature cells, an observation of major importance for the development of future therapeutic regimens. In MDS patients, X-inactivation analyses revealed reversion to polyclonal hematopoiesis following low-dose ara-C treatment, supporting the notion that even at low dosages cytarabine acts primarily as a cytotoxic agent (Janssen et al. 1989).

Prognostic Value of Oncogene Amplification in Solid Tumors

Quantitative changes of proto-oncogenes have been implicated with bad prognosis of solid tumors. Cases in point are the amplification and/or increased expression of the

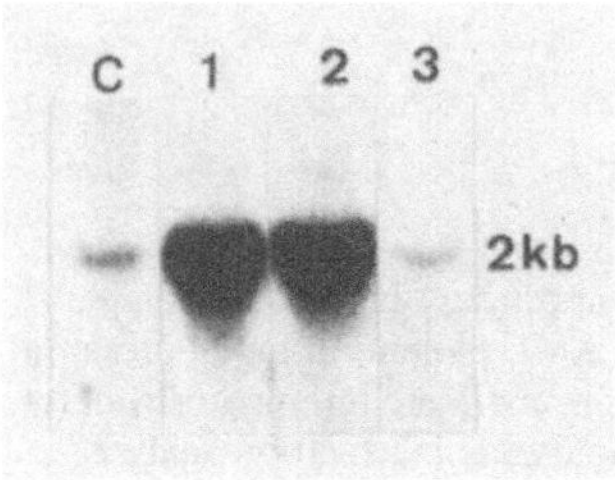

Fig. 4. Monitoring of therapeutic effectiveness in a patient with stage IV neuroblastoma characterized by a 40-fold N-*myc* amplification in tumor *(1)* and bone marrow *(2)* samples prior to chemotherapy. Southern blot analysis of bone marrow specimen obtained after treatment *(3)* reveals a single copy pattern. Placenta control in *lane C*

N-*myc* gene in neuroblastoma and of the *c-erbB*$_2$ gene in breast carcinoma. The *c-erbB*$_2$ gene, also called *HER*$_2$ or *neu*, is related to *erbB*, which encodes the epidermal growth factor receptor. Approximately 35% of human breast carcinomas are characterized by an overexpression of the erbB$_2$ protein due to gene amplification or other mechanisms. This increased expression appears to be correlated with poor prognosis and may be a stronger predictor of tumor progression than other prognostic factors including hormonal-receptor or nodal status (Slamon et al. 1987; Berger et al. 1988).

Similarly a key role of N-*myc* amplification in determining the aggressiveness of neuroblastoma has been suggested (Seeger et al. 1985). In a recent analysis of 45 patients treated by the German Neuroblastoma Study Group we confirmed that amplification and/or overexpression of N-*myc* are (a) more frequently found in stages III and IV than in less advanced stages and (b) in general are associated with a bad prognosis (Bartram and Berthold 1987). Figure 4 illustrates the value of Southern blot analysis using N-*myc* sequences in estimating the extent of bone marrow infiltration in a patient prior to and after chemotherapy. However, I would like to emphasize that we observed exceptions from the postulated rule of close correlation between N-*myc* amplification and rapid tumor progression. Thus, an 80-fold amplification was found in a stage IV neuroblastoma, while the patient is in disease-free survival for more than 3 years following chemotherapy (Bartram and Berthold 1987). Therefore, N-*myc* amplification appears to be a potent, but not infallible, prognostic factor. Other parameters including the tumor karyotype (Christiansen and Lampert 1988) are at least of equal importance for any decision of clinical treatment.

Immunogenotype of Lymphoid Neoplasias

The analysis of immunoglobulin (Ig) and T-cell receptor (TCR) gene structure and transcriptional regulation as well as the developmental hierarchy of genetic rearrangements occurring during B- and T-cell maturation has been of great value in (a) defining the lineage (B or T cell) and stage of maturation of lymphoid neoplasias, (b) determining the clonality of abnormal lymphocyte proliferation, (c) diagnosing and monitoring the therapy of leukemias/lymphomas, and (d) unravelling the molecular mechanisms of chromosomal aberrations associated with lymphoid malignancies (Haluska et al. 1987; Korsmeyer 1987; Waldmann 1987).

While the assignment of a given neoplastic cell population to a specific state of maturation is, due to the promiscuity of the recombinase system, only possible in

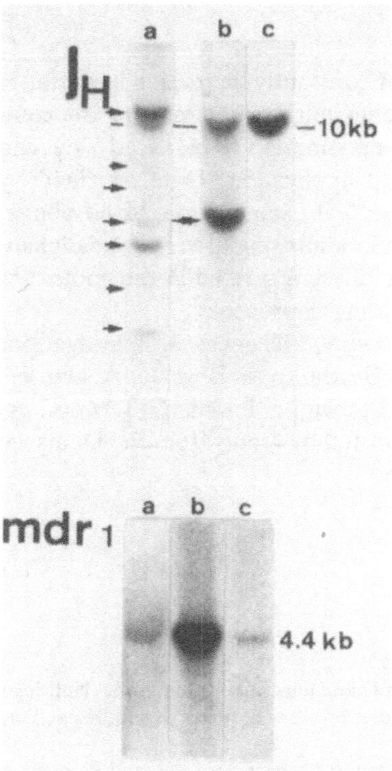

Fig. 5. Southern blot analysis of peripheral blood DNA obtained from an AUL patient characterized by an oligoclonal disease prior to therapy *(lane a)* indicated by multiple rearranged DNA fragments after hybridization to an immunoglobin heavy chain *(JH)* probe. In relapse *(lane b)* only one subclone reemerged. Rehybridization of the *Hin*dIII digests to mdr_1 sequences (kindly provided by Dr. Roninson) demonstrates a concurrent mdr_1 amplification in the subclone *(lane b)*. Placenta DNA served as control *(lances C)*

combination with morphological, cytochemical, and immunologic parameters, *Ig* and *TCR* gene rearrangements offer a unique opportunity to study individual leukemic cell clones during the course of the disease and to evaluate the remission status of a patient (Zehnbauer et al. 1986).

Our recent investigation of acute undifferentiated leukemias (AULs) may illustrate this advantage of immunogenotyping. AUL blasts are derived from B-cell precursors. In extension of a previous study (Raghavachar et al. 1986), we analyzed 31 AUL patients and found an oligoclonal pattern of *Ig* gene rearrangement in 30% of cases. Concurrent cytogenetic analyses suggested that in those patients multiple subclones originated from a common ancestor by clonal evolution. Preliminary data suggest that AULs characterized by oligoclonal disease have worse prognosis and relapse earlier than monoclonal cases. Reexamination of leukemic cells in relapse was thus far performed in two patients. In both cases reemergence of a single subclone of the oligoclonal cell population, visible at first presentation, could be demonstrated (Fig. 5). As a possible clue to the mechanisms involved in the predominance of one specific subclone in relapse we observed concurrent amplification of mdr_1 sequences in one of the patients (Fig. 5). Increased expression of *mdr* genes has been implicated with acquisition of resistance to multiple chemotherapeutic agents (Pastan and Gottesman 1987).

Concluding Remarks

Undoubtedly, molecular genetic approaches are of constantly increasing importance for clinical oncology. While the potential of these techniques in dissecting the complex pathways of carcinogenesis can hardly be overestimated, a balanced view and use of these methods is recommended in clinical application. Data obtained by molecular genetic techniques, as illustrated in the few examples discussed above, have improved the diagnosis, subclassification, and monitoring of various malignancies. However, any of these results has to be carefully interpreted in the context of clinical findings and data derived from complementing approaches.

I gratefully acknowledge the contribution of many colleagues in investigations summarized in this chapter, namely R. Arnold, F. Berthold, M. Buschle, A. Ganser, H. Heimpel, J. W. G. Janssen, M. Layton, W. D. Ludwig, J. Lyons, G. J. Mufti, A. Raghavachar, and E. Thiel. Our own work is supported by grants from the Deutsche Forschungsgemeinschaft and Deutsche Krebshilfe.

References

Barbacid M (1987) Ras genes. Ann Rev Biochem 56:779–827

Bartram CR (1988) Molecular genetic analyses of chronic myeloid leukemia. In: Huhn D, Hellriegel KP, Niederle N (eds) Chronic myelocytic leukemia and interferon. Springer, Berlin Heidelberg New York, pp 19–26

Bartram CR (1988) Rearrangement of the *c-abl* and *bcr* genes in Ph-negative CML and Ph-positive acute leukemias. Leukemia 2:63–64

Bartram CR, Berthold F (1987) Amplification and expression of the *N-myc* gene in neuroblastoma. Eur J Pediatr 146:162–165

Bartram CR, Arnold R, Kubanek B (1986) Diagnostic value of *bcr* sequences (letter). Leuk Res 10: 697–699

Bartram CR, Bross-Bach U, Schmidt H, Waller HD (1987) Philadelphia-positive chronic myelogenous leukemia with breakpoint 5′ of the breakpoint cluster region but within the *bcr* gene. Blut 55:505–511

Berger MS, Locher GW, Saurer S, Gullick WJ, Waterfield MD, Groner B, Hynes NE (1988) Correlation of *c-erb B-2* gene amplification and protein expression in human breast carcinoma with nodal status and nuclear grading. Cancer Res 48:1238–1243

Bos JL, Verlaan-de Vries M, van der Eb AJ, Janssen JWG, Delwel R, Löwenberg B, Colly LP (1987) Mutations in *N-ras* predominate in acute myeloid leukemia. Blood 69:1237–1241

Christiansen H, Lampert F (1988) Tumour karyotype discriminates between good and bad prognostic outcome in neuroblastoma. Br J Cancer 57:121–126

Clark SS, McLaughlin J, Crist WM, Champlin R, Witte ON (1987) Unique forms of the *abl* tyrosine kinase distinguish Ph-positive CML from Ph-positive ALL. Science 235:85–88

Cooperative Study Group on Chromosomes in Transplanted Patients (1988) Cytogenetic follow-up of 100 patients submitted to bone marrow transplantation for Philadelphia chromosome-positive chronic myeloid leukemia. Eur J Haematol 40:50–57

Farr CJ, Saiki RK, Erlich HA, McCormick F, Marshall CJ (1988) Analysis of *ras* gene mutations in acute myeloid leukemia by polymerase chain reaction and oligonucleotide probes. Proc Natl Acad Sci USA 85:1629–1633

Fearon ER, Burke PJ, Shiffer CA, Zehnbauer B, Vogelstein B (1986) Differentiation of leukemia cells to polymorphonuclear leukocytes in patients with acute nonlymphocytic leukemia. N Engl J Med 315:15–24

Haluska FG, Tsujimoto Y, Croce CM (1987) Oncogene activation by chromosome translocation in human malignancies. Annu Rev Genet 21:321–345

Hermans A, Heisterkamp A, von Lindern M, van Baal S, Meijer D, van der Plas D, Wiedemann LM, Groffen J, Bootsma D, Grosveld G (1987) Unique fusion of *bcr* and *c-abl* genes in Philadelphia chromosome positive acute lymphoblastic leukemias. Cell 51:33–40

Hirai H, Kobayashi Y, Mano H, Hagiwara K, Maru Y, Omine M, Mizoguchi H, Nishida J, Takaku F (1987) A point mutation at codon 13 of the *N-ras* oncogene in myelodysplastic syndrome. Nature 327:430–432

Janssen JWG, Steenvoorden ACM, Lyons J, Anger B, Böhlke JV, Bos JL, Seliger H, Bartram CR (1987) *Ras* gene mutations in acute and chronic myelocytic leukemias, chronic myeloproliferative disorders, and myelodysplastic syndromes. Proc Natl Acad Sci USA 84:9228–9232

Janssen JWG, Buschle M, Layton M, Drexler HG, Lyons J, van den Berghe H, Heimpel H, Kubanek B, Kleihauer E, Mufti GJ, Bartram CR (1989) Clonal analysis of myelodysplastic syndromes: evidence of multipotent stem cell origin. Blood 73:248–254

Korsmeyer SJ (1987) Immunoglobulin and T-cell receptor genes reveal the clonality, lineage, and translocations of lymphoid neoplasms. In: DeVita VT, Hellman S, Rosenberg SA (eds) Important advances in oncology 1987. Lippincott, Philadelphia, pp 3–25

Layton DM, Mufti GJ, Lyons J, Janssen JWG, Bartram CR (1988) Loss of *ras* oncogene mutation in a myelodysplastic syndrome after low-dose cytarabine therapy (letter). N Engl J Med 318: 1468–1469

Liu E, Hjelle B, Morgan R, Hecht F, Bishop JM (1987) Mutations of the *Kirsten-ras* proto-oncogene in human preleukemia. Nature 300:186–188

Lyons J, Janssen JWG, Bartram C, Layton M, Mufti GJ (1988) Mutation of *Ki-ras* and *N-ras* oncogenes in myelodysplastic syndromes. Blood 71:1707–1712

Pastan J, Gottesman M (1987) Multiple-drug resistance in human cancer. N Engl J Med 316:1388–1393

Raghavachar A, Bartram CR, Ganser A, Heil G, Kleihauer E, Kubanek B (1986) Acute undifferentiated leukemia: implications for cellular origin and clonality suggested by analysis of surface markers and immunoglobulin gene rearrangement. Blood 68:658–662

Saiki RK, Gelfand DH, Stoffel S, Scharf SJ, Higuchi R, Horn GT, Mullis KB, Erlich HA (1988) Primer-directed enzymatic amplification of DNA with a thermostable DNA polymerase. Science 239:487–491

Seeger RC, Brodeur GM, Sather H, Dalton SA, Siegel SE, Wong KY, Hammond D (1985) Association of multiple copies of the *N-myc* oncogene with rapid progression of neuroblastomas. N Engl J Med 313:1111–1116

Selleri L, Narni F, Emilia G, Colo A, Zucchini P, Venturelli D, Donelli A, Torelli U, Torelli G (1987) Philadelphia-positive chronic myeloid leukemia with a chromosome 22 breakpoint outside the breakpoint cluster region. Blood 70:1659–1664

Shtivelman E, Lifshitz B, Gale RP, Roe BA, Canaani E (1986) Alternative splicing of RNAs transcribed from the human *abl* gene and from the *bcr-abl* fused gene. Cell 47:277–284

Slamon DJ, Clark GM, Wong SG, Levin WJ, Ullrich A, McGuire WL (1987) Human breast cancer: correlation of relapse and survival with amplification of the *HER-2/neu*. Science 235:177–182

Vogelstein B, Fearon ER, Hamilton SR, Preisinger AC, Willard HF, Michelson AM, Riggs AD, Orkin SH (1987) Clonal analysis using recombinant DNA probes from the X-chromosome. Cancer Res 47:4806–4813

Waldmann TA (1987) The arrangement of immunoglobulin and T-cell receptor genes in human lymphoproliferative disorders. Adv Immunol 40:247–321

Westbrook CA, Rubin CM, Carrino JJ, Le Beau MM, Bernards A, Rowley JD (1988) Long-range mapping of the Philadelphia chromosome by pulsed-field gel electrophoresis. Blood 71:697–702

Yoffe G, Blick M, Kantarjian H, Spitzer G, Gutterman J, Talpaz M (1987) Molecular analysis of interferon-induced suppression of Philadelphia chromosome in patients with chronic myeloid leukemia. Blood 69:961–963

Zehnbauer BA, Pardoll DM, Burke PJ, Graham ML, Vogelstein B (1986) Immunoglobulin gene rearrangements in remission bone marrow specimens from patients with acute lymphoblastic leukemia. Blood 67:835–838

Summary of Discussion: Session 5

C. Unger

It was asked whether there is a relation between the receptor-mediated gene expression caused by tumor necrosis factor α and its in vivo antitumoral action. Dr. Nagel stated that receptor-negative cells do not respond to therapy at all. Furthermore, in commercially available cell lines there is a correlation between the receptor expression and in vitro response. So far as c-*myc* gene expression is concerned, no data are available.

Another discussant asked about the advantages of alpha interferon over conventional chemotherapy in chronic myeloid leukemia (CML). Dr. Niederle replied that in CML patients a median survival time of about 40 months can be seen after conventional chemotherapy. However, it seems impossible to eliminate the Philadelphia chromosome or to achieve distinct changes at the molecular level of the disease. In contrast, treatment of CML patients with alpha interferon at sufficient dosages in an early stage of the disease leads to a clearcut elimination of the Philadelphia chromosome in about 30% of the treated patients. In the first study, Dr. Niederle added, patients were treated with minimal effective dosages, but this regimen always led to secondary resistance and recurrence of the disease. Thus, in order to be successful, one has to treat the patients with maximum tolerable dosages. It was asked if the next step should be a bone marrow transplant or at least freezing of Philadelphia chromosome-negative cells. Dr. Niederle answered that it is wise to harvest bone marrow or peripheral stem cells during remission and give these back in the accelerating phase.

With respect to the micronucleus assay as a simple test for cytogenetic damage, questions were raised about the term "micronucleus." Dr. Streffer said that unlike the nucleolus, which is within the cell nucleus, the micronucleus is outside the cell nucleus and represents chromosomal material released from the cell nucleus during mitosis. A high incidence of micronuclei before radiation therapy indicates lability of the cellular genome and predicts cell loss in a tumor. It seems possible to measure radiation response quickly when the frequency of micronuclei formation increases.

It was asked whether, in CML patients, the polymerase chain reaction technique was applied on RNA extracted from peripheral blood cells or from bone marrow. Dr. Bartram said that in those patients RNA was extracted from both.

With respect to patients with myelodysplastic syndrome, Dr. Bartram pointed out that this disease was ignored for decades. The impression that myelodysplastic syndrome is on the increase was explained by the fact that more effort is now being put into its diagnosis.

SESSION 6

Bone Marrow Transplantation

Chairman: T. M. Fliedner

Allogeneic Marrow Transplantation in Acute Leukemia and Chronic Myelogenous Leukemia – Johns Hopkins Experience*

G. W. SANTOS for the Johns Hopkins Bone Marrow Transplantation Program

Allogeneic bone marrow transplantation (BMT) is increasingly becoming an accepted and rational therapeutic procedure in the acute leukemias and in chronic myelogenous leukemia (CML). Most of the problems of leukemic relapses, graft-versus-host disease (GVHD), viral infections, and graft rejection have been identified and solutions to these problems are being actively pursued in many centers around the world.

We wish to report our updated experience in allogeneic BMT in acute lymphoblastic leukemia (ALL), acute nonlymphoblastic leukemia (ANLL), and CML. We will also give our current approaches to some of the remaining problems.

Allogeneic Transplantation for ALL

From January 1980 to March 1988, we performed 70 marrow transplants using genotypic HLA-identical sibling donors (69) and 1 phenotypic identical parent (father) donor in patients with ALL who were in complete remission CR1 (18) with a median age of 24 years (5–36 years), CR2 (36) with a median age of 13.5 years (3–33 years), and CR3 (16) with a median age of 10 years (6–36 years). All patients were prepared with cyclophosphamide (Cy) (50 mg/kg daily × 4) followed by total body irradiation (TBI) (300 rad/day × 4 days with lung shielding for the third dose). Following transplantation, prophylaxis for GVHD included Cy, Cy and prednisolone, cyclosporine (CSA) and prednisolone, or CSA depending on what our current prophylaxis study was at the time of transplant.

Eight of 18 patients transplanted 1–17 months (median 3 months) after attaining CR1 survive in continuous remission from 2 to 68 months (median, 50 months) with an actuarial disease-free survival of 40% ± 12.5% and actuarial relapse rate of 20%. Seventeen of 18 patients had one or more poor risk factors: age ≥ 20 years ($N = 15$), initial leukocyte count ≥ 20000 ($N = 10$), chromosomal translocations ($N = 3$), delay in attaining CR > 6 weeks ($N = 8$), and nonlymphohematopoietic disease ($N = 1$).

The median duration of the first remission was 14 months (range, 1–67 months) for 36 patients in CR2. Twenty-five of these 36 patients relapsed while on their initial therapy and 11 relapsed off therapy. Twenty patients are in continuous remission at a median of 37 months (range 4–100 months) with an actuarial disease-free survival of 45% ± 9% and an actuarial relapse rate of 24%.

* Supported in part by grants (CA-15396 and CAO-6973) from the National Cancer Institute, Department of Health and Human Services, and by a grant from an anonymous donor

Sixteen patients were transplanted in CR3. The median duration of CR1 was 24 months (range, 3–60 months). Ten patients had their initial relapse on therapy and six relapsed after completion of initial therapy. Four of these 16 patients survive in continuous complete remission for a median of 64 months (range, 53–98 months). The actuarial disease-free survival is 20% ± 9.6% with an actuarial relapse rate of 47%. One patient who relapsed at 16 months achieved a fourth remission with chemotherapy and then received a second marrow transplant from the same donor following preparation with busulfan (Bu) and Cy. This patient survives free of disease 53 months after the second and 73 months after the first transplant.

Allogeneic Transplantation for ANLL

One-hundred and three patients with ANLL in first remission (50 patients) and second, third remission and early relapse 1–4 (53 patients) received HLA-identical sibling transplants following treatment with Bu 1 mg/kg orally four times daily for four consecutive days (total dose, 16 mg/kg). This was immediately followed by Cy given i.v. at a dose of 50 mg/kg daily for four consecutive doses. Post-transplantation prophylaxis was the same as outlined above for ALL. The results are displayed in Table 1.

The major contributing causes of death in patients transplanted up to 1983 were GVHD and viral infections (predominantly CMV interstitial pneumonitis). These entities accounted for 67% of deaths. Since that time we have significantly decreased these major complications to about 10%. The major changes were the institution of a standard protocol of i.v. cyclosporine (CSA) for 21 days and the oral administration of CSA for 6 months, the use of CMV seronegative blood donors for patients who were seronegative and had seronegative donors (about 30% of patients), and the use of high doses of acyclovir given i.v. until discharge from the hospital.

The actuarial disease-free survival of the 23 patients transplanted in CR1 since the institution of the above changes is 69% ± 11% and the actuarial relapse rate is 13% ± 9%. The improvement in disease-free survival was primarily due to the improvement in disease-free survival of patients aged 21–48 years, such that, in this small series, age ≤ 20 versus > 20 years did not carry a risk factor as it did when the total population of 50 patients in CR1 was analyzed.

Although the risk of fatal GVHD and viral infections was significantly decreased, in the 26 patients in CR2, CR3, and early relapse transplanted with the above prophylactic changes, the actuarial relapse was increased to about 50%. The overall result, therefore, showed no significant changes in the actuarial disease-free survival of these more recently transplanted patients.

Table 1. Allogeneic BMT in ANLL

Remission	Number of patients	Median (range), patient age (years)	Actuarial relapse rate	Actuarial disease-free survival	Median (range), disease-free survival (months)
First	50	25 (1.5–48)	13%	46%	37 (2–111)
Second, third and early relapse	53	30 (3–52)	38%	28%	56 (3–96)

Table 2. Allogeneic transplantation in CML

Median (range), age in years	Nonleukemic deaths	Actuarial relapse	Actuarial survival	Actuarial DF survival	Median (range), DF survivors in months
34 (5–50)	19 (35%)	15%	63%	53%	20 (1–36)

Table 3. Second transplants with Bu-Cy

UN[a]	Age (years)	Days to relapse after 1st BMT	Time, 2nd BMT after relapse	Days in DFS after 2nd BMT	Total days survival from 1st BMT
494	15	194	33	1375+	1602+
544	44	819	543	17+	1379+
717	34	409	49	318+	776+

[a] Unique no. (= Identification no.)

Allogeneic Transplantation for CML

Fifty-four patients with CML in the chronic phase were transplanted with HLA-identical sibling donors following the same Cy TBI regimen employed for ALL. Table 2 gives our results as of 15 June 1988.

Further analysis suggested that 19 patients who were 30 years or less (median age, 22 years with range of 5–30 years) had a better actuarial disease-free survival (85%) than the 35 patients older than 30 years (median age of 35 years with range of 31–50 years) who showed an actuarial disease-free survival of 40%. In addition, 42 patients transplanted within 2 years of their diagnosis fared better that the 12 patients who were transplanted after 2 years from their date of diagnosis. The actuarial disease-free survivals were 63% and 20% respectively. These tentative findings need validation with more patients, longer follow-up, and multivariant analysis.

Three of the patients who relapsed back into the chronic phase have been retransplanted using a preparative regimen of Bu and Cy as employed with acute nonlymphoblastic leukemia but using the same donor. The data as of 30 June 1988 are shown in Table 3.

Discussion

Two groups have reported a very low relapse rate and a relatively good disease-free survival in patients with ALL transplanted in CR2. The Memorial Sloan-Kettering group employed a preparative regimen of hyperfractionated TBI for a total dose of 1320 rad delivered in 4 days followed by Cy (60 mg/kg) given on each of two consecutive days. Of 22 patients transplanted, 14 survived in complete remission with a median follow-up of 24 months. The projected actuarial 2-year disease-free survival was 62%. There were only two relapses at 9 and 15 months. Five of 15 patients transplanted in CR3 showed an actuarial projected disease-free survival of 27%. Six of 15 patients in CR3 relapsed 1–9 months after transplantation (Dinsmore et al. 1983).

Coccia et al. (1988) reported a series of 18 patients in CR2 and 2 in CR3 (median age, 7.5 years; range, 3–15 years) who were transplanted following preparation with cytosine arabinoside (3000 mg/m^2 q 12 h for 12 doses) followed by TBI (200 rad q 12 h for 6 doses). The actuarial disease-free survival was 58% and the actuarial relapse rate was 17%. The median follow-up of survivors was 58 months with a range of 12–79 months.

Our results in CR2 do not appear to quite measure up to the results reported above; however, the number of patients in each series is small and no strict comparison has been made as to the comparability of each of the patient populations. We, of course, are disturbed by the very high relapse rate of patients transplanted in CR3. For that reason we are evaluating a combination of Bu, V16 (etoposide), and Cy as outlined below for ANLL.

With the decrease of severe GVHD and fatal viral infections in our patients transplanted in CR1 for ANLL we have seen a marked increase in disease-free survival while maintaining a low relapse rate. The present results compare favorably with those of the Memorial Sloan-Kettering Series (Dinsmore et al. 1984). Most centers such as ours have reported a high relapse rate in patients transplanted after their first remission. Accordingly we now prepare patients in all but the first remission with Bu (16 mg/kg) as before but this is followed by a single dose of VP16 (escalating doses are being evaluated) and then followed by 60 mg/kg Cy given on each of two successive days. The decrease of the Cy dosage suggests that the regimen will be less toxic (Tutschka et al. 1987) and the VP16 is added because of the apparent antileukemic effect reported by Blume et al. (1978).

Our preliminary data in patients transplanted in the chronic phase of CML appear to be comparable to those reported by others in terms of disease-free survival and relapse rate. Despite the incomplete analysis of our data, there is the strong suggestion that older patients (i.e. >30 years) and patients transplanted $>$ than 2 years after diagnosis do less well. These suggestions support those made by the Seattle group (Thomas et al. 1986) but are not supported by the report of the registry (Goldman 1987). The reasons for these apparent differences are not clear at present.

We are somewhat encouraged by our results with Bu and Cy for second transplants in CML. Because of this and anecdotal personal reports from others, we have initiated a randomized study between our current Cy-TBI regimen and Bu-Cy in CML. Those patients who have the misfortune to relapse will be offered a second transplant using the same donor but prepared with the alternative regimen.

In the past 2 years, patients >30 years of age who received HLA-identical sibling transplants have had the donor marrow treated by elutriation so that patients received only 1×10^6 T-lymphocytes/kg. In addition they received a standard regimen of cyclosporine (Wagner et al. 1988). Nineteen CML patients aged 32–60 years (median, 39 years) were part of this series. Twelve of 19 (63%) have survived from 2 to 24 months (median, 13 months). There have been two relapses (11%), three deaths of severe GVHD (16%), three deaths from nonleukemic causes (16%), and one death from failure to engraft (5%). Ten (53%) have survived free of disease from 2 to 24 months (median, 11.5 months).

Currently additional patients are being treated similarly but will receive 0.5×10^6 T-lymphocytes/kg.

Summary

In the presentation of our updated results of clinical trials we have noted the improvement in reducing the risk of severe GVHD and viral infections but have concomitantly seen a higher relapse rate in some of our subsets of patient groups. The use of a new preparative to decrease the relapse rate in these groups was noted. Finally our plans to use elutriation as a means of T-cell depletion were stated.

References

Blume KG, Forman SJ, O'Donnell MR, et al (1978) Total body irradiation and high-dose etoposide: a new preparatory regimen for bone marrow transplantation in patients in with advanced hematologic malignancies. Blood 69:1015–1020

Coccia PF, Standjord SF, Warentin PI, et al (1988) High-dose cytoside arabinoside and fractionated total-body irradiation: an improved preparative regimen for bone marrow transplantation of children with acute lymphoblastic leukemia in remission. Blood 71:888–893

Dinsmore R, Kirkpatrick D, Flomenberg N, et al (1983) Allogenic marrow transplantation for patients with acute lymphoblastic leukemia. Blood 62:381–388

Dinsmore R, Kirkpatrick D, Flomenberg N, et al (1984) Allogeneic bone marrow transplantation for patients with acute nonlymphocytic leukemia. Blood 63:649–656

Goldman JM (1987) Allogeneic bone marrow transplantation for chronic myeloid leukemia. In: Baum SJ, Santos GW, Takaku F (eds) Recent advances and future directions in bone marrow transplantation. Springer, Berlin Heidelberg NewYork, pp 94–98 (Experimental hematology today 1987)

Thomas ED, Clift RA, Fefer A, et al (1986) Marrow transplantation for the treatment of chronic myelogenous leukemia. Ann Intern Med 104:155–163

Tutschka PJ, Copeland EA, Klein JP, et al (1987) Bone marrow transplantation for leukemia following a new bulsulfan and cyclophosphamide regimen. Blood 70:1382–1388

Wagner JE, Donnenberg AD, Noga SJ, et al (1988) Lymphocyte depletion of donor bone marrow by counterflow centrifugal elutriation. Results of a phase I clinical trial. Blood 72:1168–1176

Autologous Bone Marrow Transplantation*

M. Körbling, T. M. Fliedner, K. Rother, M. Wannenmacher, and W. Hunstein

Introduction

The therapeutic concept of autologous bone marrow blood stem cell-transplantation is based on dose escalation of consolidation treatment into a "supralethal" range. The conditions for that are that the tumor remaining in the patient must respond to "supralethal" dose escalation of pretransplant therapy, and the escalated dose therapy must be primarily myelotoxic, together with acceptable extramedullary toxicity. The therapeutic advantage of the *autologous* bone marrow transplantation approach is obvious:

A marrow donor is not needed

The early transplant-related death rate is low due to the lack of "graft-versus-host" disease, due to the low incidence of interstitial pneumonitis, and due to the fact that there is no rejection of the graft.

In the *allogeneic* transplant situation, on the other hand, the marrow graft is free from clonogenic tumor cells, and the relapse rate is low due to – at least in part – the "graft-versus-leukemia" effect. The essential parts of autologous bone marrow transplantation are "purging" the autograft ex vivo from residual clonogenic tumor cells and the "supralethal" dose pretransplant therapy of the patient.

"Supralethal" Pretransplant Therapy

Hagenbeck et al. (1987) have calculated the log leukemic cell kill of different pretransplant regimens in a BN-AML rat leukemia model. The classic cyclophosphamide (CY)/total body irradiation (TBI) regimen kills leukemic cells in a range of 8–9 log, the busulfan (BU)/CY regimen, recently introduced by Santos et al. (1983), up to more than 10 log. It is interesting to see that the sequence TBI/CY with a 9–10 log cell kill is more effective than the sequence CY/TBI. This could be connected to the cell cycle characteristics of the patient's hematopoietic cell system at the time of CY treatment. The "supralethal" conditioning regimen the Heidelberg transplant group has used since 1984 consists of a myeloablative dose of TBI, superfractionated over 4 days at 120-rad single doses up to a total of 1440 cGy (lungs, 900 cGy). A linear accelerator is used as a radiation source. The dose rate lies between 5 and 17 cGy/

* Supported by the Tumor Center, Heidelberg, the Dreyhaupt Donation, and the Kind Philipp Foundation

min. Three single doses are administered per day at 8 a.m., noon, and 4. p.m. Following irradiation, CY (50 mg/kg) is given on each of the four consecutive days (total dose 200 mg/kg) (Santos et al. 1983). After 1 day rest, the cryopreserved hemopoietic cell suspension is thawed and injected into the patient over a central line. A similar pretransplant regimen which we use for patients with advanced multiple myeloma is based on what has been described by Barlogie et al. (1987) with TBI 1080 cGy (120 cGy × 9), followed by melphalan 180 mg/m^2 single dose. For Hodgkin's disease we use a pure polychemotherapeutic regimen with CY 1.7 g/m^2 q 4, BCNU 200 mg/m^2 q 4, and VP-16, 400 mg/m^2 q 4 (CBV regimen) (Jagannath et al. 1986).

"Purging" the Autograft

In 1980 Sharkis and Santos et al. (1980) first reported on a rat LBN-AML model where the syngeneic graft was successfully purged of residual tumor cells with the active cyclophosphamide derivative 4-hydroperoxycyclophosphamide (4-HC). Meanwhile 4-HC and mafosfamide, which is commercially available, are widely used for purging the autograft of patients with acute myelogenous leukemia in both, in first, and in subsequent complete remission. On the other hand, in acute lymphocytic leukemia and malignant lymphoma the ex vivo immunoseparation with cytotoxic monoclonal antibodies plus complement, with immunotoxins or with the latest and very efficient approach of immunomagnetic bead separation, is the treatment of choice to eliminate residual clonogenic tumor cells from the autograft. The idea behind a long-term culture of the autograft is to clean a marrow cell suspension by dying out residual tumor cells during a 6- to 8-week culture (Chang et al. 1986). In three patients with newly diagnosed chronic myelogenous leukemia and first-line interferon treatment we looked for the *abl-bcr* rearrangement before and during the period of marrow culture. As shown by Dr. Bartram from Ulm University, the gene rearrangement in all three patients was still there even if marrow cells were cultured for up to 6 weeks. Therefore, this latter approach of cleaning an autograft of residual clonogenic tumor cells does not seem to be successful.

The positive selection of hemopoietic precursor cells by using the monoclonal antibody CD34 (ICH3) has recently been reported by Bensinger et al. (1988) from Seattle and Levinsky from the United Kingdom. The CD34 antigen is present on 1%–4% of human and primate marrow cells including the majority of hematopoietic progenitor cells. After avidin-biotin immunoadsorption a cell suspension containing 73% or 67% CD34-positive cells was transplanted into two patients with breast cancer. Both patients showed evidence for myeloid and erythroid engraftment.

Blood-Derived Hemopoietic Stem Cells

The use of circulating blood as a stem cell compartment alternative to bone marrow was investigated extensively in the preclinical model by Fliedner et al. (1979). It is well known that hematopoietic precursor cells are in a dynamic equilibrium between the circulating blood and extravascular sites, and, therefore, blood-derived hemopoietic stem cells can be used for stem cell rescue after myeloablative treatment.

There are two possible advantages of using blood-derived stem cells rather than marrow-derived ones:

1. Fast hematopoietic reconstitution after myeloablative treatment and stem cell transplantation.
2. Possibly less tumor cell contamination of the autograft.

The major disadvantage of using circulating stem cells is the low concentration of hematopoietic precursor cells in the peripheral blood, which is about one-tenth of that in the bone marrow. Mobilization of hematopoietic precursor cell from the marrow site or from marginal pools into the circulating blood has been shown effective after chemotherapy-induced transient myelosuppression (Richman et al. 1976). After treatment with ara-C 100 mg/m^2/q 12 h s.c. on days 1–5 and daunorubicin 45 mg/m^2 i.v. injected on days 3, 4, transient myelosuppression is followed by an overshooting of CFU-GM up to 10-fold the pretreatment level at around 20 days after the end of prior cytotoxic treatment. Usually ten leukaphereses are performed per patient. The apheresis-derived white blood cells are frozen in a computerized device and stored in liquid nitrogen. Recently, we initiated a pilot study to mobilize hemopoietic precursor cells by continuous i.v. administration of GM-CSF (Behring-Werke, Marburg, FRG). At a dose of 250 μg/m^2/day the leukocyte count reaches up to 20000/μl 1 week after the start of GM-CSF administration; the CFU-GM concentration increases as well. On the other hand, the peripheral red blood cell and platelet concentration seems to remain unchanged. Nevertheless, for both mobilization techniques we do not know whether the early pluripotent stem cells are affected as well.

Therapeutic Benefit of Stem Cell Transplantation

For determination of the clinical efficacy of autologous bone marrow transplantation, marrow transplants between twins are a model. Results with syngeneic bone marrow transplantation represent the most that one might hope to achieve with autologous marrow uncontaminated with clonogenic tumor cells. The Seattle experience (5 out of 12 patients relapsed) and the experience which was gained in the United States and Europe, excluding the Seattle results (11 out of 23 patients relapsed),

Table 1. Disease-free survival after autologous bone marrow transplantation in patients with acute leukemia

	CR	Purged	Un-purged	Percentage, patients disease-free	(Median) disease-free follow-up
Stewart et al. (1985)	1		×	3/13 (23%)	26–50 months
Burnett et al. (1984)	1		×	7/12 (58%)	6.5–35 months
Gorin et al. (1986)	1	×		9/13 (69%)	22 months
Santos et al. (1988)	1	×		9/16 (56%)	18.8 months
Gorin et al. (1986)	2+	×		2/11 (18%)	9, 10 months
Santos et al. (1988)	2+	×		27/71 (38%)	17 months

show that the relapse rate after syngeneic bone marrow transplantation is surprisingly high. It lies in the range of 50% (Fefer 1986).

If one looks at autologous bone marrow transplantation, the updated results of the European Bone Marrow Transplant Group on disease-free survival in patients with acute myelogenous leukemia, first remission, and after TBI lie in the range of 60% with mafosfamide purging, and 30% without mafosfamide purging. The difference between both groups is significant ($P = 0.02$).

We transplanted a total of 37 patients with AML in first and subsequent complete remission, 17 in first complete remission, and 20 in second, third, or fourth complete remission. The probability of disease-free survival in those patients lies in the range of 60% for first remission and 30% for second, third, and fourth remission at a median follow-up of 22 months or 21 months, respectively. It should be mentioned that the disease-free survival plateau in first remission patients is very stable, whereas late relapses have been observed in high-risk AML patients. Table 1 shows what has been recently published about disease-free survival from single institutions.

If one looks at disease-free survival in patients with acute lymphocytic leukemia, transplanted in our institution in first complete remission under high-risk conditions, eight out of ten patients live in unmaintained complete remission at a median follow-up of 28 months. When autologous bone marrow transplantation has been performed in second or subsequent remission, 5 out of 13 patients are presently in complete remission at a median follow-up of 8 months.

In Hodgkin's lymphoma, the entry criteria for our study were early relapse within 12 months after COPP/ABVD and responsive to rescue treatment. Four out of nine patients are in unmaintained complete remission at 1, 2, 8, and 20 months after transplantation.

The fact that the duration of remission after autologous bone marrow transplantation exceeds that of the remission duration prior to ABMT speaks for the therapeutic benefit of this transplantation approach. Forty percent of all AML patients transplanted in second, third, or fourth remission show such an inversion.

In autologous *blood stem cell transplantation,* the median follow-up of AML patients is still too short to draw only conclusions. Nine out of 18 patients transplanted in first remission of AML live in unmaintained complete remission at a median follow-up of 7 months. One patient with Burkitt's lymphoma has survived autologous blood stem cell transplantation almost 3½ years, for the longest period of time known in the literature without any signs of disease (Körbling et al. 1986). One patient with progressive multiple myeloma, refractory to standard treatment, was treated with TBI/melphalan and eventually transplanted with blood-derived hemopoietic stem cells 6 months ago. This patient has gone into complete remission with recalcification of multiple bone lesions and no more detectable light chains.

Hemopoietic Reconstitution

Hematopoietic reconstitution after autologous bone marrow transplantation is characterized by a slow platelet recovery. In our study the probability of reaching a stable 20000/μl peripheral platelet concentration for 50% of patients was within the range of 50 days; about 10% of patients have not reached this level of platelet concentration even 200 days after transplantation. That means prolonged platelet support, the risk of immunization, and high costs. On the other hand, hemopoietic reconstitution after blood stem cell transplantation occurs very fast; the pretransplant level of white blood cell concentration is already reached after 2 weeks. Some patients only needed one or two platelet transfusions to keep their peripheral platelet concentration above 20000/μl. The reason for such a fast hemopoietic reconstitution is probably due to the fact that together with early pluripotent stem cells many more mature hemopoietic precursor cells are transplanted, giving rise to a first transient peak which is followed by the hemopoietic reconstitution from early pluripotent stem cells. This early peak decreases the time of total aplasia and therefore the risk of bleeding and infection.

If one compares both the bone marrow graft and the blood stem cell graft, disease-free survival after transplantation as well as hemopoietic reconstitution might depend on the cell composition of the graft. The bone marrow graft is mostly depleted of T cells by mafosfamide purging (Körbling et al. 1982), whereas the blood stem cell graft is characterized by high T-cell contamination, nonpurging, and the fact that stem cell harvest is performed during stem cell "overshooting" or under GM-CSF infusion. Further studies have to be performed to evaluate the role of T cells in hematopoietic reconstitution and disease-free survival, as well as the role of cell cycle characteristics of the stem cell graft.

Autologous Versus Allogeneic Marrow Transplantation

If we compare autologous versus allogeneic transplantation – at least under high-risk conditions – the difference in disease-free survival between both approaches is not clearly significant. Santos et al. (1983), Yeager et al. (1985) compared 25 autologous bone marrow transplantations with 19 allogeneic bone marrow transplantations at high risk, and did not find a significant difference in disease-free survival following relapse and transplantation. Kersey et al. (1987) made the same observation in high-risk refractory ALL patients, but in this study the statistical power to prove significance was low because of the small sample size.

Future Aspects of Autologous Stem Cell Transplantation

Certain aspects of autologous stem cell transplantation require investigation in the near future: The toxicity of the pretransplant regimen in most studies has reached a limit. Adding some more radiation or chemotherapy would definitely harm the patient. Therefore, to improve therapeutic efficacy it would probably help to add immune modulation measures or, as proposed by Hess et al. (1985), the induction of an autologous graft-versus-host disease-like syndrome.

It seems that it is possible to expand the stem cell pool of the autograft ex vivo by using human recombinant growth factors like GM-CSF or interleukin-3 (Fabian et al. 1987). Purging the autograft can be performed by positive stem cell purification with monoclonal antibodies. The prophylactic stem cell cryopreservation could be performed in persons who are at risk from severe radiation exposure or in patients where stem cell harvest is performed in first remission of acute leukemia, or transplantation on the other hand, in second or third remission.

References

Barlogie B, Alexanian R, Dicke KA, et al (1987) High dose chemoradiotherapy and autologous bone marrow transplantation for resistant multiple myeloma. Blood 70:869–872

Bensinger WI, Berenson RJ, Andrews RG, et al (1988) Proceedings of XIVth Annual Meeting of the European Cooperative Group for Bone Marrow Transplantation, Chamonix, France, 10–13 April 1988

Chang J, Coutinho L, Morgenstern G, et al (1986) Reconstitution of haemopoietic system with autologous marrow taken during relapse of acute myeloblastic leukaemia and grown in long-term culture. Lancet I:294–295

Fabian I, Bleiberg I, Riklis I, et al (1987) Enhanced reconstitution of hematopoietic organs in irradiated mice following their transplantation with bone marrow cells pretreated with recombinant interleukin 3. Exp Hematol 15:1140–1144

Fefer A (1986) Current status of syngeneic marrow transplantation and its relevance to autografting. Clin Haemtaol 15:49–65

Fliedner TM, Calvo W, Körbling M, et al (1979) Collection, storage and transfusion of blood stem cells for the treatment of hemopoietic failure. Blood Cells 5:313–328

Hagenbeck A, Martens CM (1987) Conditioning regimens before bone marrow transplantation in acute myelocytic leukemia. In: Dicke KA, Spitzer G, Jagannath S (eds) Autologous bone marrow transplantation. Proceedings of the third international symposium. University of Texas MD. Anderson Hospital and Tumor Institute, Houston, pp 99–103

Hess AD, Horwitz L, Beschorner WE, Santos GW (1985) Development of graft-versus-host disease like syndrome in cyclosporine-treated rats after syngeneic bone marrow transplantation. J Exp Med 161:718–730

Jagannath S, Dicke KA, Armitage JO, et al (1986) High dose cyclophosphamide, carmustine, and etoposide and autologous bone marrow transplantation for relapsed Hodgkin's disease. Ann Intern Med 104:163–168

Kersey HJ, Weisdorf D, Nesbit ME, et al (1987) Comparison of autologous and allogeneic bone marrow transplantation for treatment of high-risk refractory acute lymphoblastic leukemia. N Engl J Med 317:461–467

Körbling M, Hess AD, Tutschka PJ, et al (1982) 4-Hydroperoxycyclophosphamide: a model for eliminating residual human tumour cells and T-lymphocytes from the bone marrow graft. Br J Haematol 52:89–96

Körbling M, Dörken B, Ho AD, et al (1986) Autologous transplantation of blood-derived hemopoietic stem cells after myeloablative therapy in a patient with Burkitt's lymphoma. Blood 67:529

Richman CM, Weiner RS, Yankee RA, et al (1976) Increase in circulating stem cells following chemotherapy in man. Blood 47:1031–1034

Santos GW, Tutschka PJ, Brookmeyer R, et al (1983) Marrow transplantation for acute nonlymphocytic leukemia after treatment with busulfan and cyclophosphamide. N Engl J Med 309:1347–1353

Sharkis SJ, Santos GW, Colvin M (1980) Elimination of acute myelogenous leukemic cells from marrow and tumor suspensions in the rat with 4-hydroperoxycyclophosphamide. Blood 55:521–523

Yeager AM, Kaizer H, Santos GW, et al (1985) Autologous bone marrow transplantation in patients with acute nonlymphocytic leukemia, using ex vivo marrow treatment with 4-hydroperoxycyclophosphamide. N Engl J Med 315:141–147

Summary of Discussion: Session 6

H.-J. Kolb

Following the review of allogeneic bone marrow transplantation by G. W. Santos, questions were raised regarding the distinction of cytogenetic from hematologic relapse of chronic myelogenous leukemia. In contrast to hematologic relapse, cytogenetic relapse is confined to reoccurrence of the Philadelphia chromosome, without any clinical signs of chronic myelogenous leukemia. The distinction is important, since a proportion of patients with reappearing Philadelphia-positive cells after allogeneic marrow transplantation may again lose these cells later on. G. W. Santos explained that cytogenetic analyses were done in his patients at 1, 3 and 6 months and every 6 months thereafter and patients with Philadelphia-positive cells were scored as relapsing, even when the Philadelphia-positive cells were only transiently detected. Patients with a relapse of chronic myelogenous leukemia late after allogeneic marrow transplantation may profit from a second transplant.

W. Wilmanns asked whether the rate of relapse was influenced by the degree of graft-versus-host disease. There was little doubt, G. W. Santos felt, that graft-versus-host disease decreased the rate of relapses following allogeneic marrow transplantation, but patients may not reap any benefit from this, since the graft-versus-host disease itself may be like a fire that burns up the patient. At present there is no way to keep the flame of graft-versus-host disease without risking the fire.

Another point of discussion was the handling of enlarged spleens in patients with chronic myelogenous leukemia prior to transplantation. Some transplant centers consider a very large spleen to be an indication that the patient is no longer in chronic phase. G. W. Santos and H.-J. Kolb agreed that a large spleen is not an indication of accelerated phase unless the size of the spleen does not respond to systemic treatment. H.-J. Kolb referred to a study of J. M. Goldman published in the *Lancet* in which splenectomy, irradiation of the spleen, and no treatment to the spleen were compared. This study found no differences between when the spleen was treated additionally and when it was not. Another study of the European cooperative group for bone marrow transplantation (EBMT), coordinated by A. Gratwohl, compares splenic irradiation and no treatment to the spleen in a randomized multicenter trial which is still ongoing.

Questions regarding preparative regimens were raised by T. M. Fliedner, particularly as to the advantages of busulfan over total body irradiation. Like radiation, busulfan is highly toxic to hemopoietic stem cells and may provide the "space" necessary for the allogeneic graft to take. In Baltimore busulfan was chosen instead of total body irradiation at a time when there was no suitable radiation set-up for patients. At present, the major advantage of busulfan is its practicality in administration, since it keeps the transplant center independent from the radiotherapy department and can be given on weekends and so on. Further advantages may emerge in randomized studies comparing busulfan and total body irradiation.

In patients receiving second transplants after a second conditioning treatment, damage to the hemopoietic microenvironment may be expected. However, most patients receiving second transplants showed uneventful engraftment and hemopoietic recovery. Although repeated conditioning treatment for transplantation may damage the microenvironment, this damage appears not to be so severe as to prevent full hemopoietic recovery.

Autologous bone marrow transplantation was reviewed by M. Körbling and future directions were discussed. A positive selection of hemopoietic stem cells for transplantation may be achieved by the use of CD34 monoclonal antibodies. However these monoclonal antibodies should not be used in myelogenous leukemias, since cells of these leukemias also express the CD34 antigen. G. W. Santos reported a monoclonal antibody against acute myelogenous leukemia cells which crossreacts with rat acute myelogenous leukemia. This antibody is presently being tested in the rat and may be used for purging marrow from leukemia cells prior to autologous transplantation. Another new development at the Johns Hopkins University Hospital is the detection of cytotoxic T cells against autologous Ia antigens following autologous marrow transplantation and cyclosporin treatment. This autoreactivity may be used for an antileukemic effect in the former situation.

The possibility of using peripheral blood stem cells instead of marrow was discussed. One reason was a suspected lower contamination of blood with residual leukemic cells. An interesting case of a patient with multiple myeloma transplanted with peripheral blood stem cells was reported by M. Körbling. However, the criteria for bone marrow transplantation in patients with multiple myeloma are yet to be defined. Similarly, the indication for autologous bone marrow transplantation in the treatment of solid tumors is a matter of controversy. The largest group of patients studied have been patients with small cell lung cancer, and outcome was variable.

When should the marrow be harvested after chemotherapy? For practical reasons, it should be harvested as soon as possible after recovery from marrow depression. The use of granulocyte-monocyte-colony stimulating factor (GM-CSF) prior to collection of peripheral blood stem cells does not increase the number of pluripotent stem cells such as colony-forming unit-granulocytes-erythrocytes-monocytes-megakaryocytes (CFU-GEMM) in the blood. GM-CSF may be also used after autologous transplantation in order to speed up hemopoietic recovery. However, M. Körbling reported on a patient with acute lymphoblastic leukemia following transplantation who was given GM-CSF, but in whom he did not see an improvement of hemopoietic recovery. G. W. Santos quoted D. Metcalf on this point, who had observed an increase in granulocyte counts but no increase in pluripotent stem cells of the blood, nor any improvement of thrombocytopoiesis.

T. M. Fliedner suggested that transfusion of red cells in large amounts may speed up recovery of granulopoiesis and thrombocytopoiesis by relieving a competitive differentiative pathway for the pluripotent stem cells.

SESSION 7

Antibody Guided Therapy

Chairman: P. Bannasch

Predictive Pharmacology of Monoclonal Antibodies

J. N. WEINSTEIN and K. FUJIMORI

Introduction

High specificity and affinity are useful only if an administered antibody or antibody conjugate reaches the intended target and interacts with it effectively. Pharmacologic factors at several hierarchical levels – whole-body, regional, local, cellular, and molecular – all operate to determine whether effective delivery is, in fact, achieved. Studies in animal models and in humans over the last several years have shown that monoclonal antibodies tend to accumulate heterogeneously in tumors after intravenous administration. Part of that heterogeneity relates to nonuniform distribution of antigen among tumor cells and among regions of a tumor (Schlom et al. 1983). A second part relates to nonuniform access from the bloodstream.

To study the problem of access, we have developed an integrated approach to pharmacological modeling: the global pharmacokinetics are interfaced with microscopic issues related to passage across endothelial boundaries, "percolation" through the tumor to antigenic sites, and metabolic handling by the target cells. The database for analysis derives in part from our experiments in rodents, in part from clinical trials in patients with lymphoma or melanoma, and in part from *in vitro* studies. These experimental and theoretical analyses reveal a set of complex trade-offs: for example, antibodies optimized for diagnosis by gamma scintigraphy are unlikely to be most favorable for therapy; antibody/antigen pairs favorable for treatment with gamma-emitter conjugates may not be suitable for treatment with immunotoxins. Early results of this work have been described elsewhere (Weinstein et al. 1986, 1987a, b).

There are two stages of tumor growth in which the ability of antibody to percolate through tumors may become rate-limiting to effective antibody distribution: (1) at an early stage, in which the nodule (or *in vitro* tumor cell spheroid) is nonvascular and less than about 2 mm in diameter; (2) at a later stage, when the tumor has developed its own blood vessels and then has begun to outgrowth them. We will focus here on the first of those stages and, for simplicity, will treat the tumor as a simple, uniform sphere of cells through which antibody must diffuse toward the center. We will ask how uniform the concentration is predicted to be as a function of various parameters of the system and at various time points. Elsewhere, we will consider more complex cases, such as that in which the tumor is nonuniform and in which convection dominates the transport properties (Swabb et al. 1974). The problem becomes even more complex for vascularized tumors sufficiently large to develop internal hydrostatic pressure gradients (Jain 1987).

Regardless of the specific geometry, a major concern is what we have termed the "binding site barrier" – the prediction that bindable immunoglobulin (or other ligand) will be retarded in its diffusion (or convection) through tumor by the very fact of its successful binding. Nonuniformity of distribution will tend to be increased by a high density of antigenic sites, a low diffusion coefficient, and high binding affinity. To illustrate the pattern of this analysis, we will focus here on the effect of one parameter, antibody dose, on the distribution of immunoglobulin G in a hypothetical tumor spheroid of diameter 0.6 mm (600 μm). At this size, cells in the center are becoming poorly supplied with oxygen and other nutrients.

Method

Calculations were performed on a CRAY X-MP computer using a program package that we call PERC and using standard sets of parameter values described elsewhere (K. Fujimori, D. G. Covell, J. E. Fletcher, and J. N. Weinstein, in press, 1989). Diffusion of antibody through spheroids has also been analyzed mathematically by McFadden and Kwok (1988) for the special case of nonsaturating, irreversible binding.

Results and Discussion

Figure 1a shows the radial distribution of a relatively high-affinity antibody (assumed to have $K_d = 10^{-9} M$) at a high antigen density of $10^{-6} M$ with respect to interstitial space. The effective diffusion coefficient is taken as 1.0×10^{-8} cm^2/s. The antibody concentration at the outer edge of the "tumor nodule" is assumed to be in equilibrium with plasma levels after a bolus dose of 100 mg in the standard 70-kg man (Eger et al. 1987). Figure 1b shows the results for a bolus dose of 50 mg. Clearly, the distribution is more uniform at the higher dose, as antibody saturates and overwhelms binding sites at the margin of the nodule. More extensive calculations to be presented

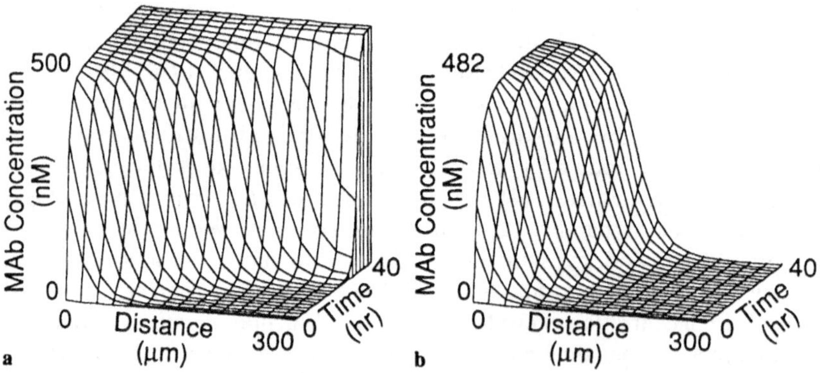

Fig. 1a, b. Calculated distribution of monoclonal immunoglobulin G in a microscopic "tumor nodule" as a function of (bolus) dose administered intravenously to the standard 70-kg man. See text for explanation of the calculation and the parameter values used. (**a**) 100-mg dose; (**b**) 50-mg dose. The larger dose partially overcomes the "binding site barrier" and produces more uniform antibody distribution

elsewhere (K. Fujimori, D. G. Covell, J. E. Fletcher, and J. N. Weinstein, in press, 1989) indicate in detail the relationship between antibody dose and the binding site barrier.

The calculations presented here must be considered as predictions from a mathematically abstract case. However, over the last few years, a number of studies have demonstrated at least qualitatively the nonuniformity of antibody distributions in tumors (Meeker et al. 1985; Abrams and Oldham 1985; Jones et al. 1986; Sutherland et al. 1987). The empirical correlations will be considered in more detail elsewhere.

Acknowledgements. We are grateful to Dr. David G. Covell and Dr. John E. Fletcher for their efforts in development of the computer packages used for these calculations.

References

Abrams PG, Oldham RK (1985) Monoclonal antibody therapy of solid tumors. In: Foon KA, Morgan AC Jr (eds) Monoclonal antibody therapy of human cancer. Nijhoff, Boston, pp 103–120

Eger RR, Covell DG, Carrasquillo JA, Abrams PG, Foon KA, Reynolds JC, Schroff RW, Morgan AC, Larson SM, Weinstein JN (1987) Kinetic model for the biodistribution of an ^{111}In-labeled monoclonal antibody in humans. Cancer Res 47:3328–3336

Fujimori K, Covell DG, Fletcher JE, Weinstein JN (1989) A modeling analysis of the global and microscopic distribution of IgG, F(ab')2, and Fab in tumors. Cancer Res (in press)

Jain RK (1987) Transport of molecules in the tumor interstitium: a review. Cancer Res 47:3039–3051

Jones PL, Gallagher BM, Sands H (1986) Autoradiographic analysis of monoclonal antibody distribution in human colon and breast tumor xenografts. Cancer Immunol Immunother 22:139–143

McFadden R, Kwok CS (1988) Mathematical model of simultaneous diffusion and binding of antitumor antibodies in multicellular human tumors spheroids. Cancer Res 48:4032–4037

Meeker TC, Lowder J, Maloney DG, Miller RA, Thielemans K, Warnke R, Levy R (1985) A clinical trial of anti-idiotype therapy for B cell malignancy. Blood 65:1349–1363

Schlom J, Colcher D, Hand PH, et al (1983) Antigenic heterogeneity, modulation and evolution in breast cancer lesions as defined by monoclonal antibodies. In: Rich M, Hager J, Furmanski P (eds) Understanding breast cancer: clinical and laboratory concepts. Dekker, New York, pp 315–358

Sutherland R, Buchegger F, Schreyer M, Vacca A, Mach J-P (1987) Penetration and binding of radiolabeled anti-carcinoembryonic antigen monoclonal antibodies and their antigen binding fragments in human colon multicellular tumor spheroids. Cancer Res 47:1627–1633

Swabb EA, Wei J, Gullino PM (1974) Diffusion and convection in normal and neoplastic tissues. Cancer Res 24:2814–2822

Weinstein JN, Black CDV, Barbet J, Eger RR, Parker RJ, Holton OD III, Mulshine JL, Keenan AM, Larson SM, Carrasquillo JA, Sieber SM, Covell DG (1986) Selected issues in the pharmacology of monoclonal antibodies. In: Tomlinson E, Davis SS (eds) Site-specific drug delivery. Wiley, New York, pp 81–91

Weinstein JN, Covell DG, Barbet J, Eger RR, Holton OD III, Talley MJ, Parker RJ, Black CDV (1987a) Local and cellular factors in the pharmacology of monoclonal antibodies. In: Bonavida B, Collier RJ (eds) Membrane mediated toxicity. Liss, New York, pp 279–289

Weinstein JN, Eger RR, Covell DG, Black CDV, Mulshine J, Carrasquillo JA, Larson SM, Keenan AM (1987b) The pharmacology of monoclonal antibodies. Ann NY Acad Sci 507:199–210

A New Approach in the Treatment of Advanced Ovarian Cancer and Brain Glioma Using Radiolabelled Monoclonal Antibodies

G. B. Sivolapenko, H. P. Kalofonos, and A. A. Epenetos

Introduction

Administration of a lethal dose of radiation to tumor cells while sparing normal tissue is the ideal aim in radiotherapy. The closest we come to this ideal is in the treatment of thyroid carcinoma, where tumor cells take up and concentrate iodine 131. Although thyroid carcinoma is not particularly radiosensitive, the dose is so great that the tumor cells are destroyed with minimal toxicity to normal tissue. Unfortunately, no other tumor behaves quite like this, and we must rely on external beam irradiation, where the tolerated dose is much less. Chemotherapy generally shows good results, but anti-neoplastic drugs cannot discriminate between cancer cells and rapidly proliferating normal cells, and therefore the side effects can be considerable.

The major aim in improving the treatment of cancer must be to find reagents that act more specifically against tumor cells, leaving the surrounding normal tissue intact.

The innovative idea of the "magic bullet", suggested by Paul Ehrlich at the beginning of this century (Ehrlich 1957), was revived in 1975, when Köhler and Milstein described a method for production of unlimited amounts of antibodies with predefined specificity (Köhler and Milstein 1975). Such monoclonal antibodies (MAbs) are used for the detection, analysis, characterization and manipulation of various substances. In clinical medicine they are particularly useful for the diagnosis and treatment of many diseases. Cancer is no exception. Indeed, as the number of tumor-associated MAbs used by various investigators increases each year, more clinical trials and more promising clinical results are added to the fight against cancer.

Monoclonal antibodies have been administered alone or conjugated to toxins or drugs with very promising results in many in vitro and in vivo experiments (Duerst et al. 1986; Herlyn et al. 1980; Miller and Levy 1981; Blackey et al. 1987; Combes et al. 1986; Dillman et al. 1986). It has been apparent for several years that radioisotopes conjugated to tumor-associated MAbs could provide a powerful tool for the diagnosis and management of neoplastic diseases. This technique may allow clinicians to identify primary and metastatic tumor lesions in patients without having to undertake intensive surgical procedures. Areas of intense radioactivity in certain regions of the body, as seen using a gamma-camera, may indicate the presence of tumor. Many investigators all over the world are successfully using radiolabelled tumor-associated MAbs for the localization or detection of neoplastic lesions (Epenetos et al. 1985; Critchley et al. 1986; Granowska et al. 1986; Pawlikowska and Epenetos 1986). Nevertheless, one of the main goals of MAb research is not only the early detection but also the therapy of cancer. Radiolabelled antibodies administered intravenously have, so far, been of limited value in the treatment of malignant melanoma, lymphoma, and neuroblastoma (Sedlacek et al. 1988). Because the amount of label reaching the tumor after intravenous administration of MAb is insufficient (Epenetos et al. 1986), we have investigated alternative routes of administering radiolabelled antibodies regionally.

Ovarian cancer is the fifth most common cancer in the human population, and it is the second most common cause of death due to cancer in women. Most patients at the time of diagnosis have tumor outside the pelvis (stage III, FIGO classification). After initial cytoreductive surgery, treatment includes systemic chemotherapy for advanced disease, producing dramatic reduction in tumor size (Griffiths et al. 1979), but the overall survival has improved only marginally (Neijt et al. 1984), as relapses occur even after complete remission. A major cause of treatment failure in these patients is the inability to control the disease within the peritoneal cavity. Radiotherapy, either by external beam irradiation to the entire abdomen or by intracavitary administration of radiocolloids, has had some beneficial effect (Dembo 1985).

Brain gliomas, comprising of about 60% of all primary CNS tumors, have a very poor prognosis despite advances in surgery, radiotherapy and chemotherapy. Postoperative irradiation may improve the quality of life and extend survival (Bloom 1975).

This report outlines our experience using MAbs labelled with iodine 131 in the treatment of patients with stage III ovarian cancer and minimal residual disease, and in patients with recurrent brain gliomas resistant to conventional treatment. The efficacy of this new method is assessed, as well as the side effects due to the radioactivity or the MAbs administered.

Patients, Materials and Methods

Patients

Thirty six patients aged 36–75 years (mean, 58 years), with residual ovarian cancer following cytoreductive surgery and chemotherapy, were eligible to enter the trial of intraperitoneal radiolabelled MAb therapy. Before antibody-guided treatment, fresh frozen or formalin-fixed, paraffin-embedded tissue sections of the tumor were tested (using the indirect immunoperoxidase technique) for antibody reactivity. A peritoneal catheter was inserted into the abdomen and its position verified by infusion of 1 mCi of technetium 99m. The labelled antibody was infused into the peritoneal cavity with 1 l 0.9% saline and the peritoneal catheter removed. Patients received potassium iodide to decrease the thyroid incorporation of iodine 131. The amount of tumor present in the peritoneal cavity was classified as follows: macroscopic disease (nodules >2 cm in diameter), minimal residual disease (nodules <2 cm in diameter) and microscopic disease. The amount of MAb administered was 10–30 mg, labelled with 80–150 mCi iodine 131.

Seven patients, aged 14–63 years (mean, 34 years), with recurrent grade III or IV glioma resistant to conventional treatment, who showed good antibody localization in external body scintigraphy, underwent treatment. Radiolabelled MAb was delivered to the tumor area by infusion into the internal carotid artery ($n = 4$) or by intravenous administration ($n = 3$). The dose of MAb given was 10–20 mg, labelled with 40–140 mCi iodine 131.

Monoclonal Antibodies

1. HMFG1 and HMFG2 are mouse IgG1 directed against a high molecular weight mucin expressed by the majority (more than 90%) of ovarian, breast and other carcinomas (Taylor-Papadimitriou et al. 1981).
2. AUA1 is a mouse IgG1 directed against an antigen (40 kDa molecular weight glycoprotein) expressed by a wide range of adenocarcinomas, including the majority of carcinomas of the ovary (Arklie et al. 1981; Spurr et al. 1986).
3. EGFR1 is a mouse IgG1 directed to the native folded external domain of the human epidermal growth factor receptor (Waterfield et al. 1982).
4. H17E2 is a mouse IgG1 directed against placental alkaline phosphatase (Travers and Bodmer 1984). This is expressed as a surface membrane antigen on many neoplasms, including ovarian cancer, testicular tumors, gliomas, etc.

Radiolabelling

Iodine 131 was coupled to immunoglobulins using iodogen-coated tubes (Fraker et al. 1978). The mixture was incubated for 5 min and the radiolabelled antibody separated from the free radioiodine by gel filtration on Sephadex G50. Iodine 131 is an isotope with high energy γ rays (364 KeV), which allows detection by gamma-camera but also, because of its β emission, is suitable for therapy. Immunoreactivity of the antibody was tested before and after radiolabelling in a direct radioimmunoassay, including competition with unlabelled MAb, as previously described (Epenetos et al. 1986).

Dosimetry

In order for the treatment to be effective, the dose of radiation to the target relative to whole body or other sensitive organs should be very high. To calculate appropriate doses it is necessary to know the proportion of the administered activity going to the target and other relevant organs, the time course of the activity in the target and through the body, and the volume of distribution of the activity in the target. Volumes for the major organs of the body have been tabulated for reference and assumed to be sufficiently accurate for most calculations of doses (Snyder et al. 1978). Radiation doses for patients with large volume disease would be lower. These dosimetry calculations have been reported in detail elsewhere (Myers et al. 1986).

Response Evaluation

The presence of ovarian cancer was histologically confirmed before antibody therapy by performing a second-look laparotomy or laparoscopy with peritoneal washings.

After therapy, three of the patients believed to have responded favourably underwent repeat laparoscopies and peritoneal washings at 3- to 6-month intervals. All patients with glioma were subjected to a pre-therapy evaluation which included a history and a physical examination as well as determining blood count and biochemical profile and carrying out X-ray, CT and antibody scans. The response in each patient after antibody treatment was assessed clinically and radiologically. Computer tomograms were taken 4 weeks after the treatment and then at various intervals.

Kinetics

Blood samples were taken every 12 h and urine colleted for 5 days following therapy. Aliquots of the serum and urine were counted in a gamma counter along with a radioisotope standard.

Anti-MAb Response

A serum sample was obtained from every patient before and 14 days after administration of the therapeutic MAb. We examined whether the patients responded against the mouse immunoglobulin. The method followed was a well-established enzyme-linked immunosorbent assay (ELISA) described elsewhere (Courtenay-Luck et al. 1986).

Results

Patients

Twenty eight out of 36 patients with ovarian cancer have been followed up for more than 3 months and are analysed in this report. Details are shown in Table 1. Patients with macroscopic disease responded poorly to MAb therapy and died 1–19 months after treatment. Patients with minimal residual disease responded better, with one partial response (PR) and one patient free of disease at 12 months. Figure 1a shows the CT scan of a patient with ovarian cancer and Fig. 1b the antibody scan of the same patient after treatment. The arrow indicates the location of the tumor on the CT, which is confirmed by the antibody scan.

Table 1. Therapy results of patients with ovarian cancer treated with ^{131}I-labelled MAb (HMFG1)

Size of tumour	No. of patients	Response
Nodules >2 cm	8	–
Nodules <2 cm	15	1 PR, 1 CR
Microscopic disease	5	3 CR

PR, partial response; CR, complete response

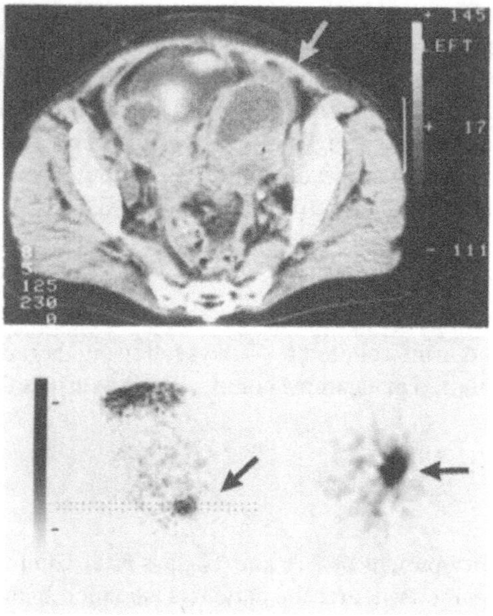

a

b

Fig. 1. a CT scan of the pelvis of a patient with ovarian cancer *(arrow)*. **b** Antibody scan *(left)* and tomogram *(right)*, confirming presence of ovarian cancer *(arrow)*

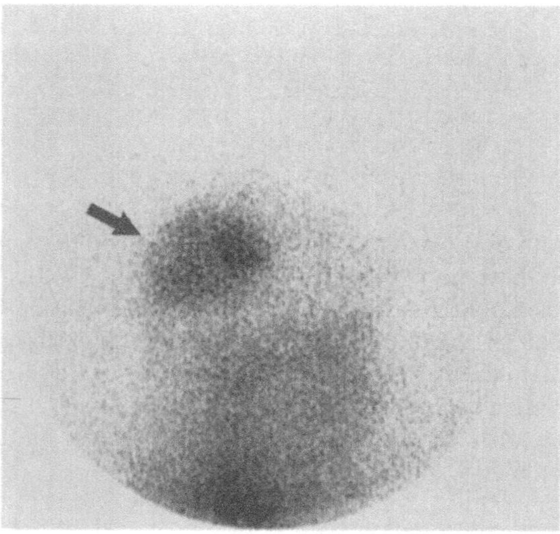

Fig. 2. Antibody scan of a patient with glioma, after intravenous administration of an ^{131}I-labelled MAb (EGFR1). Note tumor uptake *(arrow)*. Lateral view

All the other patients developed progressive disease and died. The best survival was observed in patients with microscopic disease with only two patients relapsed. Toxicity was acceptable. One patient developed subphrenic abscess and another had a perforated sigmoid colon requiring a temporary colostomy because of catheter insertion. Four patients developed pyrexia of short duration, six patients nausea and vomiting, and two patients abdominal pain with temporary peritonism. No bone marrow suppression was noted at doses below 100 mCi of ^{131}I-labelled MAb. Patients who received 150 mCi developed reversible thrombocytopenia and neutropenia.

Four out of seven patients with glioma showed clinical improvement lasting from 6 months to 3 years (Fig. 2). One patient, who was treated twice with 100 mCi each time, is continuing in complete remission 3 years after treatment, but three out of the four patients who responded initially relapsed and died 6–12 months after therapy. The patients who received more than 100 mCi also developed reversible thrombocytopenia and neutropenia.

Kinetics

The intraperitoneally administered MAb migrated slowly into the blood stream. The peak of radioactivity in the blood was observed 40 h after injection, with 26% of the injected dose in the systemic circulation. Following this peak, the iodine 131 was cleared monoexponentially from the circulation, with an effective half-life of 38–60 h (mean, 50 h). Patients receiving the first treatment excreted over 60% of the iodine 131 in the urine by 110 h after injection.

Dosimetry

Dosimetric calculations indicate that the mean radiation dose in ovarian cancer and glioma patients was 2.9 cGy and 0.7 cGy respectively per millicurie of iodine 131 administered. Bone marrow radiation dose, according to the calculations, was 1.55 cGy/mCi iodine 131.

Toxicity

The toxicity was acceptable. Abdominal pain was noted in four patients and pyrexia of up to 38°C in seven patients lasting for 4 hours. Nausea and mild vomiting were noted at 24 hours following antibody therapy and lasted for one to two days. Watery diarrhea was also noted one to three days after treatment but it was self-limiting. Two patients developed transient peritonitis within 24 hours of the treatment but this syndrome was also self-limiting within 6 hours. Finally one patient developed a subphrenic abscess within 2 weeks of the treatment, and required percutaneous drainage.

Anti-MAb Response

As expected, almost all the patients recognized the mouse immunoglobulin as foreign and responded to it. There was great variability among the responses, some patients being oversensitized to the MAb. It was also found that some patients were recognising the MAb even before administration. This is due to the presence of cross-reactive rheumatoid factors that recognise the Fc portion of the mouse immunoglobulin as well as that of the human immunoglobulin.

Discussion

In this study we showed that ^{131}I-labelled MAbs administered regionally or intravenously can achieve a therapeutic effect in patients with small-volume stage III ovarian cancer and patients with recurrent brain gliomas. A limitation of the radiolabelled MAbs is that they do not penetrate far into the tumor (Sutherland et al. 1987) and the lack of efficacy seen in patients with gross disease is therefore not surprising, although palliation of malignant effusions has been observed previously (Kalofonos and Epenetos 1987). Radiation doses delivered to solid tumor deposits were insufficient for tumour cell death in ovarian cancer and in glioma patients. However, these doses were effective in patients treated with positive washings and micrometastatic disease, as well as in one patient with glioma who was treated on two occasions with 100 mCi after conventional treatment with external beam radiotherapy. We were encouraged that four out of seven glioma patients treated showed clinical response even after one treatment.

The dose limiting organ in the radioimmunotherapy is the haemopoietic bone marrow. Bone marrow radiation dose was closely related with myelosuppression above 100 cGy. Although severe bone marrow suppression is seen with iodine 131 treatment for thyroid cancer (Dobyns and Maloof 1951), it is possible to give more than 200 mCi per treatment and more than 700 mCi total over several years without complications (Dobyns and Maloof 1951). Toxicity due to antibody-guided irradiation proved to be mild. No patient died as a result of this procedure and no patient required hospitalization for haematologic toxicity.

Despite the small number of patients in this study, we believe that we have demonstrated the potential effectiveness of this treatment. The most important parameter in achieving a useful response in ovarian cancer cases is tumour size, small-volume residual disease (nodules <2 cm in diameter and positive washings) giving the most promising results. These results may be improved if one repeatedly administers radiolabelled MAbs or more suitable isotopes such as yttrium 90 (an emitter of pure high-energy β particles; Wessels and Rogus 1984). A major problem with repeated administrations of MAbs is the development of human antimouse immunoglobulin responses (Courtenay-Luck et al. 1986). The use of antibody $F(ab')_2$ fragments could reduce toxicity due to non-specific uptake by normal tissues, particularly by the reticuloendothelial system (Lubech et al. 1985), as they are cleared from the circulation faster than the intact antibody (Colcher et al. 1983; Kalofonos et al. 1988).

In order to reduce the excess of circulating radioactivity non-specifically irradiating normal tissues, we have recently used the streptavidin-biotin system, according to which the MAb is conjugated to streptavidin and administered. After a few days (allowing the antibody to localize to the tumor and its excess to be cleared), radiolabelled biotin is injected. Biotin is a small molecule with a high affinity for streptavidin. After injection, biotin which does not localize to the antibody/streptavidin-bearing tumor is cleared through the kidneys within a few minutes. Furthermore, since favourable results are obtained within a short period after the administration of radiolabelled biotin, it may in future be possible to employ radionuclides with short half-lives. In addition, this technique may avoid accumulation of radiolabel at high levels in normal organs.

The principle of selective tumor targeting using radiolabelled MAbs is a simple one with great potential and wide margins for improvement. Undoubtedly the encouraging results that have been reported at this stage will be improved by the new developments in recombinant DNA techniques, which allow genetic manipulations of immunoglobulins, toxins and chemotherapy agents (Riechman et al. 1988), making possible the creation of better molecules with desirable properties for cancer therapy. Nevertheless, randomized and multicentre clinical trials will be necessary to achieve precision in the use of radiolabelled antibodies for the treatment of cancer.

References

Arklie J, Taylor-Papadimitriou J, Bodmer WF, et al (1981) Differentiation antigens expressed by epithelial cells in the lactating breast are also detectable in breast cancer. Int J Cancer 28:23–29

Blackey DC, Watson GJ, Knowles PP, et al (1987) Effect of chemical deglycosylation of ricin A chain on the in vivo fate of cytotoxic activity of an immunotoxin composed of ricin A chain and anti-Thy 1 antibody. Cancer Res 47:947–952

Bloom HHG (1975) Combined modality therapy for intracranial tumours. Cancer 35:111–120

Colcher D, Zalutsky M, Kaplan W, et al (1983) Radiolocalization of human mammary tumours in athymic mice by a monoclonal antibody. Cancer Res 43:736–742

Combes RC, Buckman R, Forrester JA, et al (1986) In vitro and in vivo effects of a monoclonal antibody-toxin conjugate for use in autologous bone marrow transplantation for patients with breast cancer. Cancer Res 46:4217–4220

Courtenay-Luck NS, Epenetos AA, Moore R, et al (1986) Development of primary and secondary immune responses to mouse monoclonal antibodies used in the diagnosis and therapy of malignant neoplasms. Cancer Res 46:6489–6493

Critchley M, Browyless S, Patter M, et al (1986) Radionuclide imaging of epithelial ovarian tumours with ^{123}-iodine labelled monoclonal antibody (H317) specific for placental-type alkaline phosphatase. Clin Radiol 37:1207–1212

Dembo AJ (1985) Abdominopelvic radiotherapy in ovarian cancer. A 10 year review. Cancer 55: 2285–2290

Dillman RO, Shawler DL, Johnson DF, et al (1986) Preclinical trials with combinations and conjugates of T101 monoclonal antibody and doxorubicin. Cancer Res 46:4886–4891

Dobyns BS, Maloof F (1951) The study and treatment of 119 cases of carcinoma of the thyroid with radioactive iodine. J Clin Endocrin 11:1323–1360

Duerst RE, Ryan DH, Frants CN (1986) Variable affecting the killing of culture human neuroblastoma cells with monoclonal antibody and complement. Cancer Res 46:3420–3425

Ehrlich P (1957) The collected papers of Paul Ehrlich. In: Himmelweit F (ed) Immunology and cancer research, vol 2. Pergamon, London

Epenetos AA, Courtenay-Luck NS, Pickering D, et al (1985) Antibody guided irradiation of brain glioma by arterial infusion of radioactive monoclonal antibody against epidermal growth factor receptor and blood group A antigen. Br Med J 290:1463–1466

Epenetos AA, Snook D, Durbin H, et al (1986) Limitations of radiolabelled monoclonal antibodies for localization of human neoplasms. Cancer Res 46:3183–3191

Epenetos AA, Munro AJ, Stewart JSW, et al (1987) Antibody-guided irradiation of advanced ovarian cancer with intraperitoneally administered radiolabelled monoclonal antibodies. J Clin Oncol 5:1890–1899

Fraker PJ, Speck JC (1978) Protein and cell membrane iodination with sparingly soluble chloramide, 1,3,4,6-tetrachloro-5,6-diphenyl-glycouril. Biochem Biophys Res Commun 80:849–854

Granowska M, Britton KE, Shepherd JH, et al (1986) A prospective study of ^{123}iodine labelled monoclonal antibody imaging in ovarian cancer. J Clin Oncol 4:730–736

Griffiths CT, Parker LM, Fiuler A, et al (1979) The role of cytoreductive surgical treatment of advanced ovarian cancer. Cancer Treat Rep 63:235–239

Herlyn DM, Steplewski L, Herlyn MF, et al (1980) Inhibition of growth of colorectal carcinoma in nude mice by monoclonal antibody. Cancer Res 40:717–721

Kalofonos HP, Epenetos AA (1987) Antibody guided diagnosis and therapy of patients with breast cancer. In: Ceriani RL (ed) Immunological approaches to the diagnosis and therapy of breast cancer. Plenum, New York, pp 245–257

Kalofonos HP, Sivolapenko GB, Courtenay-Luck N, et al (1988) Antibody guided targeting of non-small cell lung cancer using ^{111}In-labelled HMFG1-F(ab′)$_2$ fragments. Cancer Res 48: 1977–1984

Köhler G, Milstein C (1975) Continuous cultures of fused cells secreting antibody of predefined specificity. Nature 256: 495–497

Lubech MP, Steplewski Z, Baglia P, et al (1985) The interactions of immune subclass proteins with human monocyte Fc receptors. J Immunol 135: 1209–1304

Miller RA, Levy R (1981) Response of cutaneous T-cell lymphoma to therapy with hybridoma monoclonal antibody. Lancet 2: 226

Myers MJ, Hooker GR, Epenetos AA (1986) Dosimetry of radiolabelled monoclonal antibodies used for therapy. In: Schlalke-Stelson AT, Watson EE (eds) Fourth International Dosimetry Symposium, April 1986. Oak Ridge Associated Universities, pp 409–420

Neijt JP, Ten Bokkel Huinink WW, Van de Burg MEL, et al (1984) Randomized trial comparing two combination treatment regimens (HEXA-CAF vs CHAP-5) in advanced ovarian cancer. Lancet 2: 594–600

Pawlikowska TRB, Epenetos AA (1986) Radiolabelled monoclonal antibodies to placental alkaline phosphatase in the diagnosis and treatment of neoplasms of the testis, ovary and cervix. Clin Enzymol 3: 53–59

Riechmann L, Clark M, Waldmann H, et al (1988) Reshaping human antibodies for therapy. Nature 332: 323–327

Sedlacek HH, Schulz G, Steinstraesser A, et al (1988) In: Eckhardt S, Holzner JH, Nagel GA (eds) Monoclonal antibodies in tumour therapy. Karger, Basel, pp 68–80

Snyder WS, Ford MR, Warner GG (1978) Estimates of specific absorbed fraction for photon sources uniformly distributed in various organs of a heterogeneous phantom, vol 5. Society of Nuclear Medicine, New York

Spurr NK, Durbin H, Sheer D, et al (1986) Characterisation and chromosomal assignment of a human cell surface antigen defined by the monoclonal antibody AUA1. Int J Cancer 38: 631–636

Sutherland CA, Davis JO, Stirrat GM (1987) Penetration and binding of radiolabelled anti-carcino-embryonic antigen monoclonal antibodies and their antigen binding fragments in human colon multicellular spheroids. Cancer Res 47: 1627–1633

Taylor-Papadimitriou J, Peterson JA, Arklie J, et al (1981) Monoclonal antibodies to epithelium specific components of the human milk fat globule membrane: production and reaction with cells in culture. Int J Cancer 28: 17–21

Travers P, Bodmer WF (1984) Preparation and characterisation of monoclonal antibodies against placental alkaline phosphatase and other human trophoblast-associated determinants. Int J Cancer 33: 633–641

Waterfield MD, Mayes ELV, Strooband P, et al (1982) A monoclonal antibody to the human epidermal growth factor receptor. J Cell Biochem 20: 149–161

Wessels BW, Rogus RD (1984) Radionuclide selection and model absorbed dose calculations for radiolabelled tumour associated antibodies. Med Phys 11: 638–645

Ricin A Chain – Monoclonal Antibody 791T/36 Immunotoxin for Treatment of Colorectal and Ovarian Cancer

V. S. Byers and R. W. Baldwin

Introduction

Tumor-localizing monoclonal antibodies are being developed for targeting cytotoxic agents including radioisotopes, cytotoxic drugs and much more toxic substances, particularly plant and bacterial toxins (Baldwin et al. 1986; Baldwin and Byers 1987; Vitetta et al. 1987). With classical cytotoxic drugs such as methotrexate, antibody targeting should focus drug to malignant cells and also reduce uptake by normal tissues so lowering toxicity. It should also convert resistant cells to susceptible cells in cases where there is defective drug uptake. Toxin A chain components on the other hand have relatively low toxicity by themselves (see later) and so antibody conjugation provides a means for targeting the toxin moiety to the target cell. Providing this also results in endocytosis of the toxin A chain, the immunoconjugate should be specifically cytotoxic for the target cell which binds the antibody (Baldwin and Byers 1987).

Immunotoxins constructed by conjugating plant and bacterial toxins to monoclonal antibodies are being developed in view of the high cytotoxic potency of those ribosomal-inhibiting proteins (Baldwin and Byers 1987; Vitetta et al. 1987). Of these, ricin isolated from the beans of the plant *Ricinus communis* has been widely used for immunotoxin synthesis and clinical trials are in progress.

Ricin is a glycoprotein (mol. wt. 65000) consisting of two polypeptide chains designated A chain and B chain, both of which are important for toxin action (Olsnes and Pihl 1982, Vitetta et al. 1987). The B chain contains binding sites for galactose which enables the toxin to bind to cells. The A chain is then endocytosed by mechanisms not well understood, but thought to involve cooperation of the B chain and induces cell kill. This involves translocation of the A chain across the membrane of endocytotic vesicles to the cytosol and inhibition of cellular protein synthesis (Olsnes 1988). This is now thought to occur by A chain catalytic modification of one or two nucleoside residues in 28S ribosomal RNA (Endo and Tsurugi 1987). This process is highly efficient, one A-chain molecule inactivating 1500 ribosomes/min and so very few molecules of A chain reaching the cytoplasm are required to kill a cell.

Immunotoxins constructed by conjugating whole ricin to antibody are highly toxic, since they combine the antibody-binding capacity and the B chain, which functions both to bind the toxin to a cell and then to transfer the A chain to the internal cytosol. But the presence of a B chain leads to a lack of specificity, since many cells have receptors recognized by the B-chain galactose-containing residue. From these considerations, immunotoxins containing whole ricin have limited potential for in vivo use and attention is being given to the use of A-chain-containing immunotoxins where target cell binding is controlled by the antibody moiety (Baldwin and Byers

1987; Vitetta et al. 1987). Several factors are important in selecting antibodies for immunotoxin design. These include antibody specificity for tumour cells and the capacity of immunotoxin to be endocytosed following binding to target cells. Ideally the antibody moiety should bind to tumor cells with no binding to other tissue antigens. This criterion is most closely achieved with monoclonal antibodies reacting with melanoma-associated antigens (Spitler et al. 1987). With almost all of the other monoclonal antibodies selected for immunotoxin synthesis, e.g., antibodies reacting with colorectal, breast and ovarian tumours, there is a degree of cross-reactivity with normal tissues. This may result in immunotoxin-mediated side effects and their identification and specification is an important feature of the phase I clinical trials recently completed, or in progress (Baldwin and Byers 1987; Byers et al. 1988b; Spitler et al. 1987).

Only recently has attention been given to the important function of the antibody moiety in translocating ricin A chain to the internal milieu of the cell (Vitetta et al. 1987). In many examples, monoclonal antibodies have been found to bind to target cell antigens but have not then been endocytosed, or if so at rates too low for effective delivery of the toxin component. Accordingly conjugate endocytosis is being investigated in the pre-clinical evaluation of immunotoxins (Baldwin et al. 1988; Byers et al. 1988a; Press et al. 1988).

Immunotoxin 791T/36-RTA

Murine monoclonal antibody 791T/36 recognizes a 72-kd glycoprotein (gp72) present on tumor cells derived from colorectal and ovarian cancer tissues (Campbell et al. 1984; Price et al. 1983). Flow cytometric analysis of tumor cells derived by collagenase disaggregation of tumour tissue has been used unequivocally to establish that the gp72 antigen is expressed at the tumour cell surface. Using this technique, target cells derived from more than 80% of 50 colorectal cancers have been shown to bind monoclonal antibody 791T/36 (Durrant et al. 1986a). There is a considerable variation in the level of gp72 antigen expression, which probably reflects the heterogeneity of tumor cells within a single tumor. The design of the flow cytometry assay also allows an estimate to be given of the level of gp72 antigen expression (Roe et al. 1985). This indicates that the lower level of 791T/36 antibody binding taken as a positive reaction was equivalent to 5×10^4 antibody-binding sites/cell and up to 10^6 binding sites/cell were detected. These findings are pertinent to the view that a single molecule of ricin A chain reaching the ribosomes is sufficient to effect cell kill (Vitetta et al. 1987).

Monoclonal antibody 791T/36, unlike many other murine monoclonal antibodies, is effectively endocytosed following binding to tumour cell surface gp72 antigen (Baldwin et al. 1988). This was initially demonstrated using a technique in which monoclonal antibody 791T/36 was conjugated to a fluorescent marker tetramethylrhodamine isothiocyanate (TRITC) using a human serum albumin carrier for the TRITC component (Garnett et al. 1986). This allowed direct observation of endocytosis of 791T/36 antibody conjugate with the intracellular appearance of TRITC fluorescence. The procedure has also been used quantitatively, measuring TRITC fluorescence by flow cytometry (Byers et al. 1988a), and this has allowed the kinetics of 791T/36 endocytosis to be determined (Baldwin et al. 1988). In addition procedures have been introduced to measure the endocytosis of ^{125}I-labelled 791T/36 which take into account cell-bound product (Garnett et al. 1988). Using these procedures it has been shown that the rate of endocytosis of 791T/36 on tumor cells is relatively slow, indicating a pinocytosis pathway rather than receptor-mediated endocytosis (Baldwin et al. 1988). Nevertheless approximately 60% of cell-bound product is endocytosed over a period of 4 h, indicating that the antibody is effectively translocated into the internal milieu of the target cell.

791T/36-RTA Immunotoxin

The immunotoxin constructed by conjugating ricin A chain to monoclonal antibody 791T/36 through a disulphide bond is highly cytotoxic in vitro for tumour cells expressing the gp72 antigen (Embleton et al. 1986). Using as target tumour 791T, which expresses around 6×10^5 antibody-binding sites/cell, the dose of 791T/36-RTA producing 50% inhibition (IC_{50}) of tumor cell survival (colony formation) is 4.5×10^{-12} M in terms of ricin A chain compared with $6.3 \times 10^{-8} M$ with RTA alone (Table 1). In another study (Byers et al. 1988c) 791T/36-RTA was highly cytotoxic for ovarian tumour 429 cells (IC_{50} 0.001 μg/ml) compared with RTA (IC_{50} 2.1 μg/ml). Also the immunotoxin was some 30000 times more cytotoxic than an antimelanoma immunotoxin (XOMAZYME-MEL), which does not react with the ovarian tumor target cells (Fig. 1).

In agreement with the studies described with antibody 791T/36, the immunotoxin is effectively endocytosed (Baldwin et al. 1988). The overall pattern of endocytosis of immunotoxin, by 791T tumor cells, determined by analysis of intracellular localization of ^{125}I-labelled 791T/36-RTA, indicated an initial rapid uptake with approximately 35% of cell-bound product being internalized over the first 60-min incubation at 37°C. This is followed by a slower rate of endocytosis with approximately 50% of cell-bound immunotoxin being internalized by 2 h. Related to these findings, exposure of tumor 791T cells for 5–10 min to immunotoxin is sufficient to produce almost

Table 1. Cytotoxicity of immunotoxin 791T/36-RTA for tumour cells expressing the target gp72 antigen

Tumour cytotoxicity[a] cell line	gp72 Antigen density[b]	IC_{50} (molarity)
Sarcoma 791T	6×10^5	1.4×10^{-10}
Sarcoma 788T	3×10^5	1.6×10^{-10}
Bladder carcinoma T24	3×10^4	2.2×10^{-9}
Melanoma 2a	$<5 \times 10^3$	Not reached
Breast carcinoma BT474-3	$<5 \times 10^2$	Not reached

[a] Determined by inhibition of cell survival as assayed from incorporation of [^{75}Se]selenomethionine

[b] Mean number of antibody 791T/36 binding sites as determined by flow cytometry analysis of the reaction of fluorescence labelled 791T/36 with tumour cells

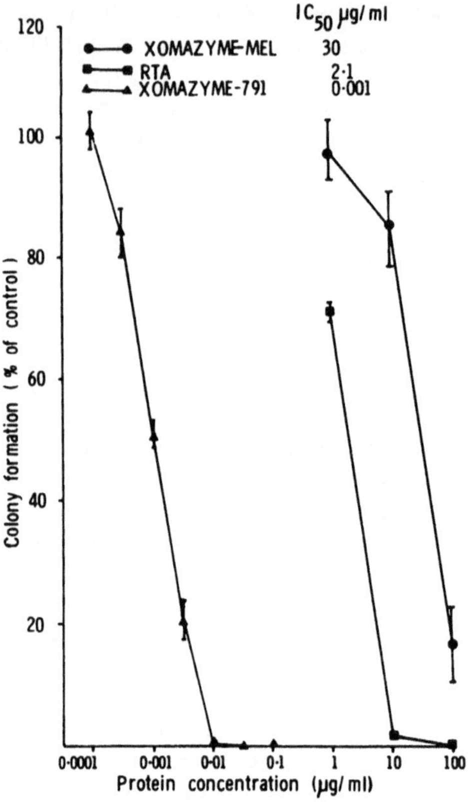

Fig. 1. Cytotoxicity of xomazyme-791 for ovarian carcinoma OVCA 429 cells: clonogenic test

Table 2. Duration of exposure of tumour 791T to immunotoxin 791T/36-RTA and cytotoxic response

Immunotoxin[a] treatment	Colony inhibition	
	Mean no. colonies/ dish	Inhibition of colony formation (%)
0 min	216.2	–
5 min	3.7	98.3
10 min	1.2	99.4
20 min	0.2	99.9
60 min	0.2	99.9
24 h	0	100.0

[a] Tumor 791T cell incubated with immunotoxin for a period of time. Cells were then washed to remove non-bound immunotoxin and colony formation assayed over 6 days

complete cell kill as measured by a colony inhibition assay which involves 5- to 6-day incubation of immunotoxin-treated cells (Table 2). This indicates that immunotoxin is rapidly bound to target tumor cells and the affinity of this binding through the antibody moiety to the target antigen is sufficiently great so that adequate amounts of cell-bound product are endocytosed to produce a cytotoxic response. The related question of how much cell-bound immunotoxin is effective has been analysed by binding 791T/36-RTA to tumor 791T cells at 4°C under conditions which do not allow endocytosis to occur. Following incubation at 37°C for various time intervals, residual surface-bound immunotoxin has been removed by papain treatment then cytotoxicity measured in the colony inhibition test. From these experiments it can be concluded that immunotoxin endocytosed over 1–2 h is sufficient to effect cell kill.

Preclinical In Vivo Studies

Immunotoxin 791T/36-RTA specifically and effectively inhibits growth of xenografts of human tumors which express the target gp72 antigen (Byers et al. 1987b). This is illustrated in Fig. 2, showing that growth of xenografts of human colon carcinoma C170 (Durrant et al. 1986b) is markedly suppressed following a schedule of daily intraperitoneal injections (5 mg/kg body wt.) of immunotoxin. Xenografts of tumors which express the gp72 antigen including sarcomas and ovarian carcinomas are also effectively suppressed by immunotoxin treatment.

Pharmacokinetic studies of 791T/36-RTA immunotoxin indicated a markedly altered biodistribution compared with that of unconjugated antibody 791T/36 (Byers et al. 1987a). The immunotoxin is rapidly eliminated from blood following injection

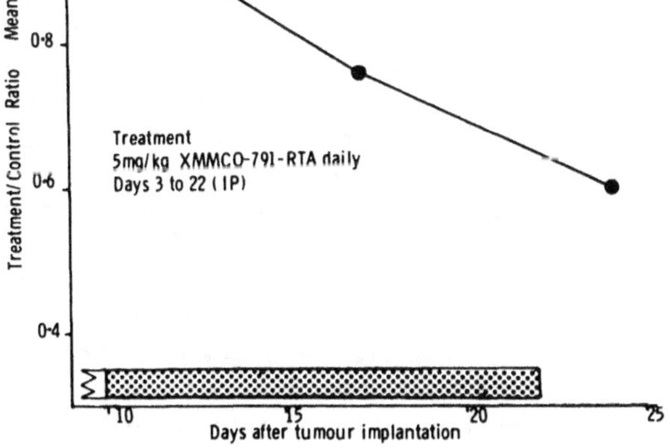

Fig. 2. Suppression of colon carcinoma C170 xenografts by XMMCO-791-RTA conjugate

into normal mice ($t_{1/2}$, 9 min) followed by a slower elimination of blood-borne product ($t_{1/2}$ B, 9.8 h). This contrasts with the relatively slow blood clearance of unconjugated 791T/36 antibody ($t_{1/2\alpha}$, 7.8 h; $t_{1/2\beta}$, 70 h) (Pimm et al. 1985). The blood clearance of 791T/36 in mice is closely similar to the pattern observed in colorectal cancer patients where the catabolic phase half-life was 44 h (Ballantyne et al. 1988).

The rapid elimination of 791T/36-RTA from the circulation is similar to the experience with many other RTA-containing immunotoxins and is largely due to its uptake by Kupffer cells in the liver (Baldwin and Byers 1987; Vitetta et al. 1987). This occurs through recognition of the RTA moiety through reaction of mannose-terminating oligosaccharide with specific receptors on Kupffer cells. Immunotoxin design, therefore, is being investigated so as to reduce hepatic uptake since this may result in improved antitumor activity. Natural ricin A chain consists of two species of molecular weight, 30 kd (RTA_{30}) and 33 kd (RTA_{33}). RTA_{33} contains approximately twice the amount of carbohydrate as RTA_{30} and so an immunotoxin has been produced by conjugating RTA_{30} to monoclonal antibody 791T/36 (J. Stoudemire et al. 1988, unpublished findings). Immunotoxin 791T/36-RTA_{30} has an increased plasma residence time compared with immunotoxin containing RTA_{33} and this results in an increased tumor localization. Another approach is to administer immunotoxin with mannose-containing agents which compete for the Kupffer cell receptors (Byers et al. 1987a). Agents such as ovalbumin, ovomucoid and more specifically designed compounds including mannosyl-lysine are effective in prolonging the blood survival of 791T/36-RTA (Byers et al. 1987a). Finally immunotoxins have been constructed using ricin A chain deglycosylated with metaperiodate and cyanoborohydride treatment (Blakey et al. 1988) and this is effective in improving immunotoxin pharmacokinetics.

Clinical Studies

Tests for cross-reactivity with normal human tissues showed that the antibody component of the immunotoxin has a low level of binding with some human tissues (Byers et al. 1988b). It binds weakly and non-specifically to human red blood cells and to macrophages. There is weak binding to granulocytes but no binding with progenitor cells or normal lymphocytes. Immunoperoxidase staining demonstrated that the antibody also binds weakly with some normal tissues, these being predominantly non-cellular stromal elements. The vascular endothelium of some capillaries and venules in various tissues are weakly reactive but most of the venules in any tissue are negative. Positive reactions with less than 10% of the glomeruli in one of four kidneys was observed and about 10% of the alveolar epithelium and macrophages were positive in lung tissue with two of four autopsy specimens.

Based upon these findings a phase I study has been carried out in patients with metastatic colorectal cancer with doses ranging from 0.02 to 0.2 mg/kg per day for a 5-day course (Byers et al. 1988b). Side effects included a reversible fall in serum albumin levels. This effect has been noted in melanoma patients receiving another immunotoxin (Spitler et al. 1987) and may represent a response, as yet undefined, to the ricin A chain moiety. Neurological symptoms in patients treated with 791T/36-RTA were mild and reversible but represented one of the more concerning side effects which may have an aetiology related to an as yet unidentified reaction of the 791T/36 antibody since similar responses were not observed in the melanoma trial (Spitler et al. 1987).

Another side effect observed with 791T/36-RTA was reversible proteinuria. This began around study day 10–16 and continued to day 30–45. The onset of proteinuria occurred around the time that anti-mouse immunoglobulin antibodies (HAMA) were detected. There was also onset of erythema and induration at the skin site used initially to test whether patients were sensitized to monoclonal antibody 791T/36. In fact none of the patients produced a positive skin test prior to immunotoxin treatment. Monoclonal antibody 791T/36 is known to localize in stromal elements of normal tissues (Armitage et al. 1984). It is possible, therefore, that antibody liberated following immunotoxin degradation may become localized in kidney as a consequence of stromal binding. In this case, the observed correlation between onset of proteinuria and HAMA response suggests kidney damage may occur as a consequence of immune complex disease. This phenomenon has been reproduced in a rat model showing that here also proteinuria occurs at the time anti-mouse immunoglobulin is produced and the lesion is enhanced by passive transfer of rat anti-791T/36 antibody.

A major side effect of immunotoxin treatment of colorectal cancer patients was the induction of antibody responses to the murine immunoglobulin 791T/36 and to the ricin A chain component (Byers et al. 1988b; Durrant et al. 1988a). The anti-mouse immunoglobulin response is quite complex and includes the generation of anti-framework, anti-isotypic and anti-combining site responses. The generation of anti-combining site antibodies was the predominant response and it could be shown that this human antibody specifically blocked the binding of monoclonal antibody 791T/36 to the target gp72 antigen.

The generation of anti-immunotoxin antibodies may impair the function of the immunotoxin by altering both its biodistribution and interaction with tumour cells. This has been shown in experimental studies in which the biodistribution of ^{111}In-labelled 791T/36 antibody is markedly altered in rats which have generated antibodies to the monoclonal antibody (Pimm et al. 1989b) and in mice immunized so as to produce anti-idiotypic antibodies (Pimm et al. 1988a).

A conclusive assessment of biological responses cannot be obtained from this phase I study. However, 2 of 16 patients with hepatic metastases had objective evidence by abdominal CT scans of decreasing size in large metastases and disappearance of smaller ones. Clinical regression of supraclavicular nodes was also noted in three patients.

Discussion

The preclinical investigations with immunotoxin 791T/36-RTA have provided the basis for initiating phase I clinical trials in patients with metastatic colorectal cancer (Byers et al. 1988b). The antibody moiety binds to a significant extent with colorectal cancer cells derived from surgically resected tumour specimens (Durrant et al. 1986a). Since a single ricin A chain molecule entering the cytosolic compartment of the cell is sufficient to cause arrest of protein synthesis, the level of antibody 791T/36 binding equivalent to between 5×10^4 and 10^6 molecules/cell should be sufficient to exert a therapeutic response. There are other factors which have to be taken into account in relation to immunotoxin cytotoxicity. At the target cell level, the immunotoxin has to be effectively endocytosed and the ricin A chain translocated across the endocytic vesicle. The overall effectiveness of the immunotoxin in vivo is influenced by a number of factors which effect its pharmacokinetics. These include the influence of ricin A chain oligosaccharide residues which results in hepatic clearance of immunotoxin. Also patient antibody responses to immunotoxin especially the murine antibody component result in modified biodistribution and pharmacokinetics.

The phase I trial of 791T/36-RTA in patients with metastatic colorectal cancer has established the side effects and clinical responses over a limited range of doses of immunotoxin. This trial has also identified factors which need to be taken into account. This includes the design of immunotoxin with RTA species which have less avidity for Kupffer cell receptors so improving their pharmacokinetics. The other major factor to be taken into consideration is the generation of anti-mouse antibody responses. Procedures being developed to abrogate HAMA responses include treatment with immunosuppressive agents such as cyclosporin A (Lederman et al. 1988; LoBuglio et al. 1988). More specific immunosuppressive methods are being sought in animal studies, and conjugates of monoclonal antibody 791T/36 with daunomycin have been used completely to abrogate anti-791T/36 immunoglobulin antibody (Durrant et al. 1988b). These approaches will allow re-treatment schedules to be used, together with improvements in immunotoxin design.

Acknowledgments. These studies were supported by a grant from the Cancer Research Campaign, United Kingdom, and Xoma Corporation, Berkeley, California, United States.

References

Armitage NC, Perkins AC, Pimm MV, Farrands PA, Baldwin RW, Hardcastle JD (1984) The localisation of an anti-tumour monoclonal antibody (791T/36) in gastrointestinal tumours. Br J Surg 71:407–412

Baldwin RW, Byers VS (1987) Monoclonal antibodies and immunoconjugates for cancer treatment. In: Pinedo HM, Longo DL, Chabner BA (eds) Cancer chemotherapy and biological response modifiers annual 9. Elsevier Science, Amsterdam, pp 409–431

Baldwin RW, Embleton MJ, Gallego J, Garnett M, Pimm MV, Price MR (1986) Monoclonal antibody drug conjugates for cancer therapy. In: Roth J (ed) Monoclonal antibodies in cancer: advances in diagnosis and treatment. Futura, New York, pp 215–257

Baldwin RW, Byers VS, Berry N, Pawluczyk IZA, Garnett MC, Robins RA, Scannon PJ (1988) Endocytosis of ricin A chain immunotoxins recognising human tumor cell surface antigens. Proc Am Assoc Cancer Res 29:423

Ballantyne KC, Perkins AC, Pimm MV, Garnett MC, Clegg JA, Armitage NC, Baldwin RW, Hardcastle JD (1988) Biodistribution of a monoclonal antibody-methotrexate conjugate (791T/36-MTX) in patients with colorectal cancer. Int J Cancer [Supp] 2:103–108

Blakey DC, Skilleter DN, Price RJ, Thorpe PE (1988) Uptake of native and deglycosylated ricin A-chain immunotoxins by mouse liver parenchymal and non-parenchymal cells in vitro and in vivo. Biochim Biophys Acta 968:172–178

Byers VS, Pimm MV, Pawluczyk, Lee HM, Scannon PJ, Baldwin RW (1987a) Biodistribution of ricin toxin A-chain monoclonal antibody 791T/36 immunotoxins and the influence of hepatic blocking agents. Cancer Res 47:5277–5283

Byers VS, Pimm MV, Scannon PJ, Pawluczyk, Baldwin RW (1987b) Inhibition of growth of human tumor xenografts in athymic mice treated with ricin toxin A-chain-monoclonal antibody 791T/36 conjugates. Cancer Res 47:5042–5046

Byers VS, Pawluczyk I, Berry N, Durrant L, Robins RA, Garnett MC, Price MR, Baldwin RW (1988a) Potentiation of anti-carcinoembryonic antigen (CEA) immunotoxin cytotoxicity by monoclonal antibodies reacting with co-expressed CEA epitopes. J Immunol 140:4050–4055

Byers VS, Rodvien R, Grant K, Durrant LG, Hudson KH, Baldwin RW, Scannon PJ (1988b) Phase I study of monoclonal antibody 791T/36-ricin A chain immunotoxin in metastatic colon cancer. Cancer Res (in press)

Byers VS, Durrant L, Embleton MJ, Marksman R, Robins RA, Powell M, Symonds M, Baldwin RW (1988c) Monoclonal antibody 791T/36-ricin A chain immunotoxin (Xomazyme-791) for treatment of ovarian cancer. Second international symposium: multimodality treatment of ovarian cancer. EORTC monograph series. Raven, New York

Campbell DG, Price MR, Baldwin RW (1984) Analysis of a human osteogenic sarcoma antigen and its expression on various human tumour cell lines. Int J Cancer 34:31–37

Durrant LG, Robins RA, Armitage NC, Brown A, Baldwin RW, Hardcastle JD (1986a) Association of antigen expression and DNA ploidy in human colorectal tumors. Cancer Res 46:3543–3549

Durrant LG, Robins RA, Pimm MV, Perkins AC, Armitage NC, Hardcastle JC, Baldwin RW (1986b) Antigenicity of newly established colorectal cell lines. Br J Cancer 53:37–45

Durrant LG, Byers VS, Scannon PJ, Rodvien R, Grant K, Robins RA, Marksman RA, Baldwin RW (1988a) Humoral immune responses to XMMCO-791-RTA immunotoxin in colorectal cancer patients. Clin Exp Immunol 75:258–264

Durrant LG, Robins RA, Marksman RA, Garnett MC, Ogunmuyiwa Y, Baldwin RW (1989) Abrogation of antibody responses in rats to murine monoclonal antibody 791T/36 by treatment with daunomycin-*cis*-aconityl-791T/36 conjugates. Cancer Immunol Immunother 28:37–42

Embleton MJ, Byers VS, Lee HM, Scannon P, Blackhall NW, Blackhall RW (1986) Sensitivity and selectivity of ricin toxin A chain-monoclonal antibody 791T/36 conjugates against human tumor cell lines. Cancer Res 46:5524–5528

Endo Y, Tsurugi K (1987) RNA N-glycosidase activity of ricin A chain. J Biol Chem 262:8128–8130

Garnett MC, Baldwin RW (1986) Endocytosis of a monoclonal antibody recognising a cell surface glycoprotein antigen visualised using fluorescent conjugates. Eur J Cell Biol 41:214–221

Garnett MC, Huehns THAY, Martin JR, Graves CRL, Smith SL (1988) Quantitation of endocytosis of antibody by a radiolabel method. Br J Cancer

Lederman JA, Begent RHJ, Bagshawe KD, Riggs SJ, Searle F, Glaser MG, Green AJ, Dale RG (1988) Repeated antitumour antibody therapy in man with suppression of the host response by cyclosporin A. Br J Cancer

LoBuglio AF, Khazaeli MB, Lee J, Haynes A, Sumeri L, Mischak R, Spitler L (1988) Pharmacokinetics and immune response to Xomazyme-Mel in melanoma patients. Monoclonal Antibody Immunoconjugates of Cancer

Olsnes S (1988) Closing in on ricin action. Nature 328:474

Olsnes S, Pihl A (1982) In: Cohen P, von Heyningen S (eds) Molecular action of toxins and viruses. Elsevier, New York, p 503

Pimm MV, Perkins AC, Armitage NC, Baldwin RW (1985) The characteristics of blood-borne radiolabels and the effect of anti-mouse IgG antibodies on localization of radiolabeled monoclonal antibody in cancer patients. J Nucl Med 26:1011–1023

Pimm MV, Durrant LG, Baldwin RW (1988a) The influence of syngeneic anti-idiotypic antibody on the biodistribution of an anti-tumour monoclonal antibody in BALB/c mice. Int J Cancer 43:147–151

Pimm MV, Perkins AC, Durrant LG, Baldwin RW (1988b) A rat model for imaging the effect of anti-mouse antibody responses on the biodistribution of radiolabelled mouse monoclonal antibodies. Eur J Nucl Med 14:507–511

Press OW, Hansen JA, Farr A, Martin PJ (1988) Endocytosis and degradation of murine anti-human CD3 monoclonal antibodies by normal and malignant T-lymphocytes. Cancer Res 48:2249–2257

Price MR, Campbell DG, Robins RA, Baldwin RW (1983) Characteristics of a cell surface antigen defined by an anti-human osteogenic sarcoma monoclonal antibody. Eur J Cancer Clin Oncol 19:81–90

Roe R, Robins RA, Laxton RR, Baldwin RW (1985) Kinetics of divalent monoclonal antibody binding to tumour cell surface antigens using flow cytometry: standardization and mathematical analysis. Mol Immunol 22:11–21

Spitler LE, Del Rio M, Kentigan A, Wedel NI, Brophy NA, Miller LL, Harkonen WS, Rosendorf LL, Shannon CE, Lee HM, Mishak RP, Kawahata RT, Stoudemire JB, Fradkin LB, Baustista EE, Dellio CL, Mendell SC, Scannon PJ (1987) Therapy of patients with malignant melanoma using a monoclonal antimelanoma antibody-ricin A chain immunotoxin. Cancer Res 47:1717–1723

Vitetta ES, Fulton RJ, May RD, Till M, Uhr JW (1987) Redesigning nature's poisons to create anti-tumor reagents. Science 238:1098–1104

Experimental Approaches to Tumor Therapy with Monoclonal Antibodies*

S. Matzku, H. Bihl, G. Moldenhauer, B. Dörken, and P. Möller

Introduction

Tumor targeting of therapeutically active substances using monoclonal antibodies (MAbs) as specific vehicles depends on a multitude of parameters, two of them being the subject of the present study: accessibility and internalization. Accessibility of vital tumor cells in solid tumor tissue is determined by (micro-)vascular permeability, by the architecture of the extravascular compartment, and by the mode of antigen expression. The intact blood-tissue barrier(s) imposes a restraint on the permeation of macromolecules, which may be abrogated by the well-documented leakiness of tumor vessels (Jain 1987). Diffusion/convection of MAbs in the extravascular space will depend on the properties of this compartment and on the mechanism of movement into densely packed tumor cell areas (Weinstein et al. 1987). Predominant intracellular antigen expression will not lead to MAb binding and retention, while antigen expression at the cell surface, and even more so antigen deposition in extracellular pools, will be highly favorable (Matzku et al. 1988). Yet, MAb binding to the tumor cell surface may not be sufficient. Quite a number of therapeutically active substances (e.g., toxins) become only active when transported into the respective target cell compartment. With radionuclides conjugated to the MAb, internalization may lead to a retention of the label, and, hence, to prolonged storage, or to degradation of the antibody and excretion of labeled products, depending on the nature of the radionuclide. Indium and iodine are the respective examples (Carrasquillo et al. 1987). Thus, the propensity of MAbs to be internalized should be analyzed in order to gain basic information as to the potential therapeutic effectiveness of a given antibody conjugate.

Internalization of Monoclonal Antibodies by B-Lymphoma Cells

We present experiments evaluating the suitability of MAbs directed against differentiation antigens on human B-lymphocytes for therapeutic application in B-lymphoma patients. MAbs and the antigens recognized by them are listed in Table 1. To characterize spontaneous internalization, the kinetics of binding of iodinated MAbs to human B-lymphoma cells (i.e., BJAB, OCI.LY1, and LICR.HMj2) were determined in vitro, discrimination between externally bound and internalized radioactivity being achieved by treatment of cells with iso-osmolar buffer of pH 2.8 (Matzku et

* The authors are supported by grants from the Tumorzentrum Heidelberg-Mannheim

Table 1. MAbs and B-cell antigens

MAb	Isotype	Antigen detected		Reference
		Designation	M_r (kD)	
HD6	IgG1	CD22	gp130/140	Moldenhauer et al. (1986)
HD39	IgG1	CD22	gp130/140	Dörken et al. (1986)
HD239	IgG2b	Switch variant of HD39		Kiesel et al. (1987)
HD37	IgG1	CD19	gp95	Pezzutto et al. (1986)
HD237	IgG2b	Switch variant of HD39		Kiesel et al. (1987)
HD28	IgG2a	CD37	gp40–52	Schwarz-Abiez et al. (1988)
HD50	IgG2b	CD23	gp45–50	Moldenhauer et al. (1987)

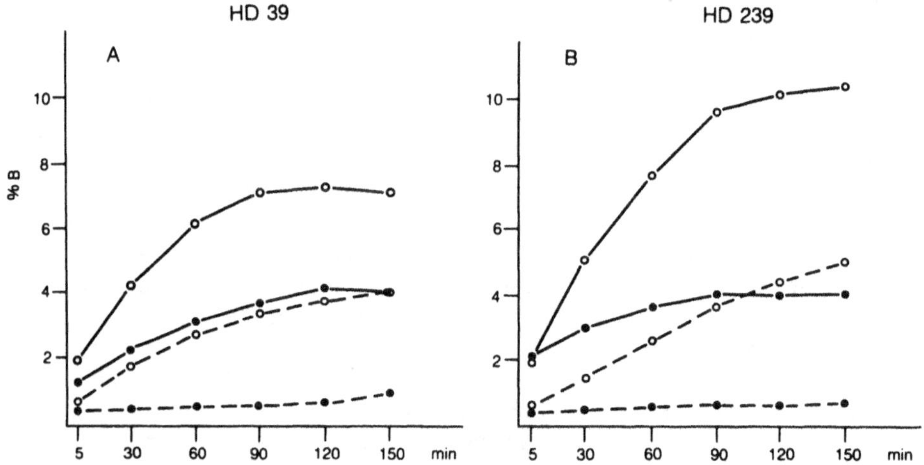

Fig. 1A, B. Time course of HD39 binding to lymphoma line BJAB. **A** Original HD39 (IgG1); **B** switch variant HD239 (IgG2b). ^{125}I-labeled MAb was incubated with lymphoma cell suspensions. At predetermined time points, aliquots were withdrawn, washed, and counted in a gamma counter. Thereafter, cells were treated with iso-osmolar buffer pH 2.8 (20 min, 0°C) to determine the internalized portion of radioactivity. Details of the procedure are given in Matzku et al. (1986). *Symbols:* ○, uptake at 37°C; ●, uptake at 0°C; *solid lines,* total radioactivity bound; *broken lines,* residual radioactivity after pH 2.8 treatment

al. 1986). As can be seen, binding at 37°C was generally superior to binding at 0°C (Figs. 1–3), which may be partly explained by a diffusion-controlled uptake process. However, acid buffer treatment revealed partial (i.e., HD39, Fig. 1) or near-total (i.e., HD6, see Fig. 4) internalization with CD22 MAbs as an additional component of temperature-dependent uptake. The other MAbs did not internalize in the short time experiment (Figs. 2, 3; data for HD28 not included), but HD37 sometimes showed moderate internalization in experiments extended to 24 h. Immunoglobulin switch variants of HD37 (HD237, IgG2b) and HD39 (HD239, IgG2b) behaved exactly like the original MAbs. To elucidate possible causes of the difference in in-

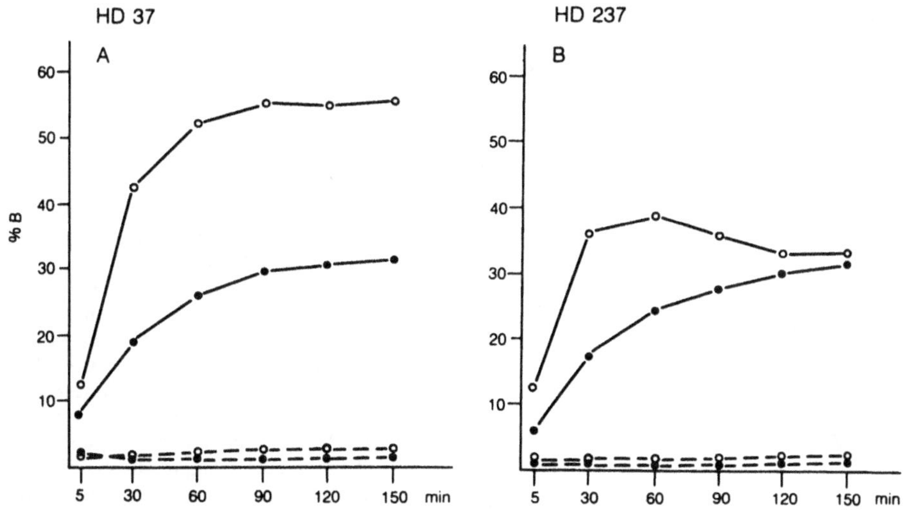

Fig. 2A, B. Time course of HD37 binding to lymphoma line BJAB. **A** Original HD37 (IgG1); **B** switch variant HD237 (IgG2b). For procedure and symbols see Fig. 1

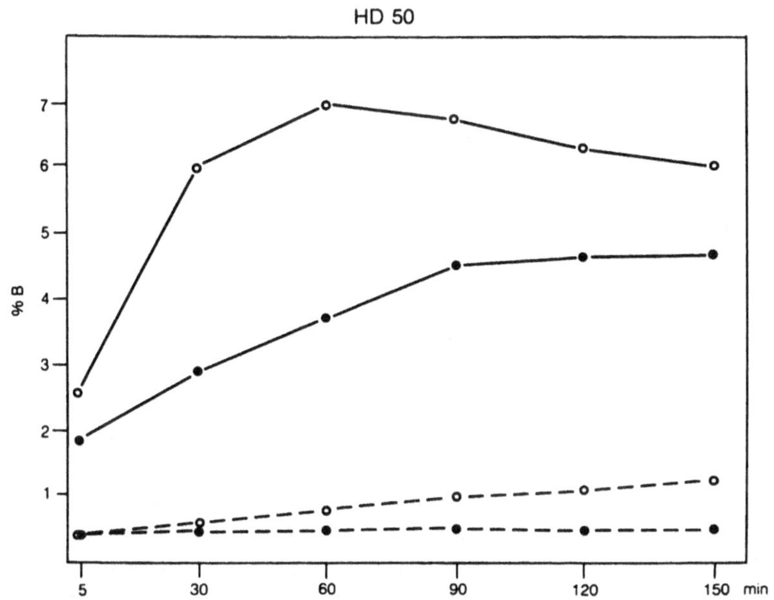

Fig. 3. Time course of HD50 binding to lymphoma line LICR.HMj2. For procedure and symbols see Fig. 1

ternalization by the CD22 MAbs, an experiment was performed in which trace amounts of labeled HD6 were mixed with an excess of unlabeled HD39 (Fig. 4). Since both MAbs bind to the same molecule, it was expected that the excess of HD39 would prevent some of the HD6 molecules from internalization. However, this was not the case. HD6 showed some reduction of binding in the presence of

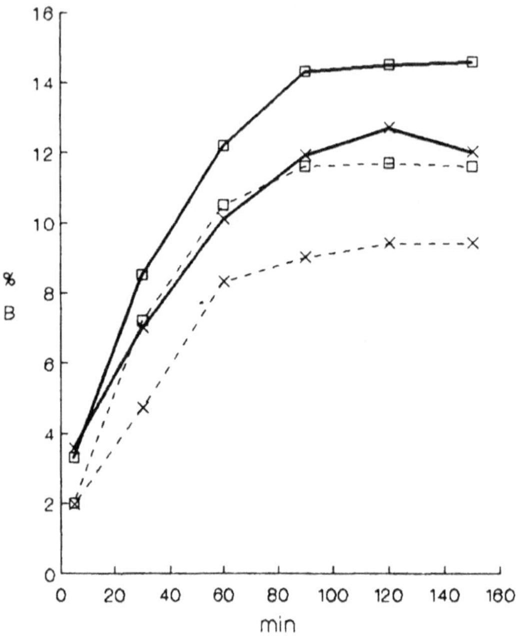

Fig. 4. Time course of binding and internalization of ^{125}I-labeled HD6 in the presence of excess unlabeled HD39. Both MAbs binding to the same surface molecule; internalization of one MAb should influence internalization of the other. However, this was not observed. □, binding of [^{125}I]-HD6 in the absence of HD39; ×, binding of [^{125}I]-HD6 in the presence of 4 μg/ml unlabeled HD39; *solid lines,* total binding; *dashed lines,* residual radioactivity after washing cells with pH 2.8 buffer. BJAB lymphoma cells

HD39, thus confirming the operational independence of the respective epitopes, but was internalized to the same extent as in the absence of HD39. The converse experiment with labeled HD39 in admixture to excess unlabeled HD6 gave corresponding results, i.e., excess HD6 was not capable of driving externally bound HD39 into the cells (data not included). Hence, HD6 and HD39 seem to act independently. But the experiment gives no explanation to the partial internalization of HD39. An obvious interpretation would be that part of HD39 antibody molecules are functionally monovalent after the iodination. This could be elucidated by changing the label attached to the antibody.

CD22 and CD19 being promising B-lymphoma markers due to their expression in most stages of B-cell differentiation (Zola 1987), both types of MAbs have been considered by other authors, too (May et al. 1986; Gethie et al. 1988). May et al. directly compared CD22(HD6) and CD19(HD37), both coupled to ricin A-chain. The cytotoxic potential of CD22(HD6)-ricin A was clearly superior to CD19(HD37)-ricin A, which may be explained by the difference in internalization. Hence, CD22 MAbs should be considered as prime candidates for therapeutic application, provided that internalization of the immune complexes would be the dominating criteria. With conjugates not relying on internalization, the amount and stability of antigen expression may be the most relevant parameter.

Accessibility of Lymphoma Cells in Nude Mouse Xenografts

When shifting to the in vivo situation, i.e., to MAb accumulation in B-lymphoma xenografts, no indication of a positive effect due to internalization was noted. The

Table 2. Distribution of MAbs in nude mice with human B-lymphoma xenografts

MAb	Lymphoma	% administered dose per gram			
		Tumor	Blood	Liver	Muscle
[^{125}I]HD6	BJAB	4.39	14.72	4.47	1.22
[^{125}I]HD39	OCI.LY1	2.84	7.41	2.84	0.52
[^{125}I]HD239[a]	BJAB	1.36	2.93	0.84	0.20
[^{125}I]HD37	BJAB	7.74	15.07	3.60	1.00
[^{125}I]HD237[a]	OCI.LY1	4.08	5.48	1.41	0.62
Control MAbs					
[^{131}I]B40 (IgG1)	BJAB	1.30	13.80	4.11	1.04
[^{131}I]142 (IgG2b)	BJAB	1.13	2.94	1.15	0.23

$n = 5$; 24 h accumulation

[a] Switch variant to IgG2b

amount of MAbs bound was moderate irrespective of specificity (Table 2), and whole body retention was such that an intratumoral degradation followed by excretion of the label was deemed unlikely. With respect to isotype switch variants, differences in the biological half-life, and, hence, in the relative accumulation in lymphoma tissue were noted.

Macroautoradiographs gave a most simple explanation to the moderate accumulation levels. Forty-eight hours after injection of iodinated MAbs, radioactivity distribution in various lymphoma xenografts was highly nonuniform. Thus, accumulation was low because substantial portions of lymphoma nodules were not reached by labeled MAbs. With Burkitt's lymphoma line BJAB, the effect was particularly obvious, because MAbs were (specifically) accumulated only in a very thin rim beneath the capsule surrounding the xenograft. The center of those nodules was essentially spared despite the absence of gross necroses. The radioactivity distribution pattern was independent of the MAb type and the antigen detected, suggesting that there exists a particular restriction of permeability in the central region, but not in the subcapsular region of the BJAB tumor. This could be most clearly illustrated by comparing the autoradiograph from a 10-μm cryostat section to an adjacent section immunohistochemically stained for mouse serum Ig of all isotypes (Fig. 5). The BJAB nodule was found to be surrounded by a thick capsular structure which – according to the impressive amounts of serum present – seems to contain a large number of microvessels directing the supply of labeled MAbs to the cell layers which are immediately underneath. The other lymphoma lines tested (i.e., OCI.Ly and Namalwa; not shown) lacked this type of capsular organization and did not show exclusively peripheral uptake of labeled MAbs. The reason why intratumoral capillaries, though present to about the same extent in all the lymphoma lines mentioned, proved to be fairly permeable in Namalwa and OCI.Ly1, but not in BJAB, is not known at the moment. Interestingly enough, ^{67}Ga (but not ^{111}In) was found to penetrate quite readily into the center BJAB xenografts (H. Bihl, unpublished data), although both nuclides are known to be transported and internalized while complexed to transferrin (Vallabhajosula et al. 1980; Chan et al. 1987). The reason why ^{67}Ga

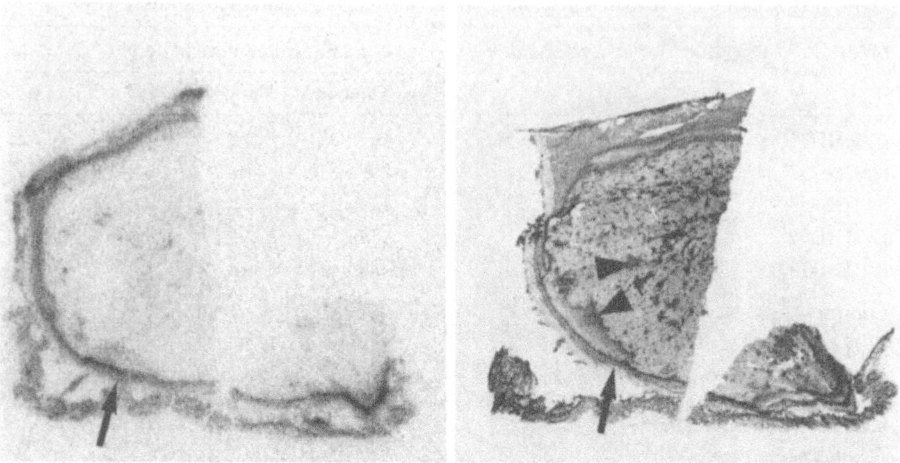
A B

Fig. 5A, B. Penetration of serum Ig and MAb HD28 into BJAB lymphoma nodules. **A** Autoradiograph obtained 48 h after administration of [^{125}I]-HD28 into a mouse with BJAB xenograft. Note exclusive MAb accumulation in the subcapsular region (→) of the nodule. **B** Adjacent section immunohistochemically stained for mouse serum Ig. *Dark structures* represent areas rich in serum Ig. Note pronounced staining in the periphery of the nodule (→), but also focal staining of more central areas (▶), indicating vessels and small necroses. Magnification, × 7.5

distributes like a low molecular weight substance while ^{111}In distributes like macromolecular antibody most likely resides in the fact that Ga binding to transferrin is much weaker than binding of In (Harris and Pecoraro 1983) so that a substantial amount of the former nuclide is available in noncomplexed form capable of crossing the blood-tissue barrier. These observations are highly encouraging for proceeding in the direction of "in vivo labeling" of tumors by the use of low molecular weight radionuclide complexes and bispecific antibody constructs, along the lines proposed by Goodwin and Meares.

Back to the aspect of therapeutic MAb administration, the lesson to be learned from xenografted lymphomas was twofold: (1) Accessibility of lymphoma cells is moderate to low, depending on the structural characteristics of lymphomas, which possibly pertain to vascular permeability and/or the texture of the extravascular compartment. However, since xenografts in the mouse are supplied by mouse vessels, it needs to be checked whether similar conditions are encountered in the human. (2) Permeability and percolation barriers may be outruled by the proper combination of a carrier protein remaining in the vascular compartment, e.g., a MAb with moderate affinity for the complexed radionuclide, and a preexistent (or preinjected) binding molecule at the level of the tumor cell, e.g., a MAb construct with specificity both for a tumor antigen and for the radionuclide complex. In this situation, the distance between the vessel and the tumor cell surface will be traversed by the released radionuclide complex as a low molecular weight species. This principle may find general application with therapeutically active substances of low molecular weight. With respect to methodology it is worth bearing in mind that the BJAB lymphoma line may be a highly sensitive indicator system for following changes in and manipulations of accessibility.

References

Carrasquillo JA, Mulshine JL, Bunn PA, Reynolds JC, Foon KA, Schroff RW, Perentesis P, Steis RG, Keenan AM, Horowitz M, Larson SM (1987) Indium-111 T101 monoclonal antibody is superior to iodine-131 T101 in imaging of cutaneous T-cell lymphoma. J Nucl Med 28:281–287

Chan SM, Hoffer PB, Maric N, Duray P (1987) Inhibition of gallium-67 uptake in melanoma by an anti-human transferrin receptor monoclonal antibody. J Nucl Med 28:1303–1307

Dörken B, Moldenhauer G, Pezzutto A, Schwarz R, Feller A, Kiesel S, Nadler LM (1986) HD39 (B3), a B lineage-restricted antigen whose cell surface expression is limited to resting and activated human B lymphocytes. J Immunol 136:4470–4479

Ghetie MA, May RD, Till M, Uhr JW, Ghetie V, Knowles PP, Relf M, Brown A, Wallace PM, Janossy G, Amlot P, Vitetta ES, Thorpe PE (1988) Evaluation of ricin-a chain-containing immunotoxins directed against cd19 and cd22 antigens on normal and malignant human b-cells as potential reagents for in vivo therapy. Cancer Res 48:2610–2617

Harris WR, Pecoraro VL (1983) Thermodynamic binding constaints for gallium transferrin. Biochemistry 22:292–299

Jain RK (1987) Transport of molecules across tumor vasculature. Cancer Metastasis Rev 6:559–593

Kiesel S, Haas R, Moldenhauer G, Kvalheim G, Pezzutto A, Dörken B (1987) Removal of cells from a malignant B-cell line from bone marrow with immunomagnetic beads and with complement and immunoglobulin switch variant mediated lysis. Leuk Res 11:1119–1125

Matzku S, Bröcker EB, Brüggen J, Dippold WG, Tilgen W (1986) Modes of binding and internalization of monoclonal anti-melanoma antibodies to human melanoma cell lines. Cancer Res 46: 3848–3854

Matzku S, Tilgen W, Bihl H, Schwechheimer K, Kalthoff H, Schmiegel W (1988) Tumor imaging: role of the target antigen. In: Gabius HJ, Nagel GA (eds) Lectins and glycoconjugates in oncology. Springer, Berlin Heidelberg New York, pp 67–76

May RD, Vitetta ES, Moldenhauer G, Dörken B (1986) Selective killing of normal and neoplastic human b-cells with anti-cd19-ricin and anti-cd22-ricin a-chain immunotoxins. Cancer Drug Deliv 3:261–272

Moldenhauer G, Dörken B, Schwarz R, Pezzutto A, Hämmerling GJ (1986) Characterization of a human B lymphocyte-specific antigen defined by monoclonal antibodies HD6 and HD39. In: Reinherz EL, Haynes BF, Nadler LM, Bernstein ID (eds) Leukocyte typing II. Springer, Berlin Heidelberg New York, pp 97–107

Moldenhauer G, Schwarz R, Dörken B, Hämmerling G (1988) Biochemical characterization and epitope analysis of B-lymphocyte-specific surface antigens defined by clustering workshop antibodies. In: McMichael A, et al (eds) Leukocyte typing III. Oxford University Press, Oxford, pp 378–382

Pezzutto A, Dörken B, Feller A, Moldenhauer G, Schwarz R, Wernet P, Thiel E, Hunstein W (1986) HD37 monoclonal antibody: a useful reagent for further characterization of "non-T-non-B" lymphoid malignancies. In: Reinherz EL, Haynes BF, Nadler LM, Bernstein ID (eds) Leukocyte typing II. Springer, Berlin Heidelberg New York, pp 391–402

Schwarz-Albiez R, Dörken B, Hofmann W, Moldenhauer G (1988) The B cell-associated CD37 antigen (gp40–52). Structure and subcellular expression of an extensively glycosylated glycoprotein. J Immunol 140:905–914

Vallabhajosula SR, Harwig JF, Siemsen JK, et al (1980) Radiogallium localization in tumors: blood binding and transport and the role of transferrin. J Nucl Med 21:650–656

Weinstein JN, Eger RR, Covell DG, Black CDV, Mulshine J, Carrasquillo JA, Larson SM, Keenan AM (1987) The pharmacology of monoclonal antibodies. Ann NY Acad Sci 507:199–210

Zola H (1987) The surface antigens of human B-lymphocytes. Immunol Today 8:308–315

Summary of Discussion: Session 7

G. Moldenhauer

Tumor targeting by antibodies alone or coupled to toxic reagents has attracted immunologists since the early days of Paul Ehrlich and his "magic bullets." Since then this concept has been further developed by using antibodies linked to radionuclides, immunotoxins, or cytostatic drugs. Powerful tools, monoclonal antibodies (MAbs) derived from hybridoma technology are expected to focus on and eliminate malignant cells in humans like missiles of destruction. However, this evocative description is at odds with our restricted knowledge of both tumor biology and the pharmacology of xenogeneic MAbs and conjugates made from them. The use of MAbs in patients causes problems at several levels. This became obvious from the speakers' contributions and the engaged and constructive discussion of the participants.

The vast majority of MAbs are directed against differentiation antigens which are not exclusively expressed on malignant cells but also on normal ones. Frequently, tumor cells carry more antigen molecules than their normal counterparts. This is reflected by the operational term "tumor-associated antigen specificity" of a MAb. Moreover, many antibodies have been shown to crossreact to some extent with unrelated tissues (e.g., connective tissue, vascular endothelium). With a few exceptions, MAbs are of murine origin and thus are recognized as foreign proteins by the human immune system. The usefulness of MAbs for in vivo administration has turned out to depend on immunoglobulin isotype, size [intact IgG $>$ $F(ab')_2$ $>$ Fab′], avidity and presensitization of the patient. These factors all influence the biological shelf life of the antibody. In general, immunoglobulins carrying the Fc portion have a long mean residence time in blood and several organs when compared to its fragments, and this is most likely due to rapid renal excretion of smaller Ig compounds.

The pharmacology of MAb conjugates is not only influenced by the antibody molecule but also by the radioactive label or toxin/drug and the stability of the complex. For example, yttrium 90 is enriched in bone marrow and high doses will cause depression of hemopoiesis. The key problem in MAb targeted therapy remains the difficulty of accumulating high amounts of cytotoxic reagent at the tumor site while at the same time minimizing background binding. Factors that account for the pharmacokinetics of MAb conjugate are specific and nonspecific binding, diffusion and convection, and metabolism, Under certain conditions, pretreatment of the patient with cold MAb can remarkably reduce nonspecific binding of the conjugate. Another strategy advised for intracavitary or locoregional therapy is the use of purified human anti-mouse antibodies (HAMA) obtained from sensitized patients. When injecting HAMA prior to or during application of radiolabeled MAb, immune complexes are formed in the blood which are catabolized rapidly in the liver, thus allowing an increase in dosage. The pharmacokinetics of ricin A chain conjugates are especially crucial, since the immunotoxin is taken up specifically into Kupffer cells in liver via mannose receptors. This interaction can be prevented either by blocking the mannose receptors with infusion of mannosylated dextran or chemically by terminal deglycosylation of the ricin A molecule.

It is assumed that only tumor-associated antigens expressed on the surface of neoplastic cells represent appropriate targets for antibody-guided therapy. They differ individually with respect to modulation following MAb binding. Three modes of action can be distinguished, namely internalization, shedding, or unchanged expression. The behavior of a particular target antigen indicates whether an MAb conjugate is therapeutically efficient or not. In the case of toxin conjugates, internalization of the complex is required, because immunotoxins act exclusively intracellularly. Shedding of antigenic material, which results in patchy deposits in tumor stroma, may lead to prolonged retention of radiolabeled MAb, and this can be beneficial for therapy (e.g., carcinoembryonic antigen in colon carcinoma).

The most critical parameters that have to be considered for therapeutic approaches are given by the architecture of the individual tumor, including vascularization, formation of tumor capsule, cell density, central necrosis, etc. Penetration and "percolation" of tumor tissue by MAb conjugates is largely dependent on the extent of vascularization, the type of endothelial layer forming the blood-tissue barrier, and the extracellular space between tumor cells. It should be noted that the development of capillaries and stroma components is induced by the tumor tissue, which more or less mimics the organ structure it has been derived from. Contradicting the commonly perpetuated opinion that high affinity MAbs will completely saturate tumor antigens, experimental evidence was provided which clearly demonstrated that this is not so. Most likely, MAbs are firmly and irreversibly bound to tumor cells located adjacent to capillaries. In consequence, they form an antibody "plug" which prevents other antibody molecules from penetrating further. Pretreatment with interleukin-2 (IL-2), which renders capillaries more leaky, was tried in order to improve extravasation of MAb conjugate. Unfortunately, IL-2 also decreases the clearance function of the kidneys, giving rise to a high background of labeled MAb. In order to analyze the accumulation of conjugate in tissue from an individual tumor, it seems advisable to take tumor biopsies for microautoradiography and/or immunohistological staining.

Detrimental side effects after systemic MAb application – often leading to severe clinical symptoms – are based on the patient's immune reaction against the foreign mouse immunoglobulin. Besides the fact that in some individuals preexisting antibodies reactive to mouse IgG can be found, generation of human anti-isotype and anti-idiotype antibodies is frequently induced after injections of MAb, particularly when they are repeated several times. These anti-mouse antibodies reduce the therapeutic efficacy either by blocking the specific recognition site of MAb (anti-idiotype) or by formating immune complexes (anti-isotype). It is noteworthy that ricin A chain conjugates were shown to preferentially induce a strong human anti-idiotype response.

To circumvent sensitization by mouse immunoglobulin, several strategies have been proposed. In animal models one can eliminate mouse immunoglobulin-reactive B lymphocyte clones using "lethal antigen", i.e., these cells are killed through the binding of radiolabeled or toxin-linked mouse immunoglobulin. Prophylactic treatment with the immunosuppressive drug cyclosporin A has also been recommended. At the moment, several laboratories are attempting to reduce immunogenicity by recombination of MAbs using genetic engineering methods. One approach is the creation of "humanized" chimeric antibodies in which the constant regions of the molecule are replaced by corresponding regions from the human immunoglobulin. This construction leaves the variable regions that are responsible for antibody specificity untouched. In the future, this development may lead to immunoreactive proteins synthesized de novo and composed of the antibody-derived variable regions, serving as recognition structure, coupled to a non-immunoglobulin carrier, e.g., an enzyme.

Looking to future prospects, we may hope that more sophisticated regimens such as two-step targeting will overcome many of the problems connected with antibody-guided therapy. One favorable concept first employs binding of streptavidin-conjugated MAb; then, after a certain time required for specific enrichment in the tumor and clearance of nonbound conjugate, ^{111}In-labeled biotin is administered as second-step reagent. An alternative strategy takes advantage of bispecific MAbs, i.e. MAbs with two different binding specificities: one binding site recognizes the tumor-associated antigen while the other is directed against a chelate molecule. At the time of maximal target concentration, radiolabeled chelate is injected and will specifically enrich in the tumor by means of the hybrid antibody.

SESSION 8

Cell Differentiation and Growth

Chairman: K. H. von Wangenheim

Induced Differentiation of Transformed Cells by Polar Compounds: From Molecular Studies to Clinical Trials*

P. A. Marks and R. A. Rifkind

Introduction

Hexamethylene bisacetamide (HMBA)-mediated conversion of murine erythroleukemia (MEL) cells (Friend et al. 1971; Reuben et al. 1976) to a terminally differentiated erythroid phenotype is a useful model to characterize molecular and cellular aspects of induced differentiation of transformed cells (Marks and Rifkind 1978; Tsiftsoglou and Robinson 1985; Marks et al. 1987). In vitro studies with HMBA induction of MEL cell and other transformed cells have also provided a basis for considering the use of this agent as an approach to therapy of various tumors (Marks and Rifkind 1984; Young et al. 1988).

Hexamethylene bisacetamide-mediated terminal cell differentiation (erythroleukemia cell line DS19) involves a latent period of approximately 10–12 h during which a number of metabolic changes occur but no commitment to terminal differentiation can be detected (Marks et al. 1987). Commitment is defined as the irreversible capacity to express characteristics of the differentiated erythroid phenotype, including loss of proliferative capacity, despite removal of the inducer (Gusella et al. 1976; Fibach et al. 1977). With continued exposure to HMBA, there is a transition from the latent period to a period of progressive recruitment of an increasing proportion of the population of cells to terminal erythroid differentiation with loss of proliferative capacity.

This review summarizes studies on: (1) the effects of inducer during the latent period of the wild-type (DS19) MEL cells, (2) the characteristics of vincristine-resistant MEL cell lines which are induced with little or no latent period, (3) HMBA-mediated terminal erythroid differentiation, and (4) the results of recent phase I clinical trials with HMBA.

Induction of MEL Cell Differentiation by Polar Compounds

Friend and colleagues (Friend et al. 1971) demonstrated that virus-transformed MEL cells in culture with dimethysulfoxide are induced to erythroid differentiation. We investigated the relationship between the structure and activity of inducing compounds (Tanaka et al. 1975) and found the polar group to be critical for inducer activity. We identified a new group of potent inducers, the polymethylene bisacetamides, of which HMBA is among the most potent (Table 1) (Tanaka et al. 1975; Reuben et al. 1976; Reuben et al. 1978).

* Studies performed in our laboratories were supported, in part, by grants from the National Cancer Institute (CA-31768 and CA-08748)

Table 1. Transformed cell lines inducible to differentiation by HMBA or other polar compounds

Cell lines
Erythroleukemia (mouse)
Teratocarcinoma (mouse)
Hepatic tumor (mouse)
Neuroblastoma (mouse)
Mammary tumor (rat) (human)
LB myeloblast (rat)
Kidney epithelial carcinoma (canine)
HL-60 promyelocytic leukemia (human)
Melanoma (human)
Colon carcinoma (human)
Bladder carcinoma (human)
Glioblastoma multiforma (human)
T cell (human)
B cell (human)
Primary cell cultures
Colon carcinoma (human)
Bladder carcinoma (human)
Acute myeloid leukemia (human)
Melanoma (human)

For references, see reviews (Marks and Rifkind 1984; Marks et al. 1987)

Hexamethylene Bisacetamide-Induced MEL Cell Differentiation; Characteristics of Latent Period

Upon addition of HMBA to MEL cells (the DS19 clone of Friend's original 745A cell line) (Chen et al. 1982), there is a latent period generally of 10–12 h during which there is no detectable commitment to terminal differentiation (Fig. 1A). This early or "latent" period is followed by a period during which an increasing proportion of the population express characteristics of terminal differentiation.

During the latent period, HMBA initiates a number of metabolic changes. Among these changes are alterations in membrane fluidity and membrane permeability to a number of ions including sodium, potassium, and, possibly, calcium (Marks et al. 1987); a prompt increase in membrane-associated protein kinase C (PKC) activity; and the appearance in the cytosol of a Ca^{2+}- and phospholipid-independent form of PKC, presumably generated by proteolytic cleavage of membrane-bound PKC and modulation in expression of a number of genes, among which are *c-myb, c-myc, c-fos,* and *p53.*

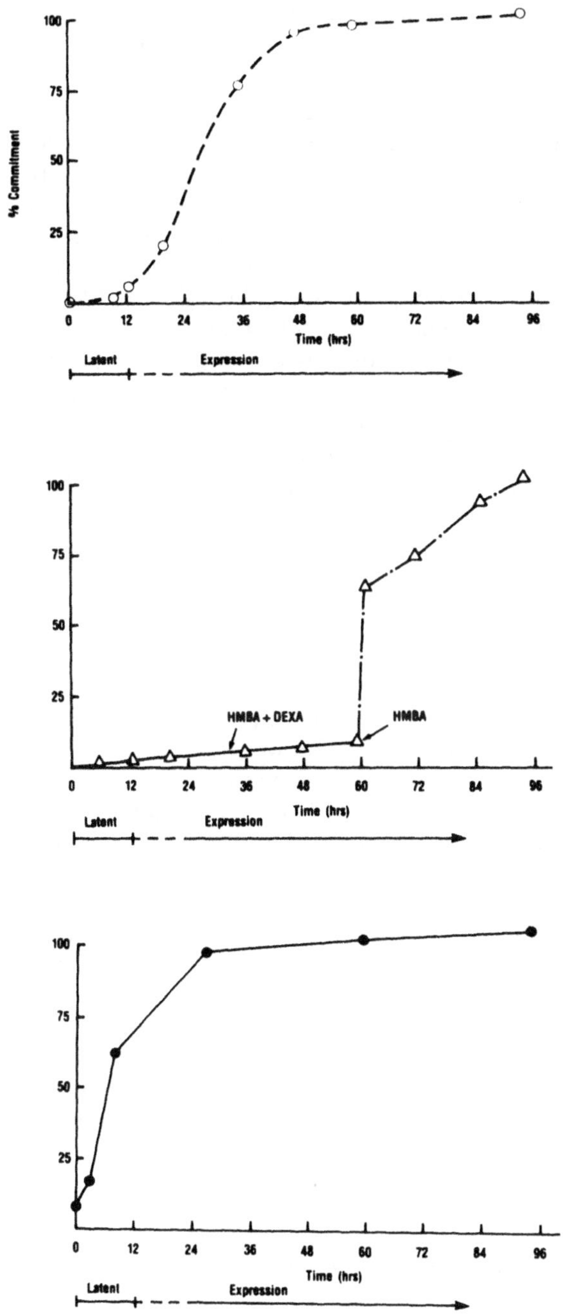

Fig. 1. a Kinetics of HMBA induction of MEL cell (DS19) to terminal differentiation. Commitment was assayed as previously described (Fibach et al. 1977). **b** Dexamethasone *(DEXA)* blocks the expression of HMBA-induced MEL cell (DS19) commitment to terminal differentiation (Chen et al. 1982). **c** Kinetics of HMBA induction of vincristine-resistant MEL cells (V3.17) to terminal differentiation (Melloni et al. 1988)

Hexamethylene Bisacetamide Effects on Protein Kinase C Activity During the Latent Period

Hexamethylene bisacetamide and related polar compounds cause a decrease in the levels of phosphatidylinositol metabolites, including inositol triphosphate and diacylglycerol, within 2 h of onset of culture (Faletto et al. 1985). PKC is a specific receptor for the tumor promotor, TPA, which can suppress HMBA-induced differentiation in MEL cells (Yamasaki et al. 1977). PKC activity appears to play a role in the signal transduction which occurs during HMBA-mediated modulation of late gene expression in MEL cell differentiation, such as increased transcription of α^1- and β-globin genes. We found that HMBA induces formation of a soluble, proteolytically activated, form of PKC that is catalytically active in the absence of Ca^{2+} and phospholipid. The protease inhibitor leupeptin blocks formation of this activated form of the kinase and inhibits HMBA-induced MEL cell hemoglobin accumulation (Melloni et al. 1987). Although TPA depletes total PKC activity and inhibits HMBA-induced MEL cell hemoglobin accumulation, it does not prevent HMBA-mediated early modulation of *c-myc, c-myb,* and *p53* gene expression.

Hexamethylene Bisacetamide Effects on Expression of *c-myb, c-myc, c-fos,* and *p53* Genes in the Latent Period

The products of the genes *c-myb, c-myc, c-fos,* and *p53* are all nuclear proteins which have been implicated in the control of cell proliferation and gene expression (Marks et al. 1987). The precise action of these proteins is not known. In MEL cells cultured with HMBA the level of *c-myc* mRNA decreases markedly within the 1st h of culture. A decrease in *c-myb* mRNA level occurs within 1–4 h. *c-fos* mRNA is almost undetectable in uninduced MEL cells and in cells cultured with HMBA begins to accumulate within about 4 h, reaching a maximum by 18–24 h. p53 protein decreases appreciably by 8 h. Dexamethasone and TPA each prevent expression of HMBA-induced MEL cell terminal differentiation (Fig. 1B) but do not modify the pattern of changes in *c-myc, c-myb, c-fos,* or *p53* gene expression during the latent period (Ramsay et al. 1986).

We have reported that DS19 cells cultured with dexamethasone and HMBA for up to 60 h do not express commitment (Chen et al. 1982). Removal of the steroid and continued culture with HMBA alone is associated with recruitment of a substantial proportion of the cells to differentiate without the characteristic latent period (Fig. 1A, B). These observations suggest that the steroid-sensitive step in HMBA-induced commitment occurs late in the latent period.

Induction of Vincristine-Resistant MEL Cells Without a Latent Period by Hexamethylene Bisacetamide

A variant MEL cell (V3.17) has been developed which is resistant to the cytotoxic effects of 2–5 ng/ml vincristine, a relatively low level of drug resistance compared with several multidrug-resistant cell lines which are 20- to several hundred-fold more resistant (Melloni et al. 1988). MEL cell line V3.17 is: (1) induced to commit with little or no latent period (Fig. 1C); (2) more rapidly induced to accumulate benzidine-reactive cells and to commit to terminal cell division than vincristine-sensitive cell lines; (3) responsive to lower concentrations of HMBA, e.g., one-tenth the concentration of HMBA optimal for inducing vincristine-sensitive MEL cells will induce over 50% of V3.17 cells; and (4) resistant to the inhibitory effects of both phorbol ester and dexamethasone on HMBA-induced differentiation. Several independently derived MEL cell lines resistant to vincristine have similar characteristics. These findings suggest that the mechanism for vincristine resistance in these cells develops in parallel or association with the mechanism which eliminates the latent period for induced differentiation. The resistance of V3.17 cells to the inhibitory effects of TPA and dexamethasone is consistent with an action of these inhibitors at a late step during the latent period. The lack of the latent period during HMBA-induced differentiation of V3.17 cells may reflect constitutive expression of a factor which circumvents HMBA-induced events in the latent period required for expression of differentiation. This factor (or factors) could, indeed, be the active product of critical latent period events.

The mechanism of vincristine resistance in V3.17 cells may involve an energy-dependent export pump which reduces intracellular levels of certain agents (Riordan and Ling 1985). Evidence for this conclusion includes: (1) accumulation of [^{3}H]vincristine in V3.17 cells is substantially lower than in DS19 cells; (2) V3.17 cells are cross-resistant to colchicine; and (3) verapamil and nephedipine, agents which reverse vincristine resistance, enhance vincristine's cytotoxic effects on V3.17 cells. Although mdr mRNA (Riordan and Ling 1985) levels are increased in certain but not all multidrug-resistant cell lines, to date we have not detected increased amounts of mdr mRNA or the *p*-glycoprotein product of this gene, compared with DS19 cells (unpublished observations).

Hexamethylene Bisacetamide-Induced MEL Cell Commitment of Differentiation

Continued culture of MEL cells with HMBA beyond the latent period results in morphological and chemical changes similar to normal terminal erythroid differentiation. These include increased expression of a number of genes, including genes for α^1- and β^{maj}-globin, the heme-synthetic enzymes, and erythroid-specific membrane proteins, as well as suppression of DNA replication and of rRNA synthesis (Marks and Rifkind 1978; Tsiftsoglou and Robinson 1985; Marks et al. 1987).

After its fall during the early latent period, the level of *c-myc* mRNA rises back toward that in uninduced cells by about 12 h and remains there for at least the ensuing 36 h; the elevated level of *c-fos* mRNA remains essentially unchanged. By comparison, by 12 h the level of *c-myb* mRNA has increased almost to control levels, from its early nadir, then falls again to an undetectable level by 24–36 h, where it remains for the duration of culture with inducer. That inducer-mediated suppression of *c-myb* mRNA may be an important factor in the recruitment of cells to commitment is suggested by several lines of evidence: (1) continued suppression of *c-myb* level is characteristic of progressive recruitment of MEL cells to terminal cell division; (2) hemin, which induces globin mRNA accumulation, but not commitment to terminal cell division, does not suppress *c-myb* mRNA; (3) dexamethasone inhibits HMBA-induced commitment and inhibits the late (>12 h) suppression of *c-myb* mRNA, but does not modify the changes in *c-myc* or *c-fos* mRNA or p53 protein which occur in response to HMBA.

We have reported that certain structural patterns of chromatin and DNA, commonly associated with actively transcribed genes, are detected in the α^1- and β^{maj}-globin gene domains of uninduced MEL cells, despite the relatively inactive transcription of these genes (Marks et al. 1987). These changes include a pattern of DNA hypomethylation of both genes, an increase (two- to threefold) in the sensitivity of the globin gene DNA domains to DNase I digestion compared with genes which are not transcribed in erythroid cells, and disruption of the normal nucleosome pattern across the α^1- and β^{maj}-globin gene transcribed regions. HMBA causes no detectable change in the pattern of methylation in the globin gene domains, but does cause certain changes in chromatin structure, including the appearance of DNase I hypersensitive sites within 100 base pairs 5′ of both the α^1 and β^{maj} genes and additional nucleosome disruption, which precede the onset of a marked increase in transcription. These changes in globin gene chromatin structure and transcription are part of the late modulation in gene expression caused by HMBA action on MEL cells.

Clinical Trials with HMBA

The evidence that HMBA can overcome the block to differentiation associated with transformation in a number of cell lines provides a basis for evaluating this agent in treatment of human neoplastic diseases (Table 2). HMBA has been evaluated in the National Cancer Institute Division of Cancer Treatment Tumor Screen Program and showed no therapeutic benefit to animals bearing several murine leukemic and solid tumors and possessed little or not cytotoxic activity against human mammary, colon, and lung xenografts in nude mice (National Cancer Institute 1984). These animal models did not, however, reproduce the in vitro conditions that appear to be critical for induced differentiation of transformed cell lines, in particular, the optimal concentration, which is about 3–5 m*M* HMBA, and the requirement for the continuous presence of the inducer over a relatively prolonged period for recruitment of transformed cells to differentiation.

At least three phase I clinical studies of HMBA have now been performed (at the University of Maryland Cancer Center, at the Johns Hopkins Oncology Center, and at the Memorial Sloan-Kettering Cancer Center) (Callery et al. 1986; Egorin et al. 1987; Rowinsky et al. 1986, 1987; Young et al. 1988). These phase I studies examined the toxicity and pharmacology of the agent, administered as a 5-day continuous infusion, repeated every 3 weeks, escalating from a starting dose of 4.8 g/m^2 per day to 40.0 g/m^2 per day. Toxicities, consisting of renal insufficiency, hyperchloremic metabolic acidemia/acidosis, and CNS toxicity characterized by agitation and delerium, limited dose escalation. Whereas these symptoms were all reversible upon cessation of the drug, the dose which was free of undesirable side effects (24 g/m^2 per day) yielded average serum concentrations of only 1.5 m*M* or lower. More recently, a 10-day continuous infusion, administered every 4 weeks, was evaluated in a phase I trial. In these studies the maximum tolerable dose was approximately 20 g/m^2 per day to avoid thrombocytopenia, which was the most prominent dose-limiting toxicity. At this dose the mean steady-state HMBA concentration among different patients

Table 2. Comparison of several differentiation induces at optimal concentration in the murine erythroleukemia system[a]

	Optimal concentration (m*M*)	Cells/ml ($\times 10^5$)	% Benzidine positive
Dimethylsulfoxide	280	1.2	67
N Methylacetamide	30	1.1	87
N;N; Dimethylacetamide	20	1.0	73
Hexamethylene bisacetamide	5	1.6	99
Butyric acid	1	1.2	42
None	–	1.4	0.5

[a] For details of the methodology of these studies see Reuben et al. (1976), Tanaka et al. (1975), Reuben et al. (1978)

ranged from a low of 0.31 to a high of 3.4 m*M*. Partial objective responses in tumor regression were noted in 5 of 29 patients in the Memorial Sloan-Kettering study (Young et al. 1988), all of whom tolerated multiple courses, from 2 to 17 cycles, of drug administration.

The potential for inducing proliferating neoplastic cells to express differentiated characteristics and decrease their rate of proliferation has important implications for cancer therapy. It is possible that such agents could prove useful in treatment of premalignant and malignant lesions. The ability to decrease the body load of cancer cells by use of an agent such as HMBA could prove valuable in conjunction with cytotoxic drugs. The in vitro studies summarized in this review suggest that to evaluate HMBA or similar agents for their potential therapeutic effectiveness it will be necessary: (1) to achieve an optimal in vivo concentration of the agent, (2) to maintain that concentration over a prolonged period, and (3) to have evaluable markers for establishing the biological activity of the agent in modulating the cancer cell phenotype.

Summary

A series of low molecular weight (generally < 400 mol. wt.) polar compounds have been shown to induce murine erythroleukemia (MEL) cells to express the differentiated erythroid phenotype, including cessation of proliferation. The structure-activity relationship of these polar compounds has been analyzed. Hexamethylene bisacetamide (HMBA) is the most effective of the compounds examined as inducers of MEL (DS19) cell differentiation. HMBA-mediated terminal differentiation of MEL cells is a multistep process. There is a latent period during which a number of changes occur including alterations in ion flux, an increase in membrane-bound RKC activity, appearance of Ca^{2+} and phospholipid-independent PKC activity in the cytosol, and modulation in expression of a number of nuclear oncogenes including *c-myc, c-myb, c-fos,* and the *p53* genes. During this latent period there is neither detectable commitment to terminal differentiation (including terminal cell division) nor increased transcription of the globin genes. HMBA-mediated commitment to terminal differentiation is first detected at about 12 h and increases in a stochastic fashion, until over 95% of the population has been recruited to terminal differentiation by 48–60 h. Commitment is associated with persistent HMBA-mediated suppression of *c-myb* gene expression. By 36–48 h, transcription of the globin genes has increased by 10- to 30-fold, whereas transcription of rRNA genes is suppressed. The steroid dexamethasone and the tumor promotor phorbol-12-myristate-13-acetate (TPA) suppress HMBA-induced MEL cell terminal differentiation. These agents appear to act at a late step during the latent period. The significance of the latent period in induced differentiation has been further examined in vincristine-resistant MEL cells. Compared with the parental strain (DS19), vincristine-resistant MEL cells are: (1) markedly more sensitive to HMBA, (2) induced to commit with little or no detectable latent period, and (3) resistant to dexamethasone- or TPA-mediated inhibition of HMBA-induced commitment. The vincristine-resistant MEL cell lines have properties consistent with the multidrug-resistant cell line phenotype. The data suggest that the mechanism of vincristine resistance is related to the mechanism of altered sensitivity to HMBA-mediated differentiation. Vincristine-resistant MEL cells may constitutively express a factor that circumvents or is the effective product of essential HMBA-mediated early events in induced differentiation. These in vitro studies of the molecular and cellular characteristics of HMBA-induced MEL cell differentiation have provided a basis for clinical trials of HMBA in human subjects with cancer. Phase I/II clinical trials with HMBA have been initiated.

References

Callery PS, Egorin MJ, Geelhaar LA, Balachandran Nayar MS (1986) Identification of metabolites of the cell-differentiating agent hexamethylene bisacetamide in humans. Cancer Res 46:4900–4903

Chen Z, Banks J, Rifkind RA, Marks PA (1982) Inducer-mediated commitment of murine erythroleukemia cells to differentiation: a multistep process. Proc Natl Acad Sci USA 79:471–475

Egorin MJ, Sigman LKM, Van Echo DA, Forrest A, Whitacre MY, Aisner J (1987) Phase I clinical and pharmacokinetic study of hexamethylene bisacetamide (NSC 95580) administered as a five-day continuous infusion. Cancer Res 47:617–625

Faletto DL, Arrow AS, Macara IG (1985) An early decrease in phosphatidylinositol turnover occurs on induction of Friend cell differentiation and precedes the decrease in c-myc expression. Cell 43:315–325

Fibach E, Reuben RC, Rifkind RA, Marks PA (1977) Effect of hexamethylene bisacetamide on the commitment to differentiation of murine erythroleukemia cells. Cancer Res 37:440–444

Friend C, Scher W, Holland J, Sato T (1971) Hemoglobin synthesis in murine erythroleukemia cells in vitro: stimulation of erythroid differentiation by dimethylsulfoxide. Proc Natl Acad Sci USA 68:378–382

Gusella JF, Geller R, Clarke B, Weeks V, Housman D (1976) Commitment to erythroid differentiation by Friend erythroleukemia cells: a stochastic analysis. Cell 9:221–229

Marks PA, Rifkind RA (1978) Erythroleukemic differentiation. Annu Rev Biochem 47:419–448

Marks PA, Rifkind RA (1984) Differentiation modifiers. Cancer 54:2766–2769

Marks PA, Sheffery M, Rifkind RA (1987) Induction of transformed cells to terminal differentiation and the modulation of gene expression. Cancer Res 47:659–666

Melloni E, Pontremoli S, Michetti M, Sacco O, Cakiroglu AG, Jackson JF, Rifkind RA, Marks PA (1987) Protein kinase C activity and hexamethylene bisacetamide induced erythroleukemia cell differentiation. Proc Natl Acad Sci USA 84:5282–5286

Melloni E, Pontremoli S, Damiani G, Viotti P, Weich N, Rifkind RA, Marks PA (1988) Vincristine-resistant erythroleukemia cells have marked increased sensitivity to hexamethylene bisacetamide induced differentiation. Proc Natl Acad Sci USA 85:3835–3839

National Cancer Institute (1984) Hexamethylene bisacetamide. National Cancer Institute, Bethesda, MD, pp 8–26

Ramsay RG, Ikeda K, Rifkind RA, Marks PA (1986) Changes in gene expression associated with induced differentiation of erythroleukemia: proto-oncogenes, globin genes and cell division. Proc Natl Acad Sci USA 83:6849–6853

Reuben R, Khanna PL, Gazitt Y, Breslow R, Rifkind RA, Marks PA (1978) Inducers of erythroleukemic differentiation: Relationship of structure to activity among planar-polar compounds. J Biol Chem 253:4214–4218

Reuben RC, Wife RL, Breslow R, Rifkind RA, Marks PA (1976) A new group of potent inducers of differentiation in murine erythroleukemia cells. Proc Natl Acad Sci USA 73:862–866

Riordan JR, Ling V (1985) Genetic and biochemical characterization of multidrug resistance. Pharm Ther 28:51–57

Rowinsky EK, Ettinger DS, Grochow LB, Brundrett RB, Cates AE, Donehower RC (1986) Phase I and pharmacologic study of hexamethylene bisacetamide (HMBA) in patients with advanced cancer. J Clin Oncol 4:1835–1844

Rowinsky EK, Ettinger DS, McGuire WP, Noe DA, Grochow LB, Donehower RC (1987) Prolonged infusion of hexamethylene bisacetamide: A Phase I and pharmacological study. Cancer Res 47: 5788–5795

Tanaka M, Levy J, Terada M, Breslow R, Rifkind RA, Marks PA (1975) Induction of erythroid differentiation in murine virus infected erythroleukemia cells by highly polar compounds. Proc Natl Acad Sci USA 72:1003–1006

Tsiftsoglou AS, Robinson SH (1985) Differentiation of leukemic cell lines: a review focusing on murine erythroleukemia and human HL-60 cells. Int J Cell Cloning 3:349–366

Yamasaki H, Fibach E, Nudel U, Weinstein IB, Rifkind RA, Marks PA (1977) Tumor promoters inhibit spontaneous and induced differentiation of murine erythroleukemia cells in culture. Proc Natl Acad Sci USA 74:3451–3455

Young CW, Fanucchi MP, Walsh TD, Baltzer L, Yaldaei S, Stevens YW, Gordon C, Tong W, Rifkind RA, Marks PA (1988) Phase I trial and clinical pharmacologic evaluation of hexamethylene bisacetamide by 10-day continuous intravenous infusion at 28 day intervals. Cancer Res 48: 7304–7309

Hematopoietic Cytokines in Cancer Therapy: Concepts and First Clinical Observations*

R. Mertelsmann, A. Lindemann, M. Wieser, W. Oster, and F. Herrmann

Introduction

The treatment options for patients with cancer are presently limited to surgical and radiotherapeutic approaches for localized disease or systemic administration of cytotoxic drugs for disseminated cancer. The molecular basis of the differential sensitivity of cancer tissues to chemotherapy compared to normal tissues remains largely undefined. It has been postulated that differences in the kinetics of cell proliferation between neoplastic cells and their normal counterparts may be the basis of this differential sensitivity. However, this has only been demonstrated for a very few neoplastic diseases and does not apply to the majority of cancers. Alternative explanations of the efficacy of chemotherapy include decreased repair capabilities of cancer cells as well as chemotherapy-induced reduction of growth factor release required for autocrine and paracrine growth of tumor cells. Overall, treatment results have remained largely disappointing and there has been little progress in recent years, especially for the more frequent cancers such as lung, breast, and colon cancer (Bailar and Smith 1986).

Current research is searching for new concepts of cancer treatment. The oncogenetic defect in neoplastic cells is a genetic alteration in a primordial cancer cell, which subsequently leads to clonal expansion and, in many instances, to clonal evolution with additional genetic alterations, giving cancer cells a proliferative advantage which tends to increase with time, e.g., by activation of drug resistance genes. The oncogenetic damage can be induced by different agents such as viruses, ionizing radiation, or other substances altering gene structure. In addition, spontaneous genetic re-arrangements leading to oncogenic growth seem to be occurring, especially in situations of proliferative stress. This oncogenetic change leads to quantitively or qualitatively abnormal production of proteins which regulate growth and differentiation. Proteins likely to be involved in this setting include growth factors and their receptors, cytoplasmic transmitter molecules or DNA-binding proteins regulating gene expression. Many of these key proteins have been identified. Aberrant expression of these proteins in various experimental systems has been shown to induce cancer, generating the term "proto-oncogenes" (Friend et al. 1988). An alternative pathway of oncogenesis is the loss of suppressor oncogene information, e.g., in retinoblastoma (Friend et al. 1988).

---

* Supported in part by the Deutsche Forschungsgemeinschaft (Grant He 1380-2/1), Deutsche Krebshilfe (Grant W 19/86/Os 1), the German Ministry for Research and Technology, and the Tumorzentrum Mainz

Once the oncogenic alteration has led to neoplastic transformation, the balance of gene expression is altered (Friend et al. 1988). The transformed cell, however, does not appear truly autonomous in its growth, but, like its normal counterpart, remains dependent on interaction with physiological regulators of the host, e.g., the dependence on growth factors and/or hormones, reminiscent of parasitic infections. Thus, the alterations leading to the malignant transformation can be very subtle and are in most instances apparently not detected by the host immune system. Only a small percentage of human cancers have been shown to be immunogenic. This appears to be the case when the malignancy-inducing mutation involves a membrane protein, or when the alteration of gene expression leads to cell surface expression of previously hidden cryptic antigens or the transfer of mutation-derived peptides to the cell surface.

Hormone-like peptides are involved in intercellular interactions of virtually all cell types, capable of modulating proliferation, differentiation, and functional activity. One promising though complex strategy for cancer treatment targets the disturbed regulation of cancer cells, aiming to restore growth and differentiation back to normal or near-normal by supplying or replacing missing regulatory factors. Other efforts focus on mobilizing host defense mechanisms against cancer, while the alleviation of chemotherapy-induced bone marrow toxicity by administration of hematopoietic growth factors has just begun to be studied.

The regulation of normal and neoplastic hematopoiesis is the best studied example of regulation of growth and differentiation which applies in principle also to all other tissues. Data obtained so far suggest that one prime difference between normal and neoplastic cells is the unstimulated production of cytokines in neoplastic cells, while normal cells require activation by extracellular signals prior to releasing cytokines (Oster et al. 1988).

Conceptually, therapeutic approaches with cytokines can be subdivided into three:

1. Stimulation of the immune system in order to increase host immunity to cancer (e.g., interleukin 2).
2. Modulation of tumor cell growth and differentiation via cytotoxic, cytostatic, or regulatory cytokines (e.g., tumor necrosis factor, interferon).
3. Stimulation of nonspecific host resistance and amelioration of the side-effects of intensive chemotherapy (e.g., colony stimulating factors, erythropoietin).

Cytokines can be produced by many cell types and their effects can be exerted on many target cells. The pleiotropic effects of cytokines complicate rational clinical approaches, since these factors can have both stimulating and inhibitory properties depending on the functional state of the target cell, receptor affinity, receptor density, and ligand concentration. While cytotoxic drugs are used at their maximum tolerated dose, the maximum tolerated dose of cytokines is frequently not the optimum biological response-modifying dose. Since the tumor-host interaction is an integral part of a co-ordinated regulatory network of cells and cytokines similar to the endocrine system, modulation of one parameter will frequently generate a broad spectrum of indirect effects via activation of target cells and secondary release of other cytokines.

Among the cytokines studied in man, interferon-α has demonstrated the most impressive clinical activity in the treatment of hairy cell leukemia (Goulomb et al. 1986)

Table 1. Cytokines involved in hematopoiesis and blood cell activation

Type	Molecules	Synonyms	Chromo-somal localization	mRNA size (kb)	Protein size (amino acids)	Molecular weight (kd)
I (growth factors)	Multi-CSF	IL-3	5q23–31	1	133	14–28
	GM-CSF	CSF-	5q23;q31	1	127	14–35
	G-CSF	CSF-	17q11;q22	2	174; 177	18–22
	M-CSF	CSF-1	5q33.1	1.5–4.5	256; 435; 554	36–90
	-receptor	c-fms	5q34			
	EPO		7q11;q22	1.6	164	34–39
II (synergizing factors)	IL-1 alpha	Hemopoietin-1	nr[a]	2.2	269; 152	31; 17
	IL-1 beta		2q14	1.6	269; 152	31; 17
	-receptor[b]		nr		319; 217	80
	IL-2	TCGF	4			
	-receptor	Tac (chain)	nr			
	IL-4	BSF-1	nr	0.9	129	15–20
	IL-5	BLGF-II, TRF	5q	1.7	134	12–18
	IL-6	IFN-2, BSF-2	7q11	1.3	212	24
III (growth factor inducing factors)	TNF-α	Cachectin	6q23;q12	1.6	157	17
	TNF-β	LT	6q23;q12	1.4	171	25
	IFN-γ	Type II IFN	12	1.7	143	15–45

[a] nr: not reported
[b] Murine

and to a lesser degree in the treatment of chronic myelogenous leukemia (Talpaz et al. 1986) and certain solid tumors refractory to chemotherapy (malignant melanoma, renal cell cancer, superficial bladder cancer, and cancer of the ovary; for overview see Faltynek and Oppenheim 1988).

Most other hematopoietic cytokines are still in the early stages of clinical evaluation (Table 1). Interleukin 2 (IL-2) and Tumor necrosis factor-α (TNF-α) have been evaluated in patients with advanced cancer, while granulocyte-macrophage colony stimulating factor (GM-CSF) and granulocyte colony stimulating factor (G-CSF) are primarily targeted at chemotherapy-induced pancytopenias. The following review will focus on IL-2, TNF-α, GM-CSF, and G-CSF, which are the agents currently most extensively studied by our department.

Interleukin-2

IL-2 is probably the most important example of an agent that acts primarily through stimulating host immunity against tumor cells. The T-cell product IL-2 is involved in proliferation and functional activation of immune competent cells which play a role in the surveillance and elimination of tumor cells. In an autocrine pathway, IL-2 is active as a growth factor and functional activator for T-helper cells. In a paracrine pathway, IL-2 stimulates natural killer (NK) cells, preactivated cytotoxic T cells, B cells and macrophages (Smith 1988). In order to exert its function, IL-2 has to bind to a specific target structure, the IL-2 receptor. The IL-2 receptor is a bimolecular structure consisting of an α chain of 55 kd and a β chain of 75 kd (Waldmann 1986; Wang and Smith 1987). Both chains together form a dimer with a 100-fold higher affinity for IL-2 than the single chains. Resting T cells or NK cells do not express high affinity IL-2 receptors and therefore do not respond to a physiological serum concentration of IL-2 unless activated. Higher concentrations of IL-2 (>100 units/ml), however, are capable of activating NK cells and T cells to synthesize α chains which then form dimers with preexisting β chains, leading to high-affinity receptors and subsequently to proliferation and activation of cytotoxic functions (Siegel et al. 1987). IL-2 activated cytotoxic T cells and activated NK cells are capable of binding to tumor target cells via nonspecific adhesion structures like CD-2 (cluster of designation), CD-16 or the leukocyte-function-associated antigen LFA-1, in addition to interaction via the antigen-specific T-cell receptor of cytotoxic T cells with its target antigen. The phenomenon of IL-2 induced lymphocyte mediated tumor lysis in vitro and in vivo has been extensively studied by Grimm and Rosenberg, who generated the term "lymphocyte activated killer cell phenomenon" for these activated NK cells (LAK; Grimm et al. 1981). Investigations in various murine models have demonstrated that administration of ex vivo activated cytotoxic cells (LAK cells) can induce tumor regressions in a variety of tumor models, especially when combined with the systemic administration of IL-2 (Mule et al. 1984). When administered at very high doses as single agent, IL-2 was also capable of inducing tumor regressions in certain model systems in vivo (Rosenberg et al. 1985). It is now clear that activated NK cells account for most of the LAK activity with high-dose administration of IL-2. The promising results which have been obtained in murine tumor models have led to the development of similar clinical strategies. First clinical studies with purified IL-2 (Lotze et al. 1985a, b; Mertelsmann et al. 1985; Kolitz et al. 1987) have not demonstrated significant tumor regressions, although immunomodulatory effects were observed. These included activation of T and NK cells and the polyclonal expansion of IL-2 receptor-positive T lymphocytes in vivo. Subsequent studies in man using high-dose recombinant IL-2 with or without simultaneous administration of ex vivo IL-2 activated LAK cells have been pursued at the National Cancer Institute and other institutions (Rosenberg et al. 1987). Other studies have investigated the combination of low-dose cyclophosphamide with IL-2. These two agents have been shown to act synergistically in the elimination of tumor metastasis in several animal models (North 1982). This approach was explored in a study at the Memorial Sloan-Kettering Cancer Center (Kolitz et al. 1988) as well as in a recently completed co-operative trial in Germany (Lindemann et al. 1988) and a trial at the University of California at Los Angeles (Mitchell et al. 1988) showing rare partial remissions in patients with malignant melanoma.

Side effects of IL-2 treatment with or without LAK cells are dose-dependent and consist of fever and chills presumably due to endogenous induction of other cytokines such as IL-1, interferon-γ and TNF (Herrmann et al. 1988d; Lotze et al. 1985a). The dose-limiting toxicity in all trials was a capillary leakage syndrome resulting in its most pronounced form in interstitial pulmonary edema. The pathophysiological basis of this IL-2 induced syndrome appears to be mediated by the nonspecific LAK cells (Ettinghausen et al. 1988). Most IL-2 associated side effects are dose dependent and rapidly reversible upon discontinuation of IL-2 administration. Biological effects include polyclonal expansion of IL-2 receptor-positive T lymphocytes, an increase in natural killer activity, and considerable bone marrow and blood eosinophilia, which is most likely caused by endogenous induction of other cytokines such as IL-3, IL-5, and GM-CSF.

Although clinical responses have been dramatic at times, overall therapeutic results have been largely disappointing. It remains to be determined whether better tolerated and more effective schedules of IL-2 administration with or without in vitro activated killer cells can be developed. Since the activated killer cells have not been shown to be responsible for killing cancer cells in vivo, but are the mediators of the major side effects of IL-2 (i.e., damage of endothelial cells and the capillary leakage syndrome; Ettinghausen et al. 1988) current efforts are focusing on the characterization and cloning of specific killer cell populations (e.g., by expanding tumor infiltrating lymphocytes; Topalian et al. 1988). Other approaches currently under investigation include the combination of IL-2 with conventional chemotherapeutic agents, with bifunctional monoclonal antibodies, and with other cytokines including interferon-α and -γ as well as TNF and IL-4.

Tumor Necrosis Factor

Tumor necrosis factor (TNF) is a cytokine demonstrating direct antitumor effects in vitro and in vivo against a broad spectrum of tumor cell types. TNF was first characterized molecularly by Carswell and colleagues in 1975 and is a product of activated macrophages. It is characterized by induction of hemorrhagic necrosis in the methylcholanthrene-induced-sarcoma model of mice. T lymphocytes, B lymphocytes and neutrophil granulocytes can also secrete TNF under appropriate induction conditions (Herrmann 1988a). Its primary physiological role appears to be the mediation of inflammatory and immune reactions. TNF can stimulate the antibody-dependent cytotoxicity of neutrophil granulocytes and activates their functional repertoire, including oxygen radical production. Furthermore, it induces cytotoxicity in monocytes and in NK cells as well as modulating IL-2 receptor expression and interferon-γ production by T cells (Philip and Epstein 1986). Other properties of TNF include induction of adhesion molecules, cell surface differentiation antigens, and major histocompatibility complex molecules, as well as of other cytokines such as IL-1, IL-6, CSF and growth- and activation-inducing factors for platelets in receptive target cells (Scheurich et al. 1987). In vivo studies in murine model systems using recombinant TNF have generated nearly identical results to those previously obtained with natural TNF. In vitro, recombinant TNF exhibits cytotoxic as well as cytostatic effects against a broad spectrum of tumor cell lines derived from different tissues. By contrast, normal diploid renal cells, melanocytes, colon epithelium, endothelial cells, and fibroblasts have been resistant in vitro. Since TNF does exert direct antitumor effects as well as serving as a co-stimulant for activated immune competent cells, the clinical evaluation in cancer patients seemed promising.

In phase I studies at M.D. Anderson Hospital in Houston, Texas (Blick et al. 1987), as well as in our own department (Mertelsmann et al. 1987), TNF-α was given in different schedules with dose escalations from 1 to 400 $\mu g/m^2$ per day. Even at lower doses, fever and chills dominated the clinical picture, while the dose-limiting toxicity was fluid retention, most likely due to a capillary leakage syndrome, similar to that described for IL-2.

In our own recently completed phase I clinical trial of recombinant human TNF-α in 65 patients with advanced cancer, the maximum tolerated dose of TNF was found to be 200 $\mu g/m^2$ b.i.d. Tumor responses were induced only sporadically. Partial remissions in a patient with colon cancer and one patient with pancreatic cancer were observed, but no significant tumor regressions were seen in a broad spectrum of other malignancies. The maximum tolerated dose for a single injection of TNF was 200 $\mu g/m^2$, while our schedule of twice daily administration allowed a total daily dose of 400 $\mu g/m^2$ given by two injections 6 h apart. When considering own data and those reported by other investigators (Blick et al. 1987; Chapman et al. 1987), it seems possible that colorectal cancers and renal cell cancers might be targets for phase II studies, although our own conclusion has been that TNF as single agent is unlikely to be of major benefit for patients with cancer. It remains to be seen whether higher doses of TNF can be administered with better control of side effects or whether combinations of TNF with IL-2 or other biological response-modifying agents will lead to more frequent and more predictable antitumor effects.

Granulocyte-Macrophage Colony-Stimulating Factor

GM-CSF is a member of the family of hematopoietic growth factors which regulates proliferation, differentiation, and functional activation of hematopoietic progenitor cells (Herrmann 1988c). Preclinical investigations of GM-CSF in a primate model (Donahue et al. 1986) have shown that GM-CSF promises to reduce the chemotherapy-associated morbidity caused by neutropenia-associated infections. In clinical situations where bone marrow toxicity is the dose-limiting side effect of chemo- and radiotherapy, GM-CSF treatment might lead to increased bone marrow tolerance allowing more frequent administration of chemotherapeutic drugs or the administration of higher doses. In the setting of autologous bone marrow transplantation, more rapid bone marrow recovery can be expected (Brandt et al. 1988). It has also been shown that GM-CSF stimulates activation of granulocytes and macrophages which might induce indirect and direct antitumor effects. In our own phase I and II clinical studies (Herrmann et al. 1988e), cancer patients refractory to chemotherapy have received recombinant GM-CSF at six dose levels ranging from 30 to 1000 $\mu g/m^2$ day in 5-day and 14-day cycles given by intravenous bolus injection, by 24-h continuous infusion, and by subcutaneous administration. A broad spectrum of reproducible and predictable hematological effects were observed. Continuous infusion of 1000 $\mu g/ml$ GM-CSF over 14 days resulted in a 17-fold increase of total white blood counts, consisting predominantly of neutrophil granulocytes as well as of increased numbers of eosinophils and monocytes, especially at higher doses of GM-CSF. Bone marrow cellularity was highly increased. In doses of 500 $\mu g/m^2$ and above an increase of circulating myeloid progenitor cells could be demonstrated. No significant effect was observed on circulating lymphocytes, platelets, or reticulocytes. Within 1 week of discontinuing GM-CSF, leukocyte counts returned to baseline. GM-CSF treatment at 500 $\mu g/m^2$ or less was associated with minor side effects.

Although objective tumor responses were not seen in patients receiving GM-CSF, our own data concerning the use of GM-CSF after chemotherapy in 15 patients, results on the use of GM-CSF after autologous bone marrow transplantation (Brandt et al. 1988), and data obtained at the Memorial Sloan-Kettering Cancer Center in a similar study with G-CSF (Gabrilove et al. 1988) strongly support the hypothesis that the administration of one of the CSFs significantly reduces chemotherapy-associated neutropenia.

Granulocyte Colony-Stimulating Factor

The second CSF, currently undergoing phase I and II clinical evaluation, is granulocyte CSF (G-CSF). This 175 amino acid protein has a molecular weight of about 18800 d. The recombinant human G-CSF produced by Amgen (Thousand Oaks, California) differs from the natural protein in one amino acid and is not glycosylated. G-CSF is a hematopoietic regulator which has the ability to promote the growth and maturation of myeloid cells and in particular the proliferation and differentiation of granulocytes both in vitro and in vivo. Human G-CSF has recently been purified (Welte et al. 1985), molecularly cloned, and successfully expressed (Souza et al. 1986), allowing production of large quantities of purified recombinant human G-CSF. Highly purified human G-CSF and rhG-CSF have identical in vitro biological activity (Souza et al. 1986). This hematopoietic regulator has effects on both immature bone marrow progenitors and terminally differentiated myeloid cells as well as on leukemic myeloid cells in vitro. In preclinical studies, rhG-CSF has been shown to induce significant rises in neutrophil counts, which are dose-dependent, reproducible, and predictable in a normal hamster model as well as in a primate model (Cohen et al. 1987; Welte et al. 1987). It has also been shown that drug-induced cytopenia in the primate model can be significantly reduced by the simultaneous or subsequent administration of G-CSF. Interestingly, G-CSF also acts to induce differentiation in malignant myeloid progenitor cells, as demonstrated in the murine WEHI-3b (D^+) myelomonocytic tumor cell line. In this model, the survival of mice was significantly prolonged when G-CSF was administered to mice with this type of leukemia (Souza et al. 1986). In our own phase I study of recombinant G-CSF, very few side effects were observed achieving neutrophil counts of up to $50000/m^3$ at doses of 30 μg/kg, while at higher doses thrombocytopenia is dose limiting. In a phase I/II study of the combination of G-CSF with chemotherapy in bladder cancer using the Methotrexate/vinblastin adriamycin cisplatin (M-VAC) protocol, prevention of neutropenia has also been demonstrated (Gabrilove et al. 1988).

Cytokines in Cancer Therapy: Outlook

While interferon-α has already found its place in the management of a small and selected group of patients with cancer, a definite role can also be predicted for the CSFs in the setting of supportive care. The use of GM-CSF and G-CSF in cancer patients is the main focus of our clinical efforts at present. Reduction of chemotherapy-associated neutropenia and morbidity has already been demonstrated. Further studies will have to analyze whether higher cure rates in chemotherapy- or radiotherapy-treated patients will be made possible by administration of CSFs in order to reduce therapy-related morbidity as well as allowing more aggressive treatment protocols. Whether erythropoietin, possibly in combination with other cytokines, will also reduce the transfusion requirements in cancer patients remains to be ascertained.

The clinical results with cytokines expected to show direct tumoristatic or tumoricidal effects have been disappointing. The intercellular network of amplifying mechanisms in vivo is insufficiently understood, resulting in unpredictable side effects and lack of predictable antitumor effects. Even the use of interferon-α in hairy cell leukemia and chronic myeloid leukemia is based on empiricism rather than on rational design.

The heterogeneity of tumors as well as of the respective hosts has to be of major relevance, since all murine in vivo results have only been reproducible in specific strains of mice and in cloned tumor cell lines not reflecting the complexity of the human setting. A definite place for IL-2 and TNF as single agents appears somewhat unlikely at this point, although remissions have been seen in a number of patients. The future for these agents, predominantly acting to suppress or kill tumor cells, will probably be in a combination setting with other cytokines or chemotherapy.

In addition, better parameters of measurement of biological responses associated with and/or leading to tumor regressions appear to be essential before the development of these agents can proceed in a more rational way. At present, the hematopoiesis stimulating factors GM-CSF, G-CSF, as well as erythropoietin, M-CSF, and IL-3, promise at least a reduction of morbidity for many cancer patients in the immediate future.

Acknowledgements. We would like to thank U. Gerhards, U. Haupt, S. Schmidt and B. Roos for data collection and preparation and M. Astheimer and C. Schumann for secretarial assistance.

References

Bailar JC III, Smith EM (1986) Progress against cancer. N Engl Med 314:1226–1232

Blick M, Sherwin SA, Rosenblum M, Gutterman J (1987) Phase I study of recombinant tumor necrosis factor in cancer patients. Cancer Res 47:2986–2989

Brandt SJ, Peters WP, Atwater SK, Kurtzberg J, Borowitz MJ, Jones RB, Shpall EJ, Bast RC, Gilbert CJ, Oette DH (1988) Effect of recombinant human granulocyte-macrophage colony-stimulating factor on hematopoietic reconstitution after high-dose chemotherapy and autologous bone marrow transplantation. N Engl J Med 318:869–876

Carswell EA, Old LJ, Kassel RL, Green S, Fiore N, Williamson B (1975) An endotoxin-induced serum factor that causes necrosis of tumors. Proc Natl Acad Sci USA 72:3666–3670

Chapman PB, Lester TJ, Casper ES, Gabrilove JL, Wong GY, Kempin SJ, Gold PJ, Welt S, Warren RS, Starnes HF, Sherwin SA, Old LJ, Oettgen HF (1987) Clinical pharmacology of recombinant human tumor necrosis factor in patients with advanced cancer. J Clin Oncol 5:1942–1951

Cohen AM, Zsebo K, Inoue H, Hines D, Boone TC, Chazin VR, Tsai L, Ritch T, Souza LM (1987) In vivo stimulation of granulopoiesis by recombinant human G-CSF. Proc Natl Acad Sci USA 84:2484–2488

Donahue RE, Wang EA, Sone DK, Kamen R, Wong GG, Sehgal PK, Nathan DG, Clark SC (1986) Stimulation of haematopoiesis in primates by continuous infusion of recombinant human GM-CSF. Nature 321:872

Ettinghausen SE, Puri KR, Rosenberg SA (1988) Increased vascular permeability in organs mediated by the systemic administration of lymphokine-activated killer cells and recombinant interleukin-2 in mice. INCI 80:177–188

Faltynek CR, Oppenheim JJ (1988) Interferons in host defense. INCI 80:10–15

Friend SH, Dryja TP, Weinberg RA (1988) Oncogenes and tumor-suppressing genes. N Engl J Med 318:618–622

Gabrilove JL, Jakubowski A, Scheer H, Sternberg C, Wong G, Grous J, Yagoda A, Fain K, Moore MAS, Clarkson B, Oettgen H, Alton K, Welte K, Souza L (1988) Effects of granulocyte colony-stimulating factor on neutropenia and associated morbidity due to chemotherapy for transitional-cell carcinoma of the urothelium. N Engl J Med 318:1414–1422

Goulomb H, Jacobs A, Fefer A, Ozer J, Thompson J, Portlock C, Ratain M, Golde D, Vardiman J, Barke JS, Brady J, Bonnem E, Spiegel R (1986) Alpha-2 interferon therapy of hairy-cell leukemia: a multicenter study of 64 patients. J Clin Oncol 4:900–905

Grimm EA, Mazumder A, Zhang HZ, Rosenberg SA (1981) Lymphokine-activated killer cell phenomenon. Lysis of natural killer-resistant fresh solid tumor cells by IL-2-activated autologous human peripheral blood lymphocytes. J Exp Med 155:1823–1841

Herrmann F (1988a) Tumornekrosefaktor. Molekularbiologische und biochemische Grundlagen, biologische Aktivität, klinische Anwendungsmöglichkeiten. Münch Med Wochenschr 128:630–632

Herrmann F (1988c) Polypeptides controlling hematopoietic growth. Blut (in press)

Herrmann F, Lindemann A, Cannistra SA, Oster W, Griffin JD, Mertelsmann R (1988b) Monocyte interleukin 1 secretion is regulated by the sequential action of gamma-interferon and interleukin 2 involving monocyte surface expression of interleukin 2 receptors. J Immunol (in press)

Herrmann F, Cannistra SA, Lindemann A, Mertelsmann RH, Rambaldi A, Griffin JD (1988d) Functional consequences of monocyte interleukin-2 receptor expression: induction of monokines by interferon-gamma and interleukin-2. J Immunol (in press)

Herrmann F, Schulz G, Lindemann A, Meyenburg W, Oster W, Krumwieh D, Mertelsmann R (1988e) Hematopoietic responses in patients with advanced malignancy treated with recombinant human GM-CSF. J Clin Oncol (in press)

Kolitz JE, Welte K, Wong GY, Holloway K, Merluzzi VJ, Enger A, Bradley EC, Konrad M, Polivka A, Gabrilove JL, Sykora FW, Miller GA, Fiedler W, Krown S, Oettgen HF, Mertelsmann R (1987) Polyclonal expansion of activated T-lymphocytes in patients treated with recombinant interleukin-2. J Biol Response Mod 6:412–429

Kolitz JE, Wong GY, Welte K, Merluzzi VJ, Engert A, Bialas T, Polivka A, Bradley EC, Konrad M, Gnecco C, Oettgen HF, Mertelsmann R (1988) Phase I trial of recombinant interleukin-2 and cyclophosphamide. Augmentation of cellular immunity and T-cell mitogenic response with long-term administration of rIL-2. J Biol Response Mod (in press)

Lindemann A, Herrmann F, Schmidt RE, Diehl V, Höffken K, Mertelsmann R (1988) A phase II study of recombinant human interleukin-2 in the treatment of metastatic renal cell carcinoma and malignant melanoma. (Submitted)

Lotze UT, Frana LW, Sharrow SO, Robb RJ, Rosenberg SA (1985a) In vivo administration of purified human interleukin-2. I. Half life and immunologic effects of the Jurkat cell line-derived interleukin-2. J Immunol 134:157–166

Lotze UT, Matory YL, Ettinghausen SE, Rayner AA, Sharrow SO, Seipp CAY, Custer MC, Rosenberg SA (1985b) In vivo administration of human interleukin-2. II. Half life, immunologic effects, and expansion of peripheral lymphoid cells in vivo with recombinant IL-2. J Immunol 135:2865–2875

Mertelsmann R, Welte K, Sternberg C, O'Reilly R, Moore MAS, Clarkson BD, Oettgen HF (1984) Treatment of immunodeficiency with interleukin 2: initial exploration. J Biol Response Mod 4:483–490

Mertelsmann R, Gamm H, Flener R, Herrmann F (1987) Recombinant human tumor necrosis factor alpha (RHTNF-alpha) in advanced cancer: a phase I clinical trial. Proc Annu Meet Am Assoc Cancer Res 28:399 (abstract)

Mitchell MS, Kempf RA, Harel W, Shau H, Boswell WD, Lind S, Bradley EC (1988) Effectiveness and tolerability of low-dose cyclophosphamide and low-dose intravenous interleukin-2 disseminated melanoma. J Clin Oncol 6:409–424

Mule JJ, Shu S, Schwarz SL, Rosenberg SA (1984) Adoptive immunotherapy of established pulmonary metastasis with LAK cells and recombinant IL-2. Science 225:1487–1489

North RJ (1982) Cyclophosphamide-facilitated adoptive immunotherapy of an established tumor depends on suppressor T-cells. J Exp Med 155:1063–1074

Oster W, Lindemann A, Mertelsmann R, Herrmann F (1988) Regulation of gene expression of M-, G-, GM-, and multi-CSF in normal and malignant hematopoietic cells. Blood Cells (in press)

Philip R, Epstein LM (1986) Tumor necrosis factor as immunomodulator and mediator of monocyte cytotoxicity induced by itself, IFN-gamma and IL-1. Nature 323:86–89

Rosenberg SA, Mule JJ, Spiess PJ, Reichert CM, Schwarz SL (1985) Regression of established pulmonary metastases and subcutaneous tumor mediated by the systemic administration of high-dose recombinant IL-2. J Exp Med 161:1169–1188

Rosenberg SA, Lotze MT, Muul LM, Chang AE, Aris FP, Leitman S, Lindeham WM, Robertson CN, Lee RE, Rubin JT, Seipp CA, Simpson CG, White DE (1987) A progress report on the treatment of 157 patients with advanced cancer using lymphokine-activated killer cells and IL-2 or high-dose IL-2 alone. N Engl J Med 316:889–897

Scheurich P, Thoma B, Ücer U, Pfizenmaier K (1987) Immunoregulatory activity of recombinant human tumor necrosis factor (TNF)-alpha: induction of TNF receptors on human T cells and TNF-alpha-mediated enhancement of T cell responses. J Immunol 138:1786–1791

Siegel JP, Sharon M, Smith PL (1987) The IL-2 receptor beta chain (p70): role in mediating signals for LAK, NK, and proliferative activities. Science 238:75–78

Smith KA (1988) Interleukin-2: inception, impact, and implications. Science 240:1169–1176

Souza LM, Boone TC, Gabrilove J, Lai PH, Zsebo KM, Murdock DC, Chazin VR, Bruszewski J, Lu H, Chenk K, Barendt J, Platzer E, Moore MAS, Mertelsmann R, Welte K (1986) Recombinant human granulocyte colony-stimulating factor: effects on normal and leukemic myeloid cells. Science 232:61–68

Talpaz M, Kantarjian HM, McCredie K, Trujillo JM, Keating MJ, Gatterman JU (1986) Hematologic remissions and cytogenetic improvement induced by recombinant human IFN-alpha in CML. N Engl J Med 314:1065–1069

Topalian SL, Solomon D, Avis FP, Chang AE, Freerksen DL, Linehan WM, Lotze MT, Robertson CN, Seipp CA, Simon P, Simpson CG, Rosenberg SA (1988) Immunotherapy of patients with advanced cancer using tumor-infiltrating lymphocytes and recombinant interleukin-2: a pilot study. J Clin Oncol 6:839–853

Waldmann TA (1986) The structure, function, and expression of interleukin-2 receptors on normal and malignant lymphocytes. Science 232:727–733

Wang HM, Smith KA (1987) The interleukin 2 receptor. J Exp Med 166:1055–1063

Welte K, Platzer E, Lu L, Gabrilove J, Levi E, Mertelsmann R, Moore MAS (1985) Purification and biochemical characterization of human pluripotent hematopoietic colony-stimulating factor. Proc Natl Acad Sci USA 82:1526–1530

Welte K, Bonilla MA, Gillio A, Boone TC, Potter GK, Gabrilove J, Moore MAS, O'Reilly R, Souza LM (1987) Recombinant human G-CSF: effects on hematopoiesis in normal and cyclophosphamide-treated primates. J Exp Med 165:941–948

Summary of Discussion: Session 8

I. L. Olsson

Cell Differentiation

Mechanistic points to attack in differentiation therapy were discussed. One possibility is to direct the malignant cells to a terminally differentiated stage so that they disappear because the probability of self renewal becomes very low. Another possibility is to convert the malignant stem cells into normal stem cells to produce normal cells. The latter phenomenon can very rarely be seen in embryonic carcinoma where a metastasis may stop growing or grow very slowly to produce normal cells. As to the Hexamethylene bisacetamide (HMBA)-treated murine erythroleukemia (MEL)-cells, the evidence indicated that the first mechanism operated to shift the cells to a more mature state. In vitro one could certainly deplete the precursor cells. The cells also lost their oncogenicity in vivo after HMBA treatment. There is no evidence of persistent stem cells, either normal or transformed. It has not been possible to identify any phenotypically normal precursor cells in the population incubated with HMBA. On the other hand, phenotypically almost normal terminally differentiated cells were produced. Differentiation of MEL cells was not compatible with long-term survival as judged by in vitro data. In vitro these cells die in 5–10 days once they are differentiated. The fate of the cells in vivo is not known. Normal bone marrow precursors were found to die in vitro as rapidly as differentiated MEL cells.

In other models for differentiation induction such as HL-60 cells, retinoic acid can prime the cells to respond with differentiation when exposed to low concentrations of various agents. The priming is in this case independent of protein synthesis, but for HMBA to be effective on MEL cells protein synthesis is necessary during the latency period. Cycloheximide effectively blocks the process; short-lived proteins not yet identified may be of importance here.

It was suggested that diamino compounds could be natural inhibitors of proliferation. It is possible to extend the life span of leukemic mice by giving them lysine. Spermine and cadaverine and all these diamines have a certain anticarcinogenic effect. The question was if HMBA is hydrolyzed in vivo so that the active form could be a free diamine. However, the free diamine is an extremely weak inducer.

As to the oncogenic expression, the early alterations seen after 3–4 h of treatment with HMBA are completely reversible if HMBA is removed; the c-*fos* mRNA disappears, c-*myc* and c-*myb* come back. If at any time during the culture HMBA is removed, c-*myb* expression reoccurs after 1–2 h. Thus, suppression of c-*myb* appears to require the continuous presence of HMBA. A high level of expression is necessary when MEL cells are transfected with the c-*myb* construct used to get inhibition of the HMBA-mediated differentiation effect.

It was suggested that a transgenic pancreatic islet tumor could be useful for studies with HMBA. If the islets are taken out at the right time they expand rapidly in vitro.

During the latency period there is a Ca^{2+} release and then Ca^{2+} is pumped out of the cell. It was not known by what mechanism Ca^{2+} goes out. There was actually a decrease in inositol 3-phosphate (IP_3) within 10–15 min of addition of HMBA. The vincristine-resistant cells did not exhibit any latency period and the question was brought up whether they showed alterations in protein kinase C activity. A slight increase in total activity of this enzyme had been found.

With respect to effects of HMBA on solid tumor cells (bladder, colon, breast), these stop growing after 10–20 days in culture in the presence of HMBA and disintegrate. The polarity of the inducing agent is of importance. The inducing activity is not as good when there are 3–4 polar groups. Compounds with longer hydrophobic chains or more polar groups tend to be more toxic, which may limit their efficacy.

Growth Factors

The efficiency of chemotherapy depends on the dosage. One question was if the use of granulocyte-macrophage-colony stimulating factor (GM-CSF) would allow a higher dose of chemotherapeutic drugs. It was pointed out that chemotherapy could be given according to schedule now, which had not been possible before. Morbidity due to chemotherapy was significantly reduced in the vast majority of patients supported with GM-CSF. The most important question is if this also translates into a higher response rate. Clinical studies are being designed to investigate where higher-dosage chemotherapy can be given over long time to increase the response rate.

In regard to combinations with GM-CSF in the treatment of acute leukemia, there is a clear risk of accelerating the leukemic stem cells as well. Actually, patient data showed evidence of expansion of the leukemic cells, as would be expected from in vitro experiments.

It was pointed out that we have to learn more about combinations of cytokines (inhibitory and stimulatory compounds) to get closer to the natural situation. Some agents have both an inhibitory and a stimulatory effect, depending on the target: tumor necrosis factor-α (TNF-α) stimulates proliferation of B-cell chronic lymphocytic leukemia. The action of these agents has to be judged both with respect to target cell and with respect to whether they induce or inhibit proliferation. For instance, in cells where differentiation is induced with G-CSF, proliferation goes down.

Combination biotherapy seems to be attractive for the future. In chronic myeloid leukemia, where there is resistance to interferon, a combination of interferon with TNF may still be active and lead to hematological remission. TNF alone has so far been rather disappointing in the therapy of malignant disorders, but the synergy between TNF and interferon may become clinically useful.

Subject Index